D1537354

EXCELLENCE IN PRACTICE Series
Katharine G. Butler, Editor

Speech, Language, and Hearing Programs in Schools

A Guide for Students and Practitioners

EXCELLENCE IN PRACTICE Series
Katharine G. Butler, Editor

Conversational Management with Language-Impaired Children
Bonnie Brinton and Martin Fujuki

Successful Interactive Skills for Speech-Language Pathologists and
Audiologists
Dorothy Molyneaux and Vera W. Lane

Communicating for Learning: Classroom Observation and Collaboration
Elaine R. Silliman and Louise Cherry Wilkinson

Hispanic Children and Adults with Communication Disorders:
Assessment and Prevention
Henriette W. Langdon with Li-Rong Lilly Cheng

Family-Centered Early Intervention for Communication Disorders:
Prevention and Treatment
Gail Donahue-Kilburg

Building Early Intervention Teams: Working Together for Children and
Families
Margaret H. Briggs

Speech, Language, and Hearing Programs in Schools: A Guide for Students
and Practitioners
Pamelia O'Connell

Dysphagia: A Continuum of Care
Barbara C. Sonies

Perspectives in Applied Phonology
Barbara Williams Hodson and Mary Louise Edwards

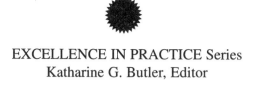

EXCELLENCE IN PRACTICE Series
Katharine G. Butler, Editor

Speech, Language, and Hearing Programs in Schools

A Guide for Students and Practitioners

Pamelia F. O'Connell, PhD
Associate Professor Emeritus
State University of New York
College at Cortland
Cortland, New York

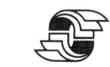

AN ASPEN PUBLICATION®
Aspen Publishers, Inc.
Gaithersburg, Maryland
1997

Library of Congress Cataloging-in-Publication Data

Speech, language, and hearing programs in schools:
a guide for students and practitioners/
[edited by] pamelia F. O'Connell
Includes bibliographical references and index.
ISBN 0-8342-0765-6 (hard cover)
1. Deglutition disorders—Treatment. 2. Deglutition disorders—Patients—Care.
I. O'Connell, Pamelia F. II. Series.
[DNLM: 1. Deglutition Disorders. WI 250 D9975 1996]
RC815.2.D97 1996
616.85'52—dc20
DNLM/DLC
for Library of Congress
96–42145
CIP

Orders: (800) 638-8437
Customer Service: (800) 234-1660

About Aspen Publishers • For more than 35 years, Aspen has been a leading professional publisher in a variety of disciplines. Aspen's vast information resources are available in both print and electronic formats. We are committed to providing the highest quality information available in the most appropriate format for our customers. Visit Aspen's Internet site for more information resources, directories, articles, and a searchable version of Aspen's full catalog, including the most recent publications: **http://www.aspenpub.com**
Aspen Publishers, Inc. • The hallmark of quality in publishing
Member of the worldwide Wolters Kluwer group

The authors have made every effort to ensure the accuracy of the information herein. However, appropriate information sources should be consulted, especially for new or unfamiliar procedures. It is the responsibility of every practitioner to evaluate the appropriateness of a particular opinion in the context of actual clinical situations and with due considerations to new developments. Authors, editors, and the publisher cannot be held responsible for any typographical or other errors found in this book.

Editorial Resources: David A. Uffelman
Library of Congress Catalog Card Number: 96-42145
ISBN: 0-8342-0765-6

Printed in the United States of America

1 2 3 4 5

Table of Contents

Contributors

Dolores E. Battle, PhD
Professor
Speech-Language Pathology Department
Buffalo State College
Buffalo, New York

Regina B. Grantham, BS, MEd
Assistant Professor
Department of Speech Pathology and
    Audiology
State University of New York College at
    Cortland
Cortland, New York

Eileen H. Gravani, PhD
Chair
Department of Speech Pathology and
    Audiology
State University of New York College at
    Cortland
Cortland, New York

Nancy P. Huffman, MS, CAS
Chair
Speech-Language and Audiology Services
Board of Cooperative Educational Services
    #1 Monroe
Fairport, New York

Jacqueline Meyer, BA, MHS, CCC-SLP
Lecturer in Speech Pathology and
    Audiology
Department of Speech Pathology and
    Audiology
State University of New York College at
    Cortland
Cortland, New York

Mary Ann O'Brien, MS, CAS
Director, Support Services
Board of Cooperative Educational Services
    #1 Monroe
Fairport, New York

Pamelia F. O'Connell, PhD
Associate Professor Emeritus
State University of New York College at
    Cortland
Cortland, New York

Mary Ann Romski, PhD
Professor
Departments of Communication,
    Psychology, and Educational Psychology
    & Special Education
Georgia State University
Atlanta, Georgia

Rose A. Sevcik, PhD
Assistant Research Professor
Department of Psychology
Georgia State University
Atlanta, Georgia

Wendy L. Sundgren, BA
Graduate Student
Georgia State University
Atlanta, Georgia

Foreword

Many of us continue to think of "schools" as we knew them as children, bringing memories of the "three Rs," desks aligned in rows, teachers talking at "the head of the class," students being required to "go to the board" and reveal their strengths or display their weaknesses for all to see. Parents, then and now, wanted, hoped, or demanded that their children do well. Grandparents informed us of their efforts in a one-room school house, and spoke of the discipline handed out to the errant scholar. If encouraged, they might render a portion of the song that identified the school as the place where "readin', writin', and 'rithmetic" were taught to "the tune of a hickory stick" while the conical dunce's cap graced a three-legged stool, always available for crowing the unprepared student who would sit in the corner where the switch reposed. In a kinder light, they might speak of the teacher whose tasks included arriving early to stoke the potbellied stove, sweep out the classroom, ring the bell announcing the beginning of class, await the children at the door, and check each child's head for lice as they entered.

Perhaps in your mind's eye you see a multi-storied building with long, dark hallways, with student monitors stationed along the way. Outside the principal's office sit students banished from their classrooms for major or even minor offenses. When asked what you liked best about school, you might have responded "recess," a common response that remains in vogue today. There's a certain unfettered sense of freedom in those all-too-brief moments on the playground, escaping from the rhythm of the instructional day, the boredom of "rest time" (if you were young) or study hall (if you were older). Moments of exhilaration were rare among the work sheets, spelling bees, assignments, and silent reading periods interspersed by teacher talk and student's brief responses. However, there were breaks in this regimen, moments of triumph or defeat. For children with speech, language, or hearing disabilities, life in and out of school brought many more of the latter.

A visit to today's classrooms reveals a very different context. Both teaching and learning are at variance with the past. The chapters that follow provide a glimpse of the schools of today and tomorrow. The authors know well the roles and responsibilities of the speech-language pathologist and educational audiologist engaged in today's service delivery models and those that hover on the horizon of the new century. They share this information and that of the dramatic societal changes occurring in the last decade of the 20th century. The authors are acutely aware of the dramatically increased provision of services over the past few decades, as well as the rapidly changing scope of practice in the schools over time. Erase from your mind the schools as they were through the first three-quarters of the 20th century, when services to children with communication disorders were sparse, and many children with severe disabilities were refused services. The year 1975 began a new era in which school services under the mantel of special education began in earnest with the promulgation of Public Law 94-142, now referenced as the Individuals with Disabilities Education Act (IDEA).

The authors provide an insightful view of the strengths and weaknesses of the current framework for the delivery of speech, language, and hearing school-based services as they now exist. They identify a number of models and provide excellent vignettes (case examples). They note emerging trends so that readers may glimpse what the schools of the future may provide for children with communication disorders through technology in the 21st century.

Readers need to know that they are entering an exciting discipline, one which provides a number of professional options. One may choose to serve in the schools in multiple ways: as a collaborator and a team member in early intervention; as a clinician who spans the continuum of services from individualized to small group to classroom; as a consultant; as a teacher of special day classes for the severely language impaired or a resource room language-learning disabilities specialist; as a specialist in pediatric dysphagia; or as a specialist in alternative and augmentative communication (AAC). In each case, if the reader chooses to select the schools as his or her context for practice, this setting provides an opportunity to help children master the yet-to-be understood miracle of spoken and written language.

The reality of the importance of the acquisition and use of language to attain literacy is the bedrock on which children move on to become productive adults in our post-industrial society. It is truly said that children spend their first years learning to use language and their later years using language to learn.

Children with language impairment are at risk for any number of academic problems. Early intervention for children zero to three can make a tremendous difference, when well done. While clinicians now inhabit classrooms and "clinical" space, such space is often carved out of a school nurse's office or a temporary structure, as student enrollment swells or decreases. Facilities and caseloads are known to be intermittent problems in a number of school settings. However, speech-language pathologists and audiologists carry with them their clinical educational experiences; those experiences enhance their ability to view the child within the context of home and school and to identify individualized assessment and intervention procedures. Their training also has stressed multiple methods of evaluation (or diagnosis). Those hours spent preparing to assess children with a variety of speech, language, and hearing problems and to measure their performance on a number of assessment procedures bears fruit in a number of ways. Whether one calls it assessment, evaluation, or diagnosis is unimportant in one sense: most qualified speech-language pathologists have an understanding of norm-based standardized instruments plus—and the plus is most important—authentic but non-standardized authentic instruments that may look at the child's functioning across modalities and across academic and social concerns. It is not good enough simply to identify academic concerns, although good speech-language assessment should take such school-based concerns into account. The task begins first with the child as a unique individual, followed by assessment of his or her speech, language, and hearing problems across contexts; and thirdly, to evaluate how the child's ability to use phonology, morphology, syntax, grammar, semantics, and pragmatics serves the child's use of language (i.e., language "processing"). Comprehension and production of appropriate language is essential to gain competency in reading and writing and, yes, arithmetic. It is also essential for interacting with others, whether they be family, school, or community based. Each child is "special" whether or not he or she is special or regular education. Clinicians not only diagnose a child's "language problem," they take a holistic view of the child. The central question is "How can I help this child whose needs extend beyond the terms used to describe a disorder, be it a phonological awareness deficit, a semantic disorder, syntactic or pragmatic difficulties, and so forth.

One of the fascinating things about dealing with human beings is their differences; such differences may be obvious but some may be subtle. The expression "alike as peas in a pod" is a saying that carries little meaning when engaged in the diagnosis and treatment of children with speech, language, and hearing disorders.

The authors of the chapters that follow take you on a journey into the land of observation, interviewing, assessment, and intervention, describing in detail the realities of that which will be encountered as one moves from the more protective area of the university clinic to the real world of the classroom and other educational settings. As one grows, so grow the challenges encountered. A companion on this journey could well be this text. Like other good companions, it will not let you down. It will show you one of the most fascinating arenas in which you can make a difference in children's lives, a difference that will reward you as nothing else can.

Katharine G. Butler, PhD
Research Professor
Communication Sciences
& Disorders
Syracuse University
Editor, *Excellence
in Practice Series*

Acknowledgments

There are always so many people to thank, as any book is the result of a myriad of experiences, all within a human context. This is especially true of a multiauthored volume like this one.

Regina B. Grantham would like to thank her husband, Robert J. Grantham, for his input, inspiration, patience, understanding, and constant support. A special thanks is also extended to the Department of Speech-Language Pathology and Audiology at the State University of New York College at Cortland for their expert help and continuous encouragement. She also thanks the national office of the American Speech-Language-Hearing Association. Eileen Gravani would like to thank Trisha Slaccus of CETRC, Helen McDonald of the New York State Health Department, and Robin Dubrovi of Special Children's Center of Cortland County. She also thanks the national office of the American Speech-Language Hearing Association (ASHA) for their help. Nancy Huffman would like to thank the audiology staff at the Board of Cooperative Educational Services (BOCES) #1 Monroe, Fairport, New York, for their advocacy and their expertise in the provision of audiology services in educational environments. Audiologists Susan Newman, CCC-A, Carol Greer, CCC-A, Janet Zieno, CCC-A, and Sarah Boser, CCC-A and audiometric technicians Sara Scott and Linda Potts are an endless source of ideas for how we can do it better. They are my best critics and my greatest inspiration, and they are full of professional energy. Jaqueline Meyer would like to thank her colleagues at SUNY Cortland for their never-ending support and encouragement, for the articles that appeared mysteriously on her desk, the sympathetic inquiries about how "the writing" was going, and their critical comments on her writing style as it evolved from journal-formal to student user-friendly. Equal thanks go to the faculty at Lyncourt School in Syracuse, New York, who exemplified every day that excellent teaching occurs in a rainbow of techniques, philosophies, and personalities. A special thanks goes to Jill Modaferri, whose collaboration, before it had a name, opened her eyes to the world of curriculum-based programming. Finally, she wishes to express gratitude to her family for their patience with a preoccupied parent, especially her daughter, Suzannah, an undergraduate in communication disorders at the College of Saint Rose, who read and criticized her mother's chapters from the vantage point of the student. Mary Ann O'Brien acknowledges John O'Brien for his excessive patience and expert editing.

The editor wishes to thank all the contributors, each of whom has produced a crucial segment or, in some cases, segments of this book. It has been my privilege to have known and worked with most of them. These associations have been one of the most positive aspects of my career in speech-language pathology. In fact, my conviction that I knew a group of remarkable professionals whose insights, ideas, and expertise needed to be brought together for the benefit of novice school practitioners served as the original impetus for this book. My sincere appreciation to all of you; you're even better than I thought you were!

Thanks, too, to Loretta Stock, Sandy Cannon, and Mary Anne Langdon of Aspen for encouragement, support, and, above all, patience. I also appreciate the gracious assistance of Susan Larson at the American Speech-Language-Hearing Association. Thank you, Diane Stumm of the Albert Carlton-Cashiers Community Library, for obtaining obscure books with efficiency and good humor.

Special thanks are due Katharine Butler for the expert guidance she provided during the creation of this book, especially the final stages. Kay's example of excellence, achievement, and professional service has been a source of continuing amazement and an animating influence. My appreciation for all her kindness and consideration and for the professional opportunities she has provided over the years runs deep indeed. Thank you, Kay.

And to Ed, for his computer skills and his unshakable determination that even I could learn at least some of them, many thanks. Not a word could have been processed without you.

Introduction

We don't receive wisdom; we must discover it for ourselves after a journey no one else can take for us or spare us.

—Marcel Proust

The professional journey taken by many in speech-language pathology and audiology will lead to the nation's schools. And if Proust is correct, only that process has the power to impart genuine wisdom. Yet the utility of guidebooks is generally unquestioned. Few of us would leave a trip to Patagonia completely to chance. Thus this book has been planned for the novice traveler in our schools, as well as for those who may return to school services after a period of absence. Consisting of many and varied components, it is unified by the recurring mention of change. Change has been a constant but it cannot completely be captured in writing, which is language made permanent. Remember, as you read, that the guidebook is not the journey.

The present volume emerged from the editor's long association with school programs for students with disorders of communication. This involvement has changed its focus a number of times since the middle 1950s, just as the nature of such school programs has altered considerably during this time. The initial role was that of a *public school speech therapist*, which was the preferred designation of that era. The term had superseded the older one of *speech correctionist*. In a schedule that was typical of the times, five elementary schools were visited, and over 100 children, primarily first and second graders, were seen twice each week.

By the early 1990s, supervision of speech-language pathology students in school practicum placements had become the window through which many school programs, urban, suburban, small town, and rural, were viewed.

Uniting these distinctly differing times and roles is the conviction that school services matter and that the school is a unique setting for service delivery. The professions of speech-language pathology and audiology are continuing to explore, expand, and refine their roles as service providers in the educational setting.

This book has been planned as a guide for students and professionals beginning their first steps toward school service. It will attempt to trace the path we have traveled from its beginnings, illuminate the various forces that have contributed to its changing directions, and provide a reasonably detailed portrait of the current scene.

That this scene is complex, multifaceted, and constantly shifting is perhaps a massive understatement. This contributed to a decision for multiple authorship. No single individual could exhibit expertise in all areas relevant to school practice. The writers assembled here are audiologists as well as speech-language pathologists, school administrators as well as academics, clinical supervisors as well as researchers. They bring special perspectives and speak with voices suited to the particular messages they seek to impart to the reader. Although many contributors have chosen the traditional third-person voice of the omniscient author, the writers of the more applied or nuts-and-bolts portions of this volume, Chapters 6, 7, and 8, have elected the more informal, personal style conferred by use of the first person. The presence of differing styles and voices serves to underscore the diversity of points from which school practice is viewed.

Along with the voices, this book represents choices; choices about what to include, what to exclude, where to supply detail, where simply to summarize, and how to achieve the most helpful focus for the beginning practitioner. The three major sections of the book are briefly discussed below, as some of the voices and choices here begin to emerge.

FOUNDATION

A number of important areas must be addressed before an informed consideration of school program implementation can take place. Chapters 1 through 5 attempt to provide the necessary foundation upon which the rest of the book will build.

An understanding of the past always enriches appreciation of the present and offers hints suggestive of possible futures. The direct antecedents of today's programs in speech and language lie in the early school programs of several large American cities begun in the early decades of this century. This

relatively short history is complemented by a summary of the much longer and quite fascinating story of the education of the deaf. For the speech-language pathologist who may be involved in providing services for deaf and hearing-impaired students, knowledge of past trends, controversies, and ideological positions is highly desirable. For the beginning professional who may serve the developmentally disabled, a historical perspective on special education is similarly useful.

The federal legislation that was initiated in 1975 and the state laws that served as precursors to national standards for the education of children with handicapping conditions are, of course, a part of the history of school services. This legislation is, in fact, such an important aspect for the school professional, such a defining factor in the everyday operations of current school programs, that Chapter 2 is completely devoted to legislative issues. Whereas Chapter 1 treats historical trends in a broad fashion, Chapter 3 supplies the details of the legislative events that have set the scene in our schools for the past 20 years.

Also contributing to the history of school programming is the national American Speech-Language-Hearing Association (ASHA). ASHA's role, as well as its relevance to the operation of school programs today and to the speech-language and hearing professionals who serve in them, is extensive. Chapter 3 offers the reader a concise yet detailed description of the organization that provides a frame and a supporting structure for school professionals in communication disorders.

Chapter 4 delineates the qualifications, roles, and services of speech-language pathologists and audiologists in schools. The two separate sections address similar but not identical areas. The speech-language pathology section outlines the qualifications for service delivery, including the requirements for the ASHA-certified practitioner, describes state licensure, and discusses the role of state educational agencies and their differing requirements. Roles and services such as screening, assessment, educational planning, consultation, counseling, and direct services are also described, but not in great detail because later chapters dealing with program implementation enlarge upon many of these areas. The section on audiology, however, offers more specific detail. It describes the qualifications and roles of audiologists in schools and includes the issues of state licensure and ASHA standards. It also contains information on the educational needs of deaf and hearing-impaired students and the range of options available to meet those needs. It includes a discussion of the role of the speech-language pathologist with respect to the hearing impaired and how this role differs from that of the audiologist, the teacher of the deaf, interpreters, and others involved in providing services for deaf and hearing-impaired students in schools.

No foundation for school programming in speech-language and hearing could be complete without consideration of the students for whom the programs exist. Every communication disorder that finds expression in individuals from birth to the age of 21 years is represented among the population to be served by school programs. The purpose of Chapter 5 is not to attempt a comprehensive account of each of these conditions; that is beyond the scope of this book. Rather, it is to offer a look at some of the groups of children who are typically represented in the school caseload of today. An emphasis is placed on those who are relatively recent entrants to such caseloads: the learning disabled, the infant-toddler-prekindergarten group, the autistic, and the traumatically brain injured.

PROGRAM IMPLEMENTATION

Chapters 6, 7, and 8 constitute the central section of the book, which lies at the heart of the enterprise. The two authors of these chapters worked together to provide a unified perspective on the actual operation of school programs for speech- and language-disordered students. They provide an insightful portrait of the professional activities performed by the speech-language specialist in today's schools.

Chapter 6 is devoted to the processes of case finding and assessment. This is the first activity for which the school speech-language pathologist is responsible. It is a process having multiple components, from the tentative identification of students who may be in need of special services to the detailed depictions of specific patterns of strengths and weaknesses that lead to decisions regarding educational planning and programming. The process involves screening, referring, observation, interviewing, formal testing and interpretation, and descriptive procedures derived from language sampling. Legal issues as well as educational relevance must be taken into account. The reader is led through the application of this complex and detailed information by the presentation of three cases. Each case represents a hypothetical child whose characteristics mirror those frequently encountered in school caseloads. For each case, a general description of the student and the presenting problem is provided. The assessment process is then described and delineated from beginning observations and teacher interviews through selection of test instruments, scoring and interpretation, language sample analyses, parent interviews, plans, and reports. Each student assessed is encountered again in Chapter 7.

The Individualized Educational Program, or IEP, is the subject of Chapter 7. The IEP is an essential component of special services for students who require them. It is a written statement of the student's needs and the means that have been chosen to meet them. Again, legal as well as educational issues are involved; parental participation is a crucial aspect of the process. The various components of the IEP are fully described, and examples are presented. The chapter culminates with IEP formulations for each of the three students assessed in Chapter 6.

With assessment results and IEP formulations in hand, the reader is presented, in Chapter 8, with descriptions and discussion of the various models of service delivery encountered in today's schools. The chapter illustrates the multiple methods available to serve the special needs of students. And our three cases are again encountered, this time with detailed information on how their needs may be addressed through differing service models.

Taken together, Chapters 6, 7, and 8 offer usable and practical guidelines for school program implementation. The stylistic distinctiveness of these chapters, the more informal tone or voice, has been adopted to make this important information as accessible as possible. Indeed, readers preparing for initial school services may feel, and we hope they will, that a wise and humane mentor has been provided to prepare them for this challenging journey.

CONTEMPORARY ISSUES

School services exist within an ever-shifting landscape. Much that is relatively new to the school scene may be ephemeral (remember "new math"?), whereas some newer trends represent concerns that will continue

and perhaps grow in importance as time progresses. Chapters 9, 10, and 11 are concerned with topics that have emerged in the relatively recent past that the editor suspects will be relevant to school practitioners for some time to come.

The increasing dominance of computers and related technology in many aspects of contemporary society does not need to be underscored. The impact on education and, more pointedly, special education cannot, however, be ignored. As more severely disabled students began to receive services in our schools, there was, quite fortunately, a rapidly evolving technology to assist the school practitioner in meeting their needs. Alternate and augmentative communication, or AAC, does not always involve advanced technology, but computer-assisted devices have played a leading role in AAC developments. Chapter 9 presents current and highly practical information on AAC and the students whose educational and communicative needs are best addressed through this means. Issues involving student eligibility, assessment, selection, and use of AAC systems are described, discussed, and illustrated through the presentation of representative cases. Basic definitions and background are also presented here.

In Chapter 10, a special education administrator with a speech-language background provides a discussion of three separate issues, united by a common thread of administrative concern. These issues, however, also affect school practitioners in many ways and may do so with even greater force in the future. They are

1. *Third-party payment for special services.* Educational and health care services have overlapped and become enmeshed, and the implications are far-ranging and perhaps a little bewildering.

2. *Supervision.* A complex process central to professional growth and development, this discussion of supervisory issues includes evaluation and mentoring.

3. *Supportive personnel.* Of particular interest here is the use of speech aides and other paraprofessionals in educational programs. Issues of quality assurance and professional autonomy meet pressures for cost containment and accountability, again raising complex issues.

Increasingly, the children in our schools are culturally and linguistically diverse. It is estimated that by the rapidly approaching year of 2020, at least half of the students in our schools will come from backgrounds that are non–Caucasian and/or non–English-speaking. Already these students constitute a significant segment of the school population. Many issues are involved in serving the needs of these students. The authors of Chapter 11 have provided a treatment that is at once comprehensive, timely, scholarly, sensitive, and practical.

In Chapter 12, the horizon is scanned for possible future trends. The users of this volume will be a vital part of that future.

Part I

Foundation

Chapter 1

History of School Services: Speech, Language, and Hearing

Pamelia F. O'Connell

The principal aim of this chapter will be to acquaint the reader with the varied and complex sources of the current patterns of school practice. It will attempt to place speech-language and hearing services within the broader context of regular and special education. It will describe early programs for the hearing impaired, the beginnings of the work with speech-handicapped children, and the burgeoning learning disability movement, with its heavy emphasis on language skills. School programs in speech, language, and hearing have been influenced by many factors. Some of these influences may be viewed as threads drawn from the fabric of general education, a cloth woven from many strands to become a large mantle that covers ever-increasing numbers of children and provides an ever-expanding variety of programs and services.

Only a little over 100 years ago, for example, "school" was held only 3 months a year in the western frontier areas of our country. Less than 50 years ago, whole counties in certain southern states provided no secondary education for African-American students. In many cities and small towns, school attendance was optional. Until the fairly recent past, children with special needs of various kinds often received no community-based public education at all. At best, services for many children were spotty and often not designed to fit their needs. In general, special education lagged behind general education in our communities.

Special education, a term coined in Germany in 1863, has three aspects, which may be viewed as stages. They are not mutually exclusive, however, and may not be successive. They are (a) treatment or education through segregation, (b) care for the physical needs of those who cannot care for themselves, and (c) instruction for the purpose of promoting inclusion into an existing social system (Heinz, 1971). Education for those with handicapping conditions has fluctuated between segregation and inclusion. The debate over the relative merits of these polarities continues and perhaps always will.

As schools grew in size and in importance, they began to address a wider variety of students in a more comprehensive manner. Threads that would eventually contribute to patterns of programs in speech, language, and hearing emerged from early services for the deaf and mentally retarded. The speech-impaired child, usually identified as the stutterer or stammerer, was the initial specific focus of the profession of speech-language pathology. Much of the impetus for the growth and development of the profession came from speech services provided for these children, and others who were deemed speech impaired, in the nation's public schools.

In tracing the history of school programs in speech, language, and hearing, then, one must examine several separate areas. Although a history of general public education in America is obviously beyond the scope of this book, it is well to remember that all services for students with special needs have been and will continue to be influenced by the context of the general education enterprise. The societal forces that shape the schools, including intellectual trends in pedagogy and politics, will affect all school programs, including those for the hearing-, speech-, and language-disabled student.

EDUCATION OF THE DEAF

All educational systems reflect the culture that supports them, and this, of course, is true of groups with special needs within general education. The history of the education of the deaf provides an excellent example of the multiple and sometimes conflicting influences of social forces and intellectual trends within the larger culture upon the education of a specific group. A detailed account of this history can be found in Moores (1987).

Early Education in Europe

Moores (1987) notes that early attitudes toward deafness were ambivalent and focused on religious and legal rights, not educational needs. This is hardly surprising because most people in early societies were unschooled. It was not until the 16th century, in Italy, that attempts to teach the deaf to read were recorded. Other early education efforts were

made in Spain and in Great Britain. Records left by a Spaniard, Juan Bonet, in the 17th century foreshadow many of the later trends in educating the deaf. These include an emphasis on early intervention, the importance of a consistent language environment, a system of manual signs, and attempts to teach speech and reading. Unfortunately, early efforts were undermined by the practice of secrecy. Methods that particular teachers found most effective were not shared and not recorded in any detail. Reports of early successes were further compromised by lack of agreement as to what constituted deafness. We know today that the effects of hearing loss on language development, speech, and literacy vary considerably with degree and type of loss, age at which the loss is incurred, and other factors. It is therefore difficult to interpret early writing on the subject. It is interesting, however, to note the beginning of continuing themes.

18th- and 19th-Century Europe

Early work with the deaf in the United States was greatly influenced by the French. Prominent French 18th-century educators included Periere, whose methods influenced Itard in his classic work with Victor, the wild child from Aveyron (Lane, 1976). The interaction between the education of the deaf and that of the mentally retarded and other special groups is illustrated here.

The work of the Abbé de L'Épée was perhaps even more influential. He stressed the importance of intellectual development in his pupils and the contribution of manual signs to this development. He was impressed by the "natural" signing systems of the Parisian deaf and devised a supplementary system of "methodological" signs, reflecting French syntax and morphology, for use alone with natural signs. De L'Épée also emphasized speech and speech reading but apparently thought these skills to be secondary to mental development.

To the present-day reader, it appears that de L'Épée was according the highest priority to language development and the use of signs to foster it. In this, his work was opposed by a well-known German educator of the period, Samuel Heinecke, who established a school for the deaf at Leipzig in 1778. Heinecke's precise methods are unknown, but his strong emphasis on teaching speech (Garnet, 1968) set the stage for the oral–manual controversy that was to inform so much of the educational debate that followed.

Early Education in the United States

In the United States, formal education of the deaf did not begin until the 19th century. The Industrial Revolution in New England created a demand for a literate work force and spurred the establishment of schools throughout the region. With recognition of the economic importance of literacy, interest in educating all children, including the deaf, grew.

Prior to the 19th century, some deaf children with wealthy parents were sent to Europe, and their educational experiences there influenced the course of development of educational programming in the United States. Many such children attended a school in Edinburgh, Scotland, established in 1767 by Thomas Braidwood. The first attempt to establish a school for the deaf in the United States was made by Francis Green, whose son attended the Edinburgh school. A later attempt was made by the Bolling family of Virginia, who also had children who attended the Braidwood school. These attempts, however, did not lead to the permanent establishment of schools.

19th-Century United States

The first permanent school for the deaf was established by Thomas Hopkins Gallaudet, a Congregational clergyman who had become interested in the education of the deaf through his relationship with the deaf daughter of a prominent physician. Gallaudet went abroad to study before accepting an offer to head his nation's first school for the deaf. While he attempted to study with the Braidwoods, his attempts were frustrated by their reluctance to share their expertise, and he studied in France instead with Sicard, the successor to de L'Épée. When he returned to the United States, he was accompanied by Laurent Clerc, a deaf teacher. In 1817, the American Asylum for the Education of the Deaf and Dumb opened with seven students in Hartford, Connecticut, supported by state-appropriated money that was supplemented by private funds. Its curriculum included English grammar, religion, and vocational training with a system of manual signs, designed by Clerc as the major method of instruction (Moores, 1987). Two other schools whose methods and curriculum were strongly influenced by the Connecticut school were established shortly thereafter, one in New York City and one in Philadelphia.

Subsequent decades saw establishment of schools in Kentucky, Ohio, Missouri, and Virginia. By the time of the Civil War, a system of schools for the deaf had spread throughout the country. One of these schools, the Columbia Institution for the Deaf and Dumb in Washington, D.C., later evolved to become the Gallaudet University, the sole liberal arts college for the deaf in the world. Most of the schools were residential, and most of them were manual, with little emphasis on speech. Some have referred to this period as a golden age for the deaf in the

United States. In the mid-19th century, however, an increased interest in oral education for the deaf emerged. Although many factors operated to encourage this interest, perhaps a key event was the tour of German institutions made by Horace Mann and Samuel Howe. These educators returned to the United States convinced that the German oral method was superior to the manual system. Other key events were the establishment of the first oral-only schools; one in Northampton, Massachusetts, the Clark Institution for Deaf Mutes, and one in New York City, now the Lexington School for the Deaf. From approximately the time of the Civil War to World War I, the education of the deaf was dominated by two figures who came to embody the controversy surrounding oral versus manual methods of instruction. They were Alexander Graham Bell and Edward Minor Gallaudet.

Gallaudet and Bell

Although Edward Minor Gallaudet is remembered as a defender of manual signs, his position was much more complex. He was an advocate of a system that combined speech training and speech reading with manual signs, a position very similar to the now-dominant total-communication philosophy. During his lengthy career at the Columbia Institution, now Gallaudet University, he argued for oral methods, and it was only when manual signing came under attack by proponents of an oral-only system that he emerged as a champion of the combined oral–manual system. Alexander Graham Bell was the son and grandson of teachers of speech, and prior to his invention of the telephone, he pursued a similar career. It is difficult to summarize his active and colorful life. He was, however, a sometime deaf educator and friend of Edward

Minor Gallaudet who became an outspoken critic of the U.S. system of deaf education of his time. He also became a strong advocate of oral-only methods. He opposed intermarriage of deaf individuals, which he believed was fostered by residential schools and the cultural isolation encouraged by manual communication. He was also opposed to deaf teachers. The oral-only position enjoyed its greatest triumph in Europe at the 1880 international convention in Milan, which sought to forbid manual systems. Although highly influential, Alexander Graham Bell was not able to ensure a similar triumph in the United States. The oral-only method increased in popularity but never completely eclipsed the combined method.

Friction and controversy between the oralists and the combined-method proponents characterized the climate in which the education of the deaf took place from the late 19th century until the fairly recent past. Also, during this time the use of manual signing declined. Many scholars believe that these events harmed the efforts to achieve the highest possible quality of education for all deaf children.

Manual Systems: Major Types

Throughout this discussion, reference has been made to manual or sign systems of communication with little specification of type of sign. Before continuing with the brief history of the education of the deaf, it is necessary to consider the type of signing system in a little more detail. Manual communication may be viewed dichotomously as systems that involve spelling a word with some type of alphabet, such as "finger spelling" (any number of these systems have existed, some using one hand and some using two), and systems that are conceptual, presenting an idea through a distinct sign. In the United States and Canada, American Sign Language (ASL), a conceptual system, is used in conjunction with a large number of other manual systems devised to parallel more closely the spoken English language.

Moores (1987) stated that Laurent Clerc was probably the strongest impetus for the development and spread of ASL, which exhibits its French influence in many ways. Clerc was called upon to create a manual system at the American School beginning in 1817, and ASL was further propagated by deaf and hearing teachers trained by him and his followers. ASL has been called the natural language of the deaf community, not only a means of communication but also a defining element of a unique culture.

As previously noted, the oral-only method of instruction was triumphant in Europe by the end of the 19th century and also became increasingly important in the United States. The emphasis on speech training came with a discouragement, in some cases a forbidding, of the use of manual signs. The influence of deaf teachers waned, and ASL became primarily a deaf-community language, one not formally taught to deaf children. Deaf children of deaf parents learned ASL at home; deaf children of hearing parents tended to learn it from their peers at the residential schools.

The Modern Period

In the 1960s and 1970s, things began to change. The linguistic revolution of the 1960s increased interest in the structure of all natural languages. Researchers also began to examine the accomplishments of deaf children of deaf parents in comparison with the achievements of deaf children of hearing parents, with findings that proved quite influential for the future of ASL. They found that in many academic areas, especially reading, children with deaf parents were significantly superior to children with hearing parents (Vernon & Koh, 1970). The growing awareness of the importance of early language stimulation for future linguistic and cognitive development, upon which academic success depends, interacted with trends toward early education for all children and early intervention for handicapped children. Manual communication systems experienced a rebirth of popularity and, paired with auditory training, speech, and speech reading, reemerged as a key component of total communication, the preferred system today.

Controversy regarding signing has continued, however, with pure ASL advocates opposing the invented systems, such as Signed English and Signing Exact English, that are more precise translations of spoken American English. The impact of the 1975 Education for All Handicapped Children Act (Pub. L. No. 94-142) was profound for all American children, including the deaf. The federal mandate for the provision of a free, appropriate public education in the least restrictive environment has led to many changes in educational programs for deaf and hearing-impaired children. There still exists, however, a mix of programs, including residential schools, both public and private; day schools; and day classes in schools that also serve hearing children. There are also programs in which deaf children attend regular classes full time and may receive support services of various kinds from specialists such as speech-language pathologists.

The trend has been toward larger enrollments in public schools, smaller ones in private schools, and increased concentration of older students in residential schools and of younger children primarily in community public schools. Interestingly, residential schools have continued to enroll a significant number of pupils, although overall residential school enrollment has shown some decline. The number of deaf teachers has increased in recent years.

Speech-Language Pathology and Audiology

Speech-language pathologists and audiologists have played significant roles in educational programs for the deaf for many years. Although speech, speech reading, and auditory training received great emphasis during the earlier years of this professional involvement, the enhancement of language development has now become the primary focus. Typically the speech-language pathologist who works with deaf students is knowledgeable about manual language systems and subscribes to the tenets of total communication. The trend has been also toward a greater integration of special speech and language teaching with overall educational goals.

The advances of technology in the area of cochlear implants and other communication devices have had an impact on educational programs and are a new source of controversy. Many members of the deaf community have been less than enthusiastic about some of the recent changes, such as more community-based schooling. Some see the cochlear implant as a threat to deaf culture. There has been a movement toward deaf pride, similar to movements within other minority groups (Solomon, 1994). It is obvious that the future will hold other changes in educational programming for the deaf. It also seems evident that the communication needs of deaf and hearing-impaired students will continue to be addressed by speech-language pathologists serving as team members in educational programs throughout the United States.

PROGRAMS FOR THE MENTALLY HANDICAPPED

As noted earlier, there is a relationship between the education of the deaf and that of the mentally retarded. The French psychologist Itard, a prominent figure in the history of special education and services for the mentally handicapped, was influenced by the methods of Periere, an early teacher of the deaf.

American Education of the Mentally Handicapped

The American educator Samuel Howe, whose trip to Germany with Horace Mann was to have a profound influence on the education of the American deaf, was responsible for the first attempt to provide educational programming for the severely retarded in the United States. In 1848, Howe requested the sum of $2,500 from the Massachusetts legislature to establish a residential school for "idiots" (Kirk & Gallagher, 1986). The request was granted, only to be vetoed by the governor. Howe's impassioned letter of response, asserting the rights of the handicapped in a democratic society, led to the overriding of the veto and the establishment of the school. Other schools were subsequently established throughout the country. By 1967, there were 167 of them in all 50 states and the District of Columbia. These institutions served over 200,000 individuals, 57% of them classified as severely retarded.

Community special education classes serving the mentally retarded began in the early 20th century. Their growth was slow, however, not sharply accelerating until the late 1950s. According to Deighton (1971), 3,600 separate programs existed in 1958, with an increase to 5,600 in 1963. Even so, not all students with special needs received appropriate services in their communities.

By the end of World War II, residential institutions became overcrowded and began to turn away potential students. In many cases, local schools as well refused these youngsters, especially the more severely impaired. Parents began to protest. This, in turn, led to an increased interest in community-based schooling and other programs, such as sheltered workshops. Association for Retarded Citizen groups began to form, and eventually these offered an array of community-based services, including prekindergarten.

Current Trends

The Education for All Handicapped Children Act of 1975 (Pub. L. No. 94-142) accelerated the trend toward community inclusion of the mentally retarded, and community school services have continued to increase. Residential institutions still exist, primarily serving the more severely handicapped. Kirk and Gallagher (1986) provided an illustration of changing enrollment patterns between 1977 and 1983 in the state of New Jersey. In 1977, residential institutions enrolled 7,932 individuals, and 705 individuals were served by community programs. In 1983, residential enrollment was down to 5,942, and community services figures rose to 3,009. This trend toward larger and larger enrollments in community-based programming has continued.

Speech and Language Services

The needs of the mentally retarded for special speech and language services were not always sufficiently recognized—or perhaps such services were not always deemed appropriate. As the final section of this chapter will show, school speech programs were initially aimed at children within the general school population who had fluency or articulation problems.

When I received my professional education in the middle 1950s, little or no emphasis was placed on the mentally retarded population. In some settings, a diagnosis of mental retardation came with the admonition that "speech therapy" was contraindicated. The communication needs of the nonspeaking mentally retarded child were frequently not addressed; indeed, the capacity to serve these children adequately did not exist.

Nevertheless, speech, language, and communication problems are very prevalent among the mentally retarded. Miller (1984) noted that all children with mental retardation have some form of language impairment. Federal government reports indicate that speech or language impairment in combination with mental retardation is the most commonly encountered of all multiple disabilities (Grossman, 1983).

Recent decades have witnessed many changes, and today programs for the mentally handicapped, whether in community schools or residential centers, invariably include speech and language and audiological services. Chapter 9 of the current volume provides detailed information on the use of augmentative and alternate communication (AAC) among retarded individuals.

PROGRAMS FOR SPEECH-IMPAIRED CHILDREN

School services for children with speech problems are more closely associated with the profession of speech-language pathology and have a shorter history. As mentioned earlier, services in schools contributed greatly to the establishment and growth of the profession. Today, the majority of speech-language pathologists are employed in the schools, although many of the services that they provide, and some of the models of service delivery, are very different from the original ones.

The early 20th century saw the establishment of speech services for schoolchildren in a number of American cities. The child labor laws may have increased interest in the speech handicapped by barring all children, those with special needs included, from the work force. In 1910, programs were initiated in Chicago and Detroit.

Early Programs

In Chicago, Ella Flagg Young, superintendent of schools, recommended the initiation of speech services in her annual report of 1910 (Moore & Kester, 1953). She had conducted a survey, following receipt of petitions and complaints from parents, of the "stammering" children in the school district. A significant number of such children were identified. She recommended that the Oral Expression Department of Chicago Teachers College select students to receive additional training. The 10 students selected would, upon completion of their training, work with the children under the department's supervision. This recommendation was followed, and 10 students received the training and were subsequently employed.

Their salaries were $65 a month. Each young teacher was assigned to several schools and traveled from school to school during each working day. This established a pattern for service delivery that was to be dominant for a long time. Not all the children with speech problems proved to be "stammerers"; children with other types of speech difficulty were identified and grouped with those who had fluency problems.

Also in 1910, the disclosure, by a survey conducted in Detroit, Michigan, of a sizable number of "stammering" children, led to the hiring of two teachers with special training who worked with them. Somewhat later, services were expanded to include children with other types of speech problems. A number of school systems in other cities soon began to hire teachers to work with speech-impaired children. They included New York, Boston, Grand Rapids, Michigan, Cincinnati, Cleveland, and San Francisco (Paden, 1970).

The University of Wisconsin was the first institution of higher learning to establish a formal educational program for those planing to work with the speech impaired. They also granted the first Ph.D. degree in the field to Sara Stinchfield Hawk, in 1921. The first state supervisor of school speech services was appointed in 1923, also in Wisconsin. Universities in other states began to establish programs somewhat later. These early programs tended to be concentrated in the Midwest, and many were located in departments of speech and theater. Other states also began to enact legislation regarding school services for speech-disordered students, but the pace was somewhat slow. By 1963, however, most of the states supported speech programs in the schools (Haines, 1965).

Growth in the Midcentury

From the 1920s through the 1960s, speech-language pathology and audiology became defined as distinct professions that experienced dynamic growth. In 1948, the American Academy of Speech Correction, established in 1926 with 25 members, changed its name to American Speech and Hearing Association (ASHA), and by 1964 there were over 11,000 members. Other significant events included the establishment of a permanent national office in 1957 and the beginning publication of a monthly professional magazine in 1959. (See Chapter 3 for more information on ASHA.)

SPEECH AND LANGUAGE

Although early school programs were designated as "speech" programs, many of the children served had language disorders. Professional interest in disorders of language as well as speech is evident from the number of early journal articles and convention papers devoted to aphasia and delayed language development. The largest number of articles and papers were on the topic of stuttering, a term that had become favored over stammering, but those on aphasia were numerous as well (Paden, 1970).

An extensive and organized knowledge base for language development and developmental disorders of language did not begin to emerge, however, until the late 1950s and 1960s (Reed, 1994), and the majority of children served in the early programs exhibited articulatory-phonological disorders. They were generally seen by individuals who were designated as *speech teachers* or *speech correctionists*, later as *speech therapists*. These professionals usually followed the model established in Chicago, frequently called the *itinerant model*, that involved traveling from school to school and working with children in small groups that met several times a week.

Recent decades have witnessed a profound shift in the relative proportion of students with language problems, as differentiated from speech problems, who receive special services in the schools. There are a number of reasons for this. Beginning in the 1960s, scholarship in all language-related fields intensified, stimulating increased attention to disordered language as well as to normal language acquisition.

There was a concomitant increase in awareness of the central role played by language in academic achievement. The expanding learning disability movement had a significant impact on language services in schools. Students with learning disabilities gained inclusion in the Education for All Handicapped Children Act of 1975, eventually becoming the largest group to receive mandated services. This legislation, Public Law No. 94-142, had far-reaching and continuing impact on all school services for handicapped children. It and other legal landmarks are described in detail in Chapter 2.

A large proportion of these services for the learning disabled have involved efforts to strengthen language skills, and these may be viewed as being within the province of the speech-language pathologist. These developments contributed to the decision to change the national organization's name once more. In 1979, language was added; the acronym ASHA now stands for *American Speech-Language-Hearing Association*.

CURRENT TRENDS

According to the ASHA 1988 Omnibus Survey, nearly 50% of ASHA members were employed in schools, most of them engaged in providing direct services to students with speech, language, or hearing disorders. Caseloads were reported to be highly variable in terms of numbers of students served. The highest number of students had language disorders, and the next highest had articulatory-phonological disorders. Although the primary disabling conditions were isolated speech and/or language impairment for the largest group, other sizable populations receiving services were the learning disabled and the mentally retarded.

Aspects of the U.S. Department of Education's annual report to Congress on the implementation of the Individuals with Disabilities Education Act of 1990 (Pub. L. No. 101-407) provides an informative summary of all current school services for special-needs students (Peters-Johnson, 1994). The total number of American students served in 1991–1992 was somewhat less than 5 million. Almost half of these were identified as learning disabled. Students with speech or language impairments were 22.9% of the total, a decrease from previous reports. This decrease probably reflects an increasing tendency to classify speech- and language-impaired students as learning disabled. Most students with disabilities, 94%, received services in regular school buildings. Students with speech or language impairment were the most integrated group, with 78% having regular class placements. In contrast, hearing-impaired students tended to be more segregated, with less than 30% in regular classes. Prevalence of various categories of exceptional children as percentages of school enrollment is shown in Table 1–1.

Schools now serve a much wider variety of students with handicapping conditions than in the past. In addition, the special speech and language services provided to these students are now more fully integrated with the total educational program. The school speech-language pathologist at this time needs to know about a large number of handicapping conditions as well as the unique educational challenges each presents. The "speech teacher" has evolved into a communications specialist in an educational setting.

STUDY QUESTIONS

1. In what ways did the oral-only position harm the education of the deaf? In what ways might it have been helpful?

2. Technological advances have been viewed in differing ways with respect to the deaf and hearing impaired. Describe these differences.

3. What groups of children received most emphasis in early speech programs? What factors may have influenced this emphasis?

4. What does language have to do with learning disability? Why is this relationship so important in school programs?

5. Trace and explain the rise and decline of residential institutions for the deaf and mentally retarded.

Table 1–1 School Enrollment by Handicapping Condition

Handicapping Condition	% of School Enrollment
Learning disability	4.57
Speech impaired	2.86
Mentally retarded	1.84
Emotionally disturbed	0.91
Hard of hearing and deaf	0.18
Orthopedically impaired	0.14
Other health impaired	0.13
Visually handicapped	0.07
Multihandicapped	0.07

Source: Reprinted from the Seventh Annual Report to Congress on the Implementation of Public Law 94-142: The Education for All Handicapped Children Act, 1985, U.S. Department of Education.

REFERENCES

Deighton, L.C. (Ed.). (1971). *The encyclopedia of education*. New York: Macmillan.

Education for All Handicapped Children Act of 1975, Pub. L. No. 94-142, (163) Sec. 121a 303. Vol. No. 163 42, Washington, D.C.: U.S. Government Printing Office.

Garnet, C. (1968). *The exchange of letters between Samuel Heinecke and Charles Michel de l'Épée*. New York: Vantage.

Grossman, H.S. (Ed.). (1983). *Classification in mental retardation*. Washington, D.C.: American Association on Mental Deficiency.

Haines, H.H. (1965). Trends in public school speech therapy. *Asha, 7*, 187–190.

Heinz, R.B. (1971). *The encyclopedia of education*. New York: Macmillan.

Individuals with Disabilities Education Act of 1990 (IDEA), Pub. L. No. 101-407, 20 U.S.C. § 1400 et seq. Formerly titled the Education for All Handicapped Children Act, originally enacted as Public Law #94-142 (1975).

Kirk, S., & Gallagher, J. (1986) *Educating exceptional children* (5th ed.) Boston: Houghton Mifflin.

Lane, H. (1976) *The wild boy of Aveyron* Cambridge, MA: Howard University Press.

Miller, J.F. (1984). Mental retardation. In W.H. Perkins (Ed.), *Language handicaps in children* (pp. 75–86). New York: Thieme-Stratton.

Moore, P., & Kester, D. (1953). Historical notes on speech correction in the pre-association era. *Journal of Speech and Hearing Disorders, 18*, 44–53.

Moores, D.T. (1987). *Educating the deaf: Psychology, principles, and practice* (3rd ed.). Boston: Houghton Mifflin.

Paden, E.P. (1970). *A history of the ASHA, 1925–1958*. Washington, D.C.: American Speech Hearing Association.

Peters-Johnson, C. (1994). Action: School services. *Language, Speech, and Hearing Services in Schools, 25*, 121–127.

Reed, V.A. (1994). *An introduction to children with language disorders*. New York: Macmillan.

Solomon, J. (1994). *Deaf is beautiful*. New York: New York Times Magazine.

Vernon, M., & Koh, S. (1970). Effects of manual communication on deaf children's educational achievement, linguistic competence, oral skills, and psychological development. *American Annals of the Deaf, 115*, 527–536.

Chapter 2

Legal Landmarks

Eileen H. Gravani

According to the *American Heritage Dictionary* (2nd ed.), a law is a rule established by authority, society, or custom. In discussing the legal history affecting special education, we will discuss several means of establishing the rights of handicapped children. One means is legislation. In our system of government, we have laws passed at the federal, state, and local levels. The laws that are passed cannot violate the U.S. Constitution or the state constitution. One example of a federal law that was passed by Congress in 1975 is the Education for All Handicapped Children Act (Pub. L. No. 94-142). We will be discussing federal law rather than laws of individual states because the purpose of this chapter is to provide you with an overview of the legislative history.

Another means of establishing law that has been important in the rights of handicapped children is case law. Case law involves the judicial system's resolving of disagreements between two parties: for example, between citizens or between a citizen and the government. The purpose of the courts is to determine facts and interpret the meaning of the law in light of these facts. There are federal, state, and local court systems. The federal court system consists of three levels: trial courts, appellate courts (U.S. appeals courts),

and the U.S. Supreme Court. State and local court systems also typically have these three levels. In this chapter, we will discuss some cases that resulted in important decisions in favor of the educational rights of children with special needs.

LEGISLATION PRIOR TO THE EDUCATION FOR ALL HANDICAPPED CHILDREN ACT OF 1975

To understand how the present legislation came about, it is important to understand some history. In the 19th century, not all children went to school. Children from poor families, some girls, and children in isolated rural areas often did not attend school or did so only for brief periods. For children with special needs, there were some special schools for the deaf or blind. Often these schools were residential. There were no facilities for children with other disabilities, so often these children did not have any type of educational program.

For several reasons, there were few programs for children with disabilities. One was the general political philosophy at that time, which emphasized the rights of the majority rather than the rights of the individual. The general welfare of the majority was strongly emphasized. A second reason was a very narrow or limited interpretation of the definition of *education*. Education was seen as strictly academic: learning to read and write, do mathematics, and so forth. Other skills, such as daily living or self-help skills, speech and language, preacademics, and vocational skills, were not seen as the responsibility of the schools.

A case that illustrates the emphasis on the general welfare is *Beattie v. State Board of Education* in 1919. The case concerned a child with normal intelligence who had cerebral palsy. The boy had attended school in a regular classroom for several years and had been able to complete the academic work. He was described in the following way:

> He has not the normal use and control of his voice, hands, feet and body. By reason of the said paralysis, his vocal cords are afflicted. He is slow and hesitant in speech, and has a peculiar high, rasping and disturbing tone of voice, accompanied with uncontrollable facial contortions, making it difficult for him to make himself understood. He also has an uncontrollable flow of saliva, which drools from his mouth onto his clothing and books, causing him to have an unclean appearance. He has a nervous and excitable nature.

The local school board would not allow him to return to school, even though he had made adequate progress. They recommended placement in a school for the deaf because this was the only "special" program available. The parents filed a lawsuit, and the case went before the State of Wisconsin Supreme Court. The ruling favored the school district and stated that it was appropriate to exclude the child because of his "depressing and nauseating effect on the teachers and school chil-

dren and . . . [because] he required an undue portion of the teacher's time." The minority could not agree because there was no proof that the boy's presence had had a harmful influence upon the rest of the class and there was no legal basis for denying education. They stated that every child has a fundamental right to attend school.

In the early 1900s, the rigid definition of *education* began to expand. One reason for this was the child labor laws that were passed first in states such as Massachusetts and then federally. As a result, children from poor families and children with some learning problems entered the schools. To serve these children, school districts began to supply some special services. In 1910, Chicago became the first school district to employ teachers to work with children demonstrating speech problems. New York City followed in 1911. Soon, services were available in several large cities. But programs varied greatly from state to state, and no programs existed in rural areas. In the 1940s and 1950s, speech programs were available in many more cities and towns. However services still varied greatly between states and even between different school districts. Services to rural areas were very limited.

Brown v. Board of Education (BOE) was a historic Supreme Court decision in 1954. This decision essentially stated that segregated education was inherently unequal. Until this decision, schools and other facilities were segregated under a Supreme Court ruling from 1896. In that case, *Plessy v. Ferguson*, the court found that separate facilities were acceptable.

Brown v. BOE actually concerned four cases that were consolidated and heard as one case. The case was based on the equal-protection clause of the Fourteenth Amendment, which says that states cannot "deny to any person within its jurisdiction the equal protection of the laws." The Supreme Court's decision indicated that segregated schools violated equal protection and denied minority students the right to an equal educational opportunity.

Brown v. BOE accomplished several things. It illustrated that the Constitution of the United States is the binding law for all government in the United States—federal, state, and local. It also was a major victory for the civil rights movement and provided the basis for school desegregation. In addition to these, it highlighted the concept of a right to education. This concept will be important later in decisions on cases concerning children with special needs.

Since *Brown v. BOE*, federal laws have been developed to ensure civil rights. Ten years after the *Brown v. BOE* decision, in 1964, the Civil Rights Act was passed. Title VI of this act has two very important components. The first is that the federal government was mandated to withhold federal funds from institutions that excluded benefits to anyone on the basis of race, color, or national origin. The second component gave the federal Office of Education the responsibility to determine if school systems were segregated.

The 1960s have been known as the decade of the civil rights movement. Although the 1970s may be remembered as the decade that emphasized rights for handicapped individuals, there was some federal legislation in the 1960s that provided support for the education of children with disabilities. One of these was Public Law No. 89-313, an amendment to an education law passed in 1950. This amendment was the beginning of federal support for the education of students with special needs. It provided grant money to state agencies for students with disabilities. This money could be used for education in state-operated or -supported schools or institutions.

In the following year, 1966, Public Law No. 89-750 was passed. This provided federal grant money for *local* school districts to educate students with special needs. This law also established the Bureau of Education for the Handicapped. Some of the purposes of the bureau were to help states to implement and evaluate programs, train teachers to work with students having special needs, and train support staff and parents. The last piece of legislation in the 1960s dealing with special education was Public Law No. 90-247. This expanded some special education services, established regional resource centers for special education, and established centers to serve deaf–blind children.

As indicated above, the 1970s may be remembered as the decade that emphasized the rights of individuals with disabilities. This emphasis can be seen in the case laws and legislation that were passed. In 1971, a class action lawsuit was filed, *Pennsylvania Association for Retarded Children (PARC) v. Commonwealth of Pennsylvania*, on behalf of 13 mentally retarded children. At that time, Pennsylvania had a policy that children needed to have a mental age of 5 years in order to enter school. As one might predict, this resulted in the exclusion of a large percentage of mentally retarded children. Like *Brown v. BOE*, the PARC case argued from the equal-protection clause of the Fourteenth Amendment. PARC also used the due-process clause from the Fourteenth Amendment and the Fifth Amendment. Additionally, testimony from legal and educational experts indicated that education was necessary for a child to function in society and that all children can learn from an education. This case was resolved the following year in federal district court by a consent decree. This was an agreement by all the parties involved and then approved by the court. It was agreed that the state and local school districts would identify all children who were excluded from school and provide all mentally retarded children with an appropriate educational program.

While the PARC case was occurring another class action suit was being filed in Washington, D.C. This case represented all out-of-school handicapped children who were excluded from school or expelled or suspended. This case represented a less specific group than the PARC case. The case, *Mills v. Board of Education (BOE)* had its name from one of the children, Peter Mills. He was a 12-year-old who had been expelled from school as a "behavior problem." Unlike the PARC case, which resulted in an agreement and did not have a judicial ruling, *Mills v. BOE* required a court decision. The court decision was against the school board and required that a list of excluded children be developed and that they be provided with a public education. Additionally, a time limit was put on the BOE so that changes would occur by given dates.

Around this time, there were a variety of similar cases, and states began to pass or revise laws that required the education of all handicapped children. Legislation in Congress used two approaches. Nondiscrimination legislation was passed as well as federal legislation concerning education. In 1973, the Rehabilitation Act (Pub. L. No. 93-112) was passed. It dealt with discrimination against people with disabilities and protected their civil rights against discrimination in civil programs. Section 504 of this law states that "no otherwise qualified handicapped individual in the United States shall, solely by reason of his [or her] handicap, be excluded from the participation in, be denied the benefits of, or be subjected to discrimination under any program or activity receiving federal financial assistance." This means that any program receiving federal funds needs to provide equal opportunity for individuals with handicapping conditions. The provision affects school districts, colleges, universities, and employers such as state and local governments and hospitals. This law has been amended several times, and its scope has been broadened. It continues today to protect people with disabilities from discrimination. It also helps to support the Individuals with Disabilities Education Act (IDEA; Pub. L. No. 101-407), passed in 1990, protecting the rights of students with special needs.

Federal legislation was also passed concerning education. In 1974, Public Law No. 93-380 was passed. It required that states begin procedures to identify and evaluate all handicapped children, establish a goal of providing full educational opportunity for all handicapped children, and submit to the federal government a plan describing how the state would meet that goal. Other sections of the law included procedural safeguards. These dealt with the evaluation and placement of students and protected families' rights by allowing parents to examine records and, if not satisfied with an educational program, to have a hearing. This procedure is called *due process*. For the first time, parents and handicapped children were allowed to question a school district's decision, using a systematic procedure and guaranteed rights.

In 1975, Congress held a series of hearings to extend and amend Public Law No. 93-380. Information was presented by parents, special educators, and professional organizations. American Speech-Hearing Association (ASHA) involvement was substantial. ASHA members testified in Washington, D.C., and in several regional hearings. They provided input to state departments of education and sent messages to the White House.

The major findings of the hearings indicated that many children aged 3 to 21 years were not receiving appropriate services. Testimony indicated that there were over 8 million children and young adults in this age range. For many of these individuals, special education needs and needs for related services such as speech-language, physical, or occupational therapy, audiology, and counseling were not being met. Many of the students who were enrolled in an educational program were not receiving appropriate services. Over 1 million of these children or young adults were excluded from public schools. Many handicapped children were placed in regular classrooms. However, their disabilities were preventing them from having a successful educational experience. Many families were forced to find services for their children independently.

THE EDUCATION FOR ALL HANDICAPPED CHILDREN ACT OF 1975

The same year, the Education for All Handicapped Children Act of 1975 was passed. The four major purposes of the act were

1. To ensure that all handicapped children would receive a "free appropriate public education." This would include special education and related services to meet their needs.

2. To ensure that the rights of handicapped children and their parents would be protected through the due-process procedure.

3. To evaluate the effectiveness of federal, state, and local efforts to educate handicapped children.

4. To provide financial assistance to state and local agencies so that they could provide full educational opportunities to all handicapped children.

Some basic elements in the act's phrase *free appropriate public education* are extremely important to educational programs. We will discuss them so that we will have a better understanding of later court cases and the guidelines that school districts follow. The word *free* means that the service is provided at no cost to the parent. This includes room and board if that is deemed appropriate. Currently, school districts are billing Medicare, HMOs, and private insurance companies for reimbursable services such as audiological evaluations, physical or occupational therapy, speech-language services, and mental health services. This will be discussed in Chapter 10. However, parents are *not* billed for services.

Another term that needs to be discussed is the word *appropriate*. This means that the special education program and related services provided for handicapped students must meet their needs *as adequately as the needs of nonhandicapped are met*. It is clear from this statement that there can be a difference between *ideal* services and *appropriate* services. How is it possible to determine what is "appropriate"?

One measure of appropriateness is that the student must be able to benefit from the program and acquire some minimum skills so that the education is considered meaningful. An early case that was concerned with this issue was *Fialkowski v. Shapp* in 1975. The case involved two brothers who were mentally retarded, with the intellectual level of preschoolers. They were placed in a classroom that emphasized reading and writing. Their lawyer argued that they were not able to find their classroom experience meaningful. We will see this issue of determining if a child is demonstrating progress in later cases. To determine what a child's needs are and to document progress, an evaluation must occur. This evaluation needs to consider all areas of suspected disability. Following this evaluation, an educational program with goals is developed. To determine progress, reevaluations need to occur. When hearing officers in due-process procedures or courts review information to determine if placements are "appropriate," records including evaluations, goals, and reevaluations are carefully reviewed.

The *least restrictive environment* is a key concept relating to the Education for All Handicapped Children Act and to later legislation and cases. According to the law, children with handicapping conditions should be educated with nonhandicapped children to the maximum extent possible. If the nature or the severity of the handicap prevents achievement in a regular classroom, then special schools are allowed. The actual wording of the law will be included when we discuss IDEA.

Because of the immense amount of planning, preparation, and paperwork involved, the Education for All Handicapped Children Act was not implemented until 1978. President Gerald Ford, who signed the legislation, was concerned that it "promised more than the federal government could deliver" (Weiner, 1985, p. 20).

The act resulted in the creation of new programs in special education and the revamping of existing programs. It has continued to have bipartisan support in Congress. In 1982, the Reagan administration proposed a series of revisions that would have weakened the guarantees of the act. Strong negative public response resulted in these proposals' being dropped. We will come back to this law when we talk about IDEA, which amended the Education for All Handicapped Children Act in 1990.

The Education of the Handicapped Amendments of 1986 (Pub. L. No. 99-457) amended the Education for All Handicapped Children Act of 1975. These amendments had two major purposes. The first was to provide funding for the education of eligible preschool children with disabilities, ages 3 to 5 years. The second was to assist states in developing programs for infants and toddlers with disabilities, focusing on early intervention for these children. For services to infants and toddlers, states were given 3 years to develop a plan and then were required to begin providing services. Public Law No. 102-119 in 1991 reauthorized these services. We will discuss the procedures used for infants and toddlers (birth to 2 years, 11 months) and preschool children (ages 3 to 5 years) in Chapter 7.

The Education for All Handicapped Children Act was amended again in 1990. At this time, its name changed to the Individuals with Disabilities Act (IDEA). IDEA has expanded the act in several areas. One of these areas is transition services, which are now part of Individualized Educational Programs (IEPs). Transition services begin when a student is 15 or 16 years old. Their purpose is to facilitate the transition into the community. They will be discussed in more detail in Chapter 7. Because transition services are now mandated, social work and rehabilitation counseling are now included under "related services." Another area that IDEA affects is assistive technology. This includes computers and electronic communication boards for augmentative communication. Additionally, changes in the law provide more services and rights to individuals with autism and traumatic brain injury.

Like other legislation that has a time component, IDEA needs to be reauthorized. Written comments from the public are requested in the *Federal Register*. For reauthorization in 1996, organizations such as ASHA have had the opportunity to present oral and written testimony to Congress. Parents, people with disabilities, and members of ASHA and other organizations have maintained pressure on Congress to support IDEA reauthorization. Phone calls, e-mail messages, letters, and telegrams have been sent by supporters of IDEA.

Some of the components of IDEA that are in danger include

- personnel standards
- personnel preparation development
- training and research funds
- full access to related services
- full access to assistive technology
- appropriate instructional programs (Rabins, 1996)

An amendment concerning the capping of related services may also be proposed (Rabins, 1996).

Another issue of concern in the bill under consideration in the U.S. House of Representatives is the possibility that 10 local education agencies may be given permission to conduct "pilot projects" that drop the requirements for free appropriate public education and the least restrictive environment (Moore, 1996).

At this time, a bill that reauthorizes IDEA has passed the House. ASHA has concerns regarding personnel standards in this bill. The Senate has not yet passed its version of IDEA reauthorization. An additional concern is that states may still cut special education funds (Moore, 1996).

It will continue to be important that ASHA, its members, other professional organizations, and families of children with special needs send strong messages to members of Congress as IDEA is reauthorized now and in the future.

According to the current law, *least restrictive environment* (LRE) specifies

1. that to the maximum extent appropriate, children with disabilities, including children in public or private institutions or other care facilities, are educated with children who are not disabled; and

2. that special classes, separate schooling or other removal of children with disabilities from the regular educational environment occurs only when the nature or severity of the handicap is such that education in regular classes with the use of supplementary aids and services cannot be achieved satisfactorily (34 C.F.R. Sec. 300.550).

IDEA requires that school districts educate students with special needs in the "least restrictive environment." This means that districts need to have a continuum of placements available and procedures to ensure that these students are educated with students without disabilities to the maximum extent possible.

The Office of Special Education and Rehabilitation Services (OSERS) responds to letters from interested parties and gives information and guidance on the implementation of IDEA. An example of this was the response to a state representative from South Carolina ("Letter to Spratt") questioning the policy of inclusion of students with special needs into general education classes. OSERS responded that a regular (or general) education classroom in a local school should be the first option when a placement decision is made for a student with disabilities. Also, a continuum of placements (discussed in Chapter 7) is an important part of IDEA. The letter noted that placement in a more restrictive setting should be made only on the basis of the educational needs of the child (OSERS, 1994, cited in Peters-Johnson, 1995).

At times it seems that the benefits of the least restrictive environment need to be compared against a specialized program with possibly more services. Because each child has individual needs and abilities, each case needs to be considered individually. However, some general principles can be followed. The Fifth Circuit Court of Appeals developed a criterion or "test" to determine if a school district had fulfilled its obligation to educate students with disabilities in the least restrictive environment. This was done in response to a case that it heard in 1989. The case, *Daniel R.R. v. State Board of Education*, concerned a child with Down syndrome with the classification of "mentally retarded." The student had been in a general education classroom for part of the day. The boy had not taken part in the classroom activities and had not mastered skills that were part of the classroom program. The school district planned to place him in a special education class. The court held that the special education class was appropriate and that this placement did not violate the least restrictive environment stipulation. The three-judge appeals court developed a two-part test to determine if a school district had attempted to educate students with special needs as much as possible with students without disabilities. The first criterion is: Can education in the general education classroom be achieved when supplementary aids and services are provided? If it cannot be achieved at a satisfactory level, then the second question is posed: Was the student mainstreamed to the maximum extent possible? In this case, the school district had supplied a continuum of placements and had provided supplementary aids and services, attempting to maintain Daniel in a general education class. The court also noted that the school district had provided mainstreaming for Daniel to the maximum extent possible.

The Fifth Circuit Court of Appeals instructed lower courts to consider five factors:

1. the student's ability to comprehend and learn the general classroom curriculum
2. the type and severity of the disability
3. the impact that the student's presence would have upon the general education classroom
4. The student's experiences with mainstream settings
5. The extent of contact that the student with special needs would have with students without disabilities

This two-part test has become a standard in cases involving the LRE. Some of the recent decisions have supported separate settings; others have supported education for some students with special needs within general education (Osborne & Dimatta, 1994).

Lisco v. Woodland Hills School District (1989) concerned a student who was classified as educable mentally retarded and socially and emotionally disturbed. This student had been in a setting with part-time mainstreaming. Testimony indicated that the student had made little academic progress in the mainstream program and did not interact or socialize with the other students. In addition, his behavior was often disruptive and affected the classroom activities and routines. The school district planned to place the student in a more restrictive setting: a special education classroom in a center. The district court approved the placement of the student in the special education program in the center and ordered some mainstreaming into a public school. The information that the school district presented on the student's academic, social, and behavioral functioning within the classroom and his impact upon the classroom was very likely a factor in the court's decision.

DeVries v. Fairfax County School Board (1989) concerned a high school student who was autistic. This student had lowered cognitive functioning, difficulty with interpersonal relationships, difficulty with communication, and immature behavior. Additionally, the student performed best in a predictable environment. The school district recommended placement in the county vocational center, but the parent wanted placement in a high school program. The district court decided that the vocational program was appropriate, and the appeals court concurred.

One of the court decisions that stresses contact with children without disabilities was *Greer v. Rome City School District* (1990). Christy Greer, a 9-year-old girl with Down syndrome, had been mainstreamed into a kindergarten program for 3 years rather than placed in a separate special education classroom. The court supported the kindergarten placement, noting that the child had made some progress and that she was not disruptive in the classroom. They did note that although the placement was appropriate at this time, it might not continue to be appropriate in future years. The court also noted that Rome City School District did not consider a range of supplementary aids and services or attempt to modify the classroom curriculum to meet Christy's needs. Additionally, the IEP was developed before the IEP meeting, and a continuum of placement options were not discussed.

It is clear that these recent court decisions do not require that *all* students with special needs be educated in general education classrooms. School districts need to make an effort to provide general education programs using supplemental aids and services for a student with special needs. If the program does not meet the student's needs in terms of academic progress and/or social interaction, or if the student is disruptive and affects the other

students' education negatively, then the school district is justified in placing the student in a more restrictive setting. The courts have also indicated that school districts' decisions may consider cost and that education in a general education classroom may not be a choice if the cost of the supplemental aids and services is excessive. At this time, the parameters for defining *excessive* have not been determined (Osborne & Dimatta, 1994).

As indicated above, one continuing legal issue for special education is that of least restrictive environment. Another issue that we may see concerns the definition of "appropriate" education, especially concerning related services. This issue relates to limited funding and the high cost of specialized services. A second issue that relates to funding is the definition of *highest standard requirements* for qualified providers. This issue will be dealt with in legislation rather than through litigation. Parental choice over educational placements will continue to be an issue, particularly with private schools. Finally, schools will need to be in compliance with the Americans with Disabilities Act of 1990.

In the first thorough analysis of litigation related to special education, it was noted that the amount of litigation had increased. Typical concerns are

- procedural issues
- liability and negligence actions
- civil rights violations
- responsibility for funding of special education
- least restrictive environment
- free appropriate public education

Overall, the school prevailed in 54.3% of the decisions. In cases involving communication disorders, parents prevailed 62.5% of the time and in 57.4% of cases related to hearing impairments (Maloney & Shenker, 1995).

Clearly, legislation and court decisions will continue to affect services provided to children with special needs in the future. It is very likely that in your own professional careers, you will see a variety of changes occurring.

STUDY QUESTIONS

1. What provided the basis of civil rights legislation and legislation for special education?

2. What were the four major purposes of Public Law 94-142?

3. What are the two areas that IDEA (Public Law 101-407) expanded services to special-needs students?

4. What is the least restrictive environment? Why is the least restrictive environment often the issue for due process hearings and legal cases?

REFERENCES

Beattie v. State Board of Education, 172 N.W. 153 (1919).

Brown v. Board of Education, 347 U.S. 483 (1954).

Daniel R.R. v. State Board of Education 874 F.2d 1036, 53 Ed.Law Rep. 824 (5th Cir. 1989).

DeVries v. Fairfax County School Board, 882 F.2d 876, 55 Ed.Law Rep. 442 (4th Cir. 1989).

Fialkowski v. Shapp, 405 F. Supp. 946 (E.D.Pa. 1976).

Greer v. Rome City School District, 762 F. Supp. 936, 67 Ed.Law Rep. 666 (N.D.Ga. 1990); affirmed 905 F.2d 688, 71 Ed.Law Rep. 647 (11th Cir. 1991); withdrawn 956 F.2d 1025, 73 Ed.Law Rep. 34 (11th Cir. 1992); reinstated 967 F.2d. 470, 76 Ed.Law Rep. 26 (11th Cir. 1992).

Letter to Spratt, 20 *Individuals with Disabilities Education Law Report* 1457 (OSERS 1994) 6/30/94, XIV 202. in Peters-Johnson, C. (1995). "Action: school services." *Language, Speech and Hearing Services in the Schools,* (1995) 26, 101.

Lisco v. Woodland Hills School District, 734 F.Supp. 689, 60 Ed.Law Rep. 47 (W.D.Pa. 1989): affirmed 902 F.2d 1561, 60 Ed.Law Rep. 1083 (3d. Cir.1990).

Maloney M. and Shenker, B. (1995). "The continuing evolution of special education law 1978 to 1995." *Individuals with Disabilities Education Law Report—Special Report no. 12.* in Peters-Johnson, C. (1996). "Action: school services." *Language, Speech and Hearing Services in the Schools,* 27, 188–189.

Mills v. Board of Education, 348 F. Supp. 866 (D.D.C. 1972).

Moore, M. (1996). "House opposes personnel standards, Senate bill gains support." *ASHA Leader,* 1, 4.

Osborne, Jr., A.G., and Dimatta, P. (1994). "The IDEA's least restrictive environment mandate: legal implications." *Exceptional Children,* 61, 6–14.

Pennsylvania Association for Retarded Children v. Commonwealth of Pennsylvania, 343 F. Supp. 279 (E.D. Pa. 1972).

Rehabilitation Act of 1973, Pub. L. No. 93-112 Sec. 504, 87 Stat. 355.

Education amendments of 1965, Pub. L. No. 89-313, Sec. 1 et seq., 79 Stat. 1158.

Civil Rights Act of 1964, Pub. L. No. 88-352, Sec. 101 et seq., 78 Stat.

Americans with Disabilities Act of 1990, Pub. L. No. 101-336 Sec. 2 et seq., Education amendments of 1974, Pub. L. No. 93-380, Sec. 101 et seq., 88 Stat. 484.

Education for All Handicapped Children Act, Pub. L. No. 94-142, Sec. 3 et seq., 89 Stat. 774.

Education of the Handicapped Act Amendments of 1986, Pub. L. No. 99-457. Sec. 101 et seq. 100 Stat. 1145.

Individuals with disabilities education act amendments of 1990, Pub. L. No. 102-119, Sec. 3 et seq., 105 Stat. 587.

Rabins, A. (1996). "Senate awaits vote, House preps for markup." *ASHA Leader,* 1, 1&6.

Weiner, R. (1985). P.L. 94-142: Impact on the schools (p. 20). Arlington, VA: Capitol Publications.

Plessy v. Ferguson, 163 U.S. 537 (1896)

Moore, M. (1996). "State funding cuts target special ed." *ASHA Leader,* 1, 12.

Chapter 3

ASHA and the Schools

Regina B. Grantham

This chapter provides information about the American Speech-Language-Hearing Association (ASHA). It presents the association's history, purpose, governance, membership, standards, code of ethics, guidelines, benefits, and support of school services. This information will be a valuable resource for practitioners and students in the field of speech-language pathology and audiology.

ASHA HISTORY

ASHA is a nonprofit, national, scientific, professional, accrediting organization. It was first established in 1925 by a group of people who were interested in the study and treatment of communication disorders. Before ASHA's founding, many professionals who worked in communication disorders were members of the National Association of Teachers of Speech (NATS). NATS provided presentation opportunities for people in the field of communication disorders and published their papers in its periodical, *Quarterly Journal of Speech Education*. NATS's membership became so large that except for business meetings and general sessions,

Special appreciation goes to ASHA's national office, for providing background information and generously giving of their time.

people began to meet in specific-interest sections to facilitate discussion. Through these special-interest discussions, the need for an organization whose total purpose was dedicated to the science of speech correction was developed (Paden, 1970).

Initially, ASHA was called the American Academy of Speech Correction (AASC). Membership was restricted to members of NATS who met specific requirements. As the professions (we say "professions" because speech-language pathology and audiology are considered two professions) grew, the Academy of Speech Correction underwent several name changes. In 1927, it was renamed the American Society for the Study of Speech Disorders and was again renamed the American Speech Correction Association in 1934. The association's name changed to the American Speech and Hearing Association (ASHA) in 1947. This new name recognized the rapid growth in aural rehabilitation. In 1978, the name was changed again to the American Speech-Language-Hearing Association, but the acronym *ASHA* was retained. This change recognized the treatment and evaluation of communication disorders in the area of language.

As of January 1, 1997, the association will be known as the *American Association of*

Speech-Language Pathology and Audiology. Again, the acronym *ASHA* will remain. The new name embraces both speech-language pathology and audiology and includes the science and research aspects of the two professions. Some ASHA members feel that this name change has moved the professions from a scientific and professional emphasis to a strictly professional one and are lobbying for another name change. Given the professions' changing scope of practice, it is my opinion that the association's name will probably continue to change to reflect the expansion of services.

ASHA PURPOSE

Although ASHA has undergone many name changes, its basic purpose has remained intact: commitment to scientific work in communication disorders. To acknowledge the dynamic nature of the field, the purpose has expanded and now includes stimulating the scientific study of communication, with special reference to speech, language, and hearing; encouraging appropriate clinical and academic preparation for the professions of speech-language pathology and audiology; maintaining the current knowledge of those within the discipline; promoting the investigation and prevention of disorders; fostering improvement of services and procedures for communication disorders; advocating for the rights and interests of people with these disorders; distributing and promoting the exchange of information; and advancing the interests of the profession and members of the association (ASHA, 1995i).

ASHA GOVERNANCE

To pursue its purposes, ASHA has a governing structure that involves its members in the decision-making process. The policy-making body for the association is the Legislative Council (LC), which is composed of ASHA members elected from each of the 50 states, the District of Columbia, members residing outside the United States, and other representatives as may be specified by ASHA's bylaws. The president of the association is the chair of the LC, with the other members of the Executive Board (EB) serving as ex officio LC members. The EB is the managing body of the association. Its composition includes officers (president and vice presidents) elected from the ASHA membership and the executive director of the association. The EB, with monitoring from the LC, supervises and directs the association's affairs, implements programs and policies, and distributes funds as appropriate. Also in this ASHA structure are numerous committees, boards, councils, task forces, and ad hoc committees composed of ASHA members. Each committee/board/council/task force/ad hoc committee has specific charges and is responsible to the LC or EB (ASHA, 1995j; Lubinski & Frattali, 1994). Figure 3–1 is a schematic representation of ASHA's governing structure. Governance structures are frequently revised, and the reader should be advised that changes may already have occurred since this chapter was written.

ASHA members who are interested in serving on committees/boards/councils should complete and submit a committee pool form. This application form is available through FAX-on-Demand, a member service established to provide immediate access to up-to-date information. Appointments will be made from among those who have applied to the committee pool, and "High priority will be given to school speech-language pathologists and audiologists, women, and federally designated ethnic minority groups"

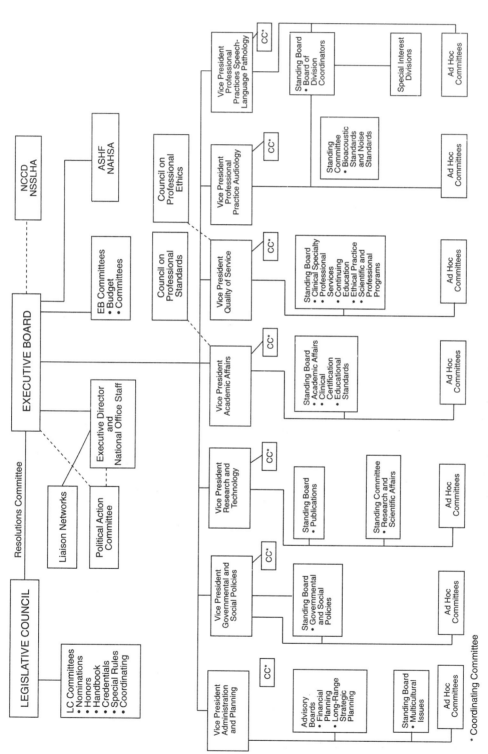

Figure 3–1 Association Governance Structure. Courtesy of the American Speech-Language-Hearing Association.

(ASHA, 1995a, p. 72). A list of the committees/boards/councils, their charges, and their members, along with complete instructions on how to become a member of these groups, is given in the journal *Asha*.

Any ASHA member can propose a new policy for the association or change an existing one. The member must propose the policy in the form of a resolution. That proposed resolution must be considered by the LC. The member should submit this resolution to a legislative councilor from his or her state or to a member of the EB for assistance. Members of the EB and LC are listed in the *Asha* journal or *Leader*.

As the services to members expanded and the officers' responsibilities increased, it became apparent that a national office was needed to augment the governing structure. This office officially opened in 1958 (Paden, 1970) and is currently located in Rockville, Maryland. The national office is managed by a dedicated, qualified staff under the direction of the executive director and the guidance of the EB.

ASHA MEMBERSHIP

ASHA's membership has increased dramatically, from 25 charter members (Paden, 1970) to over 81,000 professionals in 1995 (ASHA, 1995a). To accommodate the increased interest in the professions, ASHA offers several categories of membership: (a) membership with certification, (b) membership without certification, (c) membership without certification—research or allied professional, and (d) international affiliate. Membership with certification is for those individuals who will provide or supervise clinical services. To be eligible for this category, a person must successfully complete the requirements for the Certificate of Clinical Competence (CCC) in speech-language pathology or audiology or both. A person who holds a master's degree or its equivalent, with a major in speech-language pathology, audiology, or speech-language and hearing science, and who is not providing or supervising services, qualifies for membership without certification. An individual who holds a master's degree and demonstrates active research, interest, and performance in the professions but who does not provide or supervise clinical services is eligible for the category "membership without certification—research and allied professional." A person who resides abroad and who holds a master's degree or its equivalent may apply for international affiliate membership. Applicants for ASHA membership should carefully review all categories to determine the one that best represents their professional status (ASHA, 1995j).

ASHA BENEFITS/SERVICES

ASHA offers numerous benefits and services to its members. These services include the development of standards for clinical certification, the development of standards for accreditation of educational programs and clinical agencies, the provision of clinical and ethical guidelines for the practice of the professions, lobbying for the professions at various levels of government, the provision of opportunities for ongoing education, the provision of occasions to network professionally, and the provision of easy access to information.

Standards Program

Standards are a way of making certain that quality services and products are provided to consumers by individuals, agencies, and associations. ASHA certifies individuals and accredits graduate programs and professional service programs to make certain that these quality services are provided to the public. It should be noted that accreditation and certification are voluntary processes.

The American Board of Examiners in Speech Pathology and Audiology (ABESPA) was created in 1959 to ensure quality services for persons with communication disorders. ABESPA was replaced by the Council on Professional Standards in Speech-Language Pathology and Audiology (Standards Council) in 1980. The Standards Council was responsible for establishing and monitoring all standards programs of ASHA. The Educational Standards Board (ESB) applied the standards for graduate programs, the Professional Services Board (PSB) applied the standards for clinics and agencies, and the Clinical Certification Board (CCB) applied the standards for the Certificate of Clinical Competence (CCC). However in 1996/1997, a separate body, the Council on Academic Accreditation (CAA) in Audiology and Speech-Language Pathology, assumed the responsibilities of establishing standards as well as applying them in the accreditation of graduate programs, thus replacing ESB. This newly created council was a response to the rapid growth of the profession, which necessitated change in academic accreditation. This change also meant that the Standards Council was then dedicated to setting standards for clinical certification and accreditation of professional services programs only (ASHA, 1995d, 1995e, 1995i).

Educational Program Accreditation

In 1965, ASHA established the master's degree as the minimum level of preparation needed for entry into the professions. To ensure that certain standards were met in ob-

taining this degree, ASHA accredits master's degree programs that train speech-language pathologists and audiologists. These standards for accreditation have moved toward qualitative standards and a focus on outcomes. For example, previously an educational program had to have a student faculty ratio of 6:1 (six students for every faculty member). University programs found this ratio restrictive and often costly. To address this concern, ASHA adopted a more flexible, accommodating approach. The standard was revised to indicate that the educational programs must demonstrate sufficient faculty/staff to support the programs' goals/objectives and mission (ASHA, 1995a, 1995f).

Until 1995, the ESB interpreted and applied the standards for educational programs. As mentioned earlier, these responsibilities were assumed by CAA. When a graduate program applies for accreditation, evaluators appointed by ASHA visit the facility. The team reviews such aspects as faculty qualifications, academic course work, clinical supervision, library support, and physical space. After the site visit, the evaluators report back to CAA. If the specific criteria are met, the department is accredited. To make certain that standards are maintained, the program review cycle occurs every 8 years. Specific standards for accreditation of educational programs can be obtained from ASHA's national office.

Because of the broad range of diagnostic and remedial services associated with the practice of audiology, the LC voted in 1993 to support the professional doctorate (Au.D.) as the entry level for audiology. This is a postbaccalaureate degree that will place major emphasis on clinical training. The specific standards for accrediting this program are in process. The implementation of the new standards for the Au.D. is expected to begin in 2002 (ASHA, 1995e; Lubinski & Frattoli, 1994).

Professional Service Program Accreditation

ASHA also accredits professional service programs (clinics, hospital departments, agencies) where treatment and evaluation are provided for persons with communication disorders. The Professional Services Board (PSB) of ASHA evaluates the speech-language and hearing services of a clinic or agency that applies for accreditation. Agencies who apply for accreditation receive a site visit during which such features as the qualifications of the clinicians, the physical space, the equipment used, and the quality of clinical services provided are reviewed. If the agency/clinic meets the requirements, then the agency is accredited. Periodic reviews of service programs occur to ensure the continuation of quality services.

Most clinics/agencies that provide services for people with communication disorders will be reviewed by more than one accrediting body. Therefore ASHA has made major efforts in establishing joint programs with other accrediting organizations. For instance, an agency that desires ASHA accreditation and also needs CARF (Rehabilitation Accreditation Commission) accreditation can do both in a collaborative manner. This joint process seems most efficient for both the clinic and the accrediting organization, as it saves time and reduces both paperwork and cost (ASHA, 1995a, 1995c).

Certificate of Clinical Competence

ASHA also provides a Certificate of Clinical Competence (CCC) to individuals who provide services to persons with communication disorders. This certificate is awarded by the Clinical Certification Board (CCB). The CCB consists of ASHA members with certification in speech-language pathology and/or

audiology. This board interprets and applies the standards established by the Council on Professional Standards. A person seeking certification from ASHA in speech-language pathology or audiology must have either a master's or a doctoral degree in the field, must complete a clinical fellowship under the supervision of someone who has his or her CCC, and must pass the national exam administered by the Educational Testing Service (ASHA, 1995j). A more in-depth discussion of ASHA's certification requirements can be found in Chapter 4.

Because ASHA-accredited graduate programs will definitely provide the required academic and clinical training necessary for obtaining a CCC, prospective speech-language pathologists and audiologists should be aware of these programs. They should also be familiar with the most current CCC requirements. This information may be obtained by calling or writing ASHA's national office.

Position Statements, Guidelines, and Other Relevant Papers

In addition to setting and implementing standards for certification and accreditation, ASHA develops position statements, guidelines, definitions, bibliographies, reports, tutorial papers, and other relevant documents. The position statements specify ASHA's policy on specific matters such as issues in the delivery of service to individuals with learning disabilities, facilitated communication (Appendix 3–A), augmentative and alternative communication, social dialects, and scope of practice.

Scope of Practice

The document "Scope of Practice, Speech-Language Pathology and Audiology" (ASHA, 1990) is of particular interest to students and practitioners. It defines the range of services provided by speech-language pathologists and audiologists. This statement is a list of professional activities that specifies the broad range of services offered within the professions. Not only does it define the scope of practice for speech-language pathologists and audiologists, but it also educates consumers, the general public, and other professionals about the services provided. However, consumers and others are reminded that this statement does not guarantee the skill or proficiency of the professional but rather merely states the range of activities provided by speech, language, and hearing professionals. Because the professions are continuously developing, the Scope of Practice statement will be updated as new clinical practices emerge. To view the complete Scope of Practice statement see Appendix 3–B.

Preferred Practice Patterns

To define practices in the professions further, ASHA developed preferred practice patterns (ASHA, 1993b). These practice patterns are not official standards, but they do serve as guidelines for enhancing the quality of professional services to consumers. They represent 3 years of intensive work by the Task Force on Clinical Standards and reflect a consensus of current practices based on the most current knowledge available at the time. These practices are universally applicable across work settings. Each procedure is described, along with the professional who is responsible for the procedure, the structural requisites of the practice, the expected outcomes of the procedure, the clinical indications for performing the procedure, the clinical processes, the setting and equipment specifications, safety and health precautions, and documentation aspects. These guidelines are an education tool for professionals. However, total adherence to each step does not guarantee a specific outcome. As new proce-

dures and technology develop in the professions, the preferred practice patterns will be updated. Copies of the preferred practice patterns for articulation/phonology assessment and speech-language pathology treatment are included in Appendix 3–C.

Many of the preferred practice patterns refer to ASHA's guidelines. These practice guidelines consist of recommended sets of procedures for specific areas of practice. The procedures are based on research findings and current practice and detail the knowledge and skills necessary to perform the techniques competently. Examples of guidelines include guidelines for caseload size and speech-language service delivery in schools; suggested competencies for effective clinical supervision; guidelines for identification audiometry; and guidelines for speech-language pathologists serving persons with language, sociocommunicative, and/or cognitive communicative impairments.

Definitions of relevance to the profession (e.g., communicative disorders and variations, learning disabilities, severely hearing handicapped) along with bibliographies, reports, and other relevant papers, are also published by ASHA for professional reference (Appendix 3–D). These can be found in the *ASHA Desk Reference: Guidelines, Position Statements, Definitions, and Relevant Papers* and its 1995 supplement (ASHA, 1995l). As with all professional activity, ASHA members and certificate holders are bound by the ASHA's Code of Ethics when applying the position statements, practice guidelines, definitions, and other relevant material.

Ethics

From its inception, ASHA has made a commitment to professional ethics. In 1930, a section headed "Principles of Ethics" was added to ASHA's constitution. The principles consisted of three parts: "Duties of Members," "Secrecy," and "Unethical Practices" (Paden, 1970). In 1951, the Principles of Ethics were removed from the bylaws and became a separate document known as the Code of Ethics. This document has been revised from time to time to accommodate the changing scope of the professions.

Code of Ethics

The Code of Ethics provides guidelines for professional practice. It delineates professional boundaries and protects consumers, members, and the professions. The code is divided into two main parts: the preamble, which defines the code, and the four principles of ethics statements, which target specific audiences. Principles of Ethics 1 and 2 define a member's responsibilities to the persons served. Principle 3 outlines the responsibilities a member has to the public. The responsibilities to the professions of speech-language pathology and audiology are delineated in Principle 4. Specifically, the code incorporates high standards of integrity and is based on the following ethical principles:

1. Individuals shall honor their responsibility to hold paramount the welfare of persons they serve professionally.

2. Individuals shall honor their responsibility to achieve and maintain the highest level of professional competence.

3. Individuals shall honor their responsibility to the public by promoting public understanding of the professions, by supporting the development of services designed to fulfill the unmet needs of the public, and by providing accurate information in all communications involving any aspect of the professions.

4. Individuals shall honor their responsibilities to the professions and their rela-

tionships with colleagues, students, and members of allied professions. Individuals shall uphold the dignity and autonomy of the professions, maintain harmonious interprofessional and intraprofessional relationships, and accept the professions' self-imposed standards. (ASHA, 1995h, p. 74)

Each principle of ethics includes rules that state the minimally acceptable professional conduct. The rules include such concepts as providing services in a competent manner, not discriminating against a consumer, not guaranteeing the results of therapy, appropriately representing one's credentials, protecting the patient's confidentiality, and not engaging in dishonesty, fraud, or deceit. ASHA members and/or certificate holders, applicants for membership or certification, and persons in their clinical fellowship year are bound by the Code of Ethics (ASHA, 1995h).

Ethical decision making includes not only professional ethics (difficult decisions regarding such concerns as fees for service, qualifications, certification, advertising, available resources, and research) but clinical ethics (dilemmas involving patient care and management) as well (Sharp & Genesen, 1996). The challenges of managed care and the expansion of the professions' scope of practice have placed greater demands upon the clinical provider, thus posing difficult ethical decisions. The following are a few ethical dilemmas that have arisen in the schools:

1. Should the speech-language pathologists in schools evaluate and treat swallowing disorders?

2. Should the speech-language pathologists in schools facilitate oral feeding by changing the food texture or the student's posture, especially when the patient is aspirating?

3. Should the speech-language pathologists in schools provide evaluation and treatment for children with cognitive communication disorders that have occurred as a result of traumatic brain injury (TBI)?

4. Should the speech-language pathologists or audiologists in schools suction a child in respiratory distress?

To respond to these questions, one must use the Code of Ethics as a guideline, consult the Scope of Practice and preferred practice patterns, be cognizant of one's skills and training as well as moral values, and use an ethical decision-making process that includes the student's family and related medical and educational professionals.

Issues in Ethics

Periodically, additional instruction and analysis about specific ethical issues are necessary to assist ASHA members in the ethical decision-making process. When this occurs, statements that are illustrative of the Code of Ethics are published and entitled *Issues in Ethics Statements*. These statements are provided to heighten members' sensitivity and increased awareness about specific features of ethical conduct (ASHA, 1994a, 1995h,). A partial list of these statements and the complete Code of Ethics can be found in Appendix 3–E. When appropriate, these statements are written by either the Ethical Practice Board (EPB) or the Council on Professional Ethics in Speech-Language Pathology and Audiology (COPE).

Ethical Practice Board

EPB and COPE are two ASHA committees that are responsible for ethics. The EPB has the responsibility of interpreting and enforcing the Code of Ethics. EPB's charge is to

formulate and publish procedure that will be used for the processing of alleged violations of the Code of Ethics including a reasonable opportunity to be heard through counsel of one's own choosing; determine sanctions for violations in its discretion as it deems appropriate including revoking and/or suspending membership and/or certification. (ASHA, 1995g, p. 68)

The responsibilities of EPB are accomplished through a well-defined process that is described in the "Statement of Practice and Procedures" (ASHA, 1994c). This statement defines terms used in the process, delineates the investigative procedure, discusses sanctions or penalties of a violation, and describes the appeal process. As a reference for members, the entire statement is published in the March 1994 supplement to the journal *Asha*. It is important to note that some sanctions, such as revocation of certification, are published in *Asha*. If you think a person has violated ASHA's Code of Ethics, send a letter stating your concerns to the chair of the Ethical Practice Board (ASHA, 1995g, 1995j).

Council on Professional Ethics

COPE defines and proposes revisions to the Code of Ethics for approval by the LC. COPE develops educational programs in the area of ethics for members and certificate holders and prepares educational materials for educational programs. *Ethics: Resources for Professional Preparation and Practice* (ASHA, 1993a) is an educational tool created by COPE. This manual is a collection of materials such as the Code of Ethics; issues in ethics statements; ethical scenarios; a sample ethics curriculum for college and university instruction, including classroom exercises, overheads, and handouts; a bibliography; and ethics articles written by leading professionals. This information is helpful both to the individual and to the educational program as tools in the ethical decision-making process.

Education

ASHA provides opportunities for continuing education to keep its membership informed about clinical procedures, scientific research, and professional issues. The association has established a formal, but voluntary, continuing education program. ASHA members earn continuing educational units (CEUs) and are awarded an ACE (Award for Continuing Education) to document and reward their rigorous pursuit of additional and updated information. ACE recipients have their names published in the journal *Asha* to honor their achievements. ASHA also facilitates exchange of ideas and information, the sharing of research and materials, and the dissemination of information on recent developments and professional affairs. Distribution of information and networking occurs through such avenues as journals, conventions, workshops, seminars, and teleconferences.

Journals

In its embryonic stages, ASHA mimeographed and sold its convention papers. However, in 1936, ASHA issued its first publication, the *Journal of Speech Disorders* (Paden, 1970). Now ASHA has six publications: the *Journal of Speech and Hearing Research*; *Language, Speech, and Hearing Services in Schools*; *American Journal of Speech-Language Pathology: A Journal of Clinical Practice*; *American Journal of Audiology: A Journal of Clinical Practice*; *ASHA Leader*; and *Asha* (Uffen, 1995).

The research journal is the *Journal of Speech and Hearing Research (JSHR)*. This publication contains studies about the processes and disorders of hearing, language, and speech and about the diagnosis and treatment of these disorders. This journal is published six times annually. Effective 1997, *JSHR* will change its name to the *Journal of Speech, Language and Hearing Research*.

The *American Journal of Speech-Language Pathology (AJSLP)* is dedicated to clinical issues in speech-language pathology and is published three times a year. Articles in this journal include such topics as screening, assessment, and treatment techniques; professional issues; supervision; and administration. The journal that is dedicated to similar issues but in the field of audiology is the *American Journal of Audiology (AJA)*. This journal is also published three times a year.

Of special interest to school-based clinicians is the *Language, Speech and Hearing Services in Schools (LSHSS)* journal. *LSHSS* is concerned with all aspects of speech, language, and hearing services in the schools. Specifically, it deals with the assessment, nature, and remediation of speech, hearing, and language disorders; program organization; and management and supervision, as well as other issues related to school programming. It is published four times a year.

Asha, published four times annually, emphasizes the professional and administrative issues of ASHA and of the professions of speech-language pathology and audiology. The information is presented in the form of articles, special reports, news items, committee reports, reviews of books and materials, and letters.

The *ASHA Leader* is a brand-new publication, with its first issue occurring in January 1996. It is a newsletter that is published twice a month to keep ASHA members abreast of all "late-breaking" news. The content of *Leader* is similar to that of *Asha*. It provides information on the ever-changing health care system, professional skills, up-to-date treatment techniques and technologies, and employment. All of these publications keep ASHA members and affiliates informed and involved.

Conventions, Conferences, and Other Avenues of Information

ASHA holds annual conferences in various parts of the United States. This allows networking of colleagues and presentation of information through short courses, mini-seminars, and poster and technical sessions. The LC, the EB, and other committees/councils/boards meet at that time, and the membership has an opportunity to view the various aspects of ASHA governance at work.

ASHA gives teleconferences, regional workshops, and seminars on specific topics of interest. These sessions are usually listed in the journal *Asha*. Brochures and other professional products are available as well. Upon request, a catalogue of all ASHA products and materials can be acquired from the national office.

A new feature for ASHA is helping its membership obtain information through the Internet. The Internet offers the opportunity to send and receive electronic mail (e-mail), to join discussion groups and/or chat lines, to explore databases, and to download programs. In the journal *Asha*, there is an Internet report section that describes how members can subscribe to special-interest discussion groups (often called mailing lists) such as those on stuttering, dialect, articulation, and phonology (ASHA, 1995e, Kuster & Kuster, 1995).

ASHA also has a home page (a page of text that links you to other resources in the professions) on the World Wide Web (a system that links you to other Internet sites and resources). ASHA's website address is: http://www.asha.org. Items listed in ASHA's website include drafts of position statements, state information, other Internet resources, updated information on workshops and conferences, news releases, and answers to frequently asked questions (ASHA, 1996a).

Another way to have your questions answered is to use ASHA's Information Resource Center (IRC). Send your questions to ASHA's IRC e-mail address (irc@asha.org) and they will either respond to you directly or forward your questions to the national office for response (ASHA, 1996b).

Special Interests Divisions

In 1989, Special Interests Divisions (SIDs) were developed. SIDs are groups of ASHA members who wish to meet and share information about specific areas of study. ASHA houses 15 of these divisions, and each one has a designated number:

1. Language Learning and Education (SID 1) promotes activities in the areas of linguistic knowledge and communication interaction of infants, children, and youth from diverse cultures.

2. Neurophysiology and Neurogenic Speech and Language Disorders (SID 2) promotes the study of neurophysiologic aspects of speech, language, and cognition and the prevention, assessment, and resolution of communication disorders from central and/or peripheral nervous systems impairment.

3. Voice and Voice Disorders (SID 3) promotes the study of normal voice production and the nature, presentation, and treatment of voice disorders.

4. Fluency and Fluency Disorders (SID 4) promotes the study of characteristics and processes of normal fluency of speech and the presentation, assessment, and treatment of fluency disorders.

5. Speech Science and Orofacial Disorders (SID 5) promotes the study of the anatomy and physiology of the speech mechanisms.

6. Hearing, Its Disorders and Their Diagnosis: Electrophysiological and Psychoacoustics Testing (SID 6) promotes the study of normal and abnormal auditory functions.

7. Aural Rehabilitation and Its Instrumentation (SID 7) promotes the study, development, and application of amplification systems and assistive communication devices.

8. Hearing Conservation and Occupational Audiology (SID 8) promotes the study and application of techniques for the prevention, measurement, management, and control of noxious and toxic agents causing hearing impairment.

9. Hearing and Hearing Disorders in Childhood (SID 9) promotes the study and diagnosis of normal and abnormal auditory development in infants and children.

10. Division 1 and 10 merged in January 1994 to form the present SID 1.

11. Administration and Supervision (SID 11) promotes the study of problems, issues, and responsibilities in administration and supervision.

12. Augmentative and Alternative Communication (SID 12) promotes a leadership role within ASHA through education of the consumer, the membership, and other organizations.

13. Swallowing and Swallowing Disorders (Dysphagia; SID 13) promotes the study of anatomy, physiology, and neurophysiology of the mechanisms employed in normal and disorders of swallowing and the prevention, assessment, and treatment of swallowing disorders.

14. Communication Disorders and Sciences in Culturally and Linguistically Diverse Populations (SID 14) promotes the study and application of the knowledge of normal communication, communication disorders, and service delivery issues that affect culturally and linguistically diverse groups.

15. Gerontology (SID 15) provides information, support, and affiliation for clinical providers who work with older adults.

The SIDs often bring about immediate action on important issues. For example, in response to requests from federal legislation, the Language Learning and Education Division developed a policy statement affirming an educational continuum of services. SIDs also publish newsletters, sponsor convention short courses, and in some cases sponsor regional conferences (ASHA, 1995a, 1995e). Again, as the professions' services expand, more special interests divisions will be established so that ASHA members can engage in dialogue about specific issues.

Specialty Recognition

The Legislative Council in 1994 passed a specialty recognition plan. This plan established the Clinical Specialty Board, which will oversee the creation of ASHA's program of voluntary specialty recognition. The plan also recommended that a specific group, such as a special interest division, define its specialization and develop the mechanisms for awarding this recognition. Specialty recognition will provide opportunities for practitioners to achieve official recognition in a specific practice area, and consumers will be able to easily identify "specialists" in such areas as neurological disorders, language disorders, pediatric audiology, or geriatric audiology (ASHA, 1995b, 1995i). Of particular interest to the school clinician is the specialty recognition in child language created by Special Interest Division 1: Language Learning and Education.

Lobbying

ASHA is a strong advocate for the professions of speech, language, and hearing. It uses a proactive strategy and strives to increase awareness of the field at the public, governmental, and legislative levels. ASHA lobbies for more and better funding for research, acts as a consultant to various committees considering laws or legislation that affect the practices of speech-language pathology and audiology, and provides testimony and input to proposed legislation and regulations. It promotes the importance of the services provided by the professions to persons with communication disorders. It lobbies for recognition of these services and for better consumer protection. Three ASHA groups that are dedicated to advocacy are CAC, PAC, and ASHA-PAC.

The Congressional Action Contact (CAC) Network is ASHA's "grassroots" lobbying network. ASHA members have an opportunity through CAC to voice collectively their concerns about legislation that affects their professions. The members of CAC lobby their senators and representatives to support legislation that will improve professional opportunities for speech-language pathologists and audiologists and that would improve the education of and services to people with communication disabilities. This networking increases the legislators' knowledge of the professions and can help influence the outcomes of key legislation (ASHA, 1995a).

The American Speech-Language-Hearing Association Political Action Committee (ASHA-PAC) is a bipartisan committee of speech-language pathologists and audiologists whose main purpose is to support candidates for Congress who support ASHA positions on health care, education, and disability issues. The actions of this committee increase the visibility of the professions on Capitol Hill and allow ASHA members to be active participants in the election of supportive federal legislators. These efforts have not gone unrewarded. In 1994, 74% of ASHA-supported candidates were re-elected (ASHA, 1995a, 1995c).

The American Speech-Language Hearing Association Political Action Committee Finance Council (ASHA-PAC Finance Council) was created in 1989 by the ASHA-PAC board of directors. Its charge was to build grassroots support for ASHA-PAC in all communities and/or states and to help raise funds for the ASHA-PAC committee (ASHA, 1995a).

Consumer Services

A major thrust for ASHA has been consumer protection. To address this area, ASHA established a Consumer Affairs Division in 1988. This division's goals are to advocate on behalf of consumers and to educate them about audiology and speech-language pathology services for persons with communication disorders. The consumer can write to ASHA or call toll free (HELPLINE: 1-800-638-8255) to receive information or free educational material.

Other educational material for consumers is made available to ASHA members through "Let's Talk," published in *Asha*, and the "School Bulletin" published in *LSHSS*. "Let's Talk," in existence since 1988, discusses issues that are related to the prevention and treatment of communication disorders. Examples of topics included are hearing loss, adolescent language, bilingualism, pragmatic language tips, brain injury, autism, learning disabilities and dyslexia, deaf culture, and troubleshooting of hearing aids. Members can purchase reprints from ASHA or photocopy the newsletter directly from *Asha* and distribute copies to teachers, consumers, libraries, PTAs, day care centers, and referral sources as reference sources.

The "School Bulletin," also in existence since 1988, introduces the speech-language pathologist and audiologist as communication specialists for the schools. The bulletins give practical recommendations for both parents and teachers. Parents are given suggestions for listening to their children, reading to them, and identifying otitis media early. Teachers discover how to ask students better questions and how to identify children with potential communication disorders (ASHA, 1995d).

ASHA has produced a computerized database of nationwide audiology and speech-language pathology programs, called Professional Services (PROSERV) Database. As of May 1995, 1,803 audiology and 2,155 speech-language programs were listed. The database includes such information as basic identifying information, age groups served, types of payment accepted, program-identified areas of expertise, and other variables that might help to match consumers with a program that will meet their needs. This information is available for parents and other caregivers who are seeking speech, language, and hearing services for persons with communication disorders. Parents can contact ASHA and through this database obtain the name(s) of programs in their area that can evaluate and/or treat their child. If professionals wish to be listed in the database, they can request an application

from the ASHA national office, complete the information, and return it to ASHA's Consumer Affairs Division (ASHA, 1995a).

ASHA makes every attempt to reach out to consumers and consider their needs. Periodically, parent advocacy groups have been invited to participate in discussions about such issues as education reform, health care, and ASHA's policies. ASHA has listened to all of the concerns voiced at these discussions and has instituted responsive programs. One of ASHA's responses has been the creation of a Model Bill of Rights for People Receiving Audiology or Speech-Language Pathology Services (see Appendix 3–F; ASHA, 1995k). This model bill was developed by the Task Force on Protection of Client's Rights and is an official statement by ASHA. It provides guidance for individuals who receive services in speech-language pathology and audiology. Another ASHA consumer-sensitive response has been to place consumers on boards and task forces to represent the interests of persons receiving services in the professions of speech-language pathology and audiology. Consumer grants have been awarded to recognize self-help groups who assist people with communication disorders (ASHA, 1995d).

ASHA AND THE PUBLIC SCHOOLS

The public schools have had a major role in the provision of services for children with communication disorders. Key events in the history of these services are recounted in Chapters 1 and 2.

ASHA has been committed to and supportive of practitioners who work in the schools. In fact one of ASHA's largest memberships consists of professionals who work in the schools. A 1994 demographic profile of ASHA membership indicated that 52.8% of the speech-language pathologists and 9.5% of the audiologists listed schools as their primary site of employment (ASHA, 1995a).

In its embryonic years, ASHA established the position of Associate Secretary for School Clinic Affairs. This position was created to support school-based clinicians; act as a liaison between ASHA and clinics, schools, and other agencies in the country; and be responsible for the publication of *Speech and Hearing Services in Schools* (a journal that contained school-related issues). This person also worked closely with ASHA committees. A Committee on Speech and Hearing Services in the Schools was also created to address school-related issues (ASHA, 1970, 1974).

School Services Division

Through the years, the position of associate secretary evolved into a division known as the School Services Division (SSD) of ASHA, which was officially established in 1989. The SSD is dedicated to school issues. The mission of this division is to "provide leadership, information and support for members employed in public and private school settings on issues related to administration and delivery of service in the schools" (ASHA, 1994b, p. 5). Some of the goals and objectives of this division are providing school-based clinicians with materials and products to enhance service delivery; providing professional consultation to members, consumers, and related organizations; facilitating committee and task force activities and product development that are related to services in the schools; and developing ASHA continuing education programs to increase the members' knowledge base.

The SSD staff provides member assistance on topics germane to the practice of speech-language pathology and audiology in the schools, such as caseload issues and guidelines, service delivery models (pull-out, collaboration, consultation), public laws and mandates, assessment, education and certification requirements, use of support personnel, entry and exit criteria rating scales, and third-party reimbursement issues. The SSD staff attends professional conferences, gives presentations on school-based issues, serves as an advocate for speech-language pathologists and audiologists, and collaborates with other organizations such as the National Education Association, the National Association of Elementary School Principals, and the National School Boards Association.

The SSD develops position statements, guidelines, products, publications, and other activities to support the school-based ASHA member. It also comments on proposed changes in federal legislation and regulations. It develops testimony on issues that affect the professions or persons with communication disorders. The SSD made major contributions to the proposed reauthorization of the Individuals with Disabilities Education Act of 1990 (IDEA), the Goals 2000: Educate America Act, and the National Agenda to Achieve Better Results for Students with Disabilities (ASHA, 1994b).

SSD is responsible for Action: School Services in *LSHSS*. This article includes discussions and information about such issues as Medicaid, federal legislation, ethical considerations, and all other professional issues in speech-language pathology and audiology that are related to the provision of service for children with speech, language, and hearing disorders.

Related ASHA Committees

Many ASHA committees/task forces/ad hoc committees are relevant to school-based services. One such committee is the Ad Hoc Committee on Provision of Appropriate Technology Services and Devices to Students in Schools. This committee has been charged with developing a report that lists appropriate educational uses of technology. The report includes a list of technology services, devices, manufacturers, possible funding sources, and assessment techniques. Their charge also includes the creation of training programs and other material for continuing education.

Another committee pertinent to services in the schools is the Ad Hoc Committee on Inclusion. This committee is coordinated by SID 1 (Language Learning and Education). The committee's goals are to develop a report and eventually a position statement on inclusion as it affects children with speech, language, and hearing disorders (Peters-Johnson, 1995).

The Joint Committee of the American Speech-Language-Hearing Association and the Council on Education of the Deaf is also applicable to school-based services. This committee researches issues of concern about service delivery to persons who are deaf or hard of hearing. It publishes technical reports and is discussing the definitions of *deaf* and *hard of hearing* as well as other issues relevant to the deaf culture. The committee is also charged with the development of minimum competencies for speech-language pathologists working with persons who are deaf and hard of hearing (ASHA, 1994b).

The Ad Hoc Committee on Scope of Practice in Audiology and the Ad Hoc Committee on Scope of Practice in Speech-Language Pathology are two other committees of special interest. They have been commissioned to revise and update the professions' scope of practice. The audiology committee reviews the Scope of Practice position statement for

the profession of audiology, and the speech-language pathology committee revises the Scope of Practice position statement for the profession of speech-language pathology.

The Joint Committee on Learning Disabilities studies all aspects of the management of children with learning disabilities. Because a large percentage of the caseload of the school practitioner consists of children who have been diagnosed as having learning disabilities, information from this committee should be very valuable in the provision of assessment and treatment of children in this population who have communication disorders. Other committees of interest include the Ad Hoc Committee on Attention Deficit Hyperactivity Disorder (which delineates the role and competencies of the audiologist and speech-language pathologist for service delivery to students with attention-deficit hyperactivity disorder), the Multicultural Issues Board (which improves the availability and quality of services for persons from diverse linguistic and cultural backgrounds who have communication disorders), the Task Force on Treatment Outcome and Cost Effectiveness (which generates an efficacy database for professionals), and the Task Force on Support Personnel (which develops statements and guidelines for training, credentialing, use, and supervision of support personnel; ASHA, 1995a).

Recently, ASHA established the Ad Hoc Committee on the Roles and Responsibilities of the School-Based Speech-Language Pathologist to address the needs of the school-based clinicians. Specifically, the committee will develop guidelines in the areas of "identification, assessment, diagnosis, case selection, intervention service delivery, consultation/collaboration, legislative and regulatory mandates, and other areas" (ASHA, 1996c, p. 6). This committee is in response to the changing demographics, scope of practice, regulations, evaluations, and treatments that are occurring in the schools.

RELATED PROFESSIONAL ORGANIZATIONS

There are many related professional organizations (RPOs; see Appendix 3–G). Some of these RPOs meet in conjunction with the ASHA convention. They are separate organizations that focus on specific issues and areas of interest, but they have their own governing structure. These organizations work closely with each other and with ASHA. They provide an opportunity for networking with individuals and groups about an area of mutual interest.

The School Services Division staff are members of several of the RPOs that are related to school services. They often serve as consultants to and or liaisons for these RPOs. A partial list of these RPOs includes the National Rural and Small Schools Consortium; the National Alliance of Pupil Services Organizations; the Council of Language, Speech, and Hearing Consultants in State Education Agencies; the National Association for the Education of Young Children; the National Association of Elementary School Principals; the National School Boards Association; the American Association of School Administrators; the Council of Public School Supervisors and Administrators; and the Public School Caucus.

Public School Caucus

The Public School Caucus (PSC) is an RPO that is particularly appropriate for school practitioners. The PSC was founded in 1973 to promote the use of school-based speech-language pathologists and audiologists, to encourage and increase the involvement of public school ASHA members in ASHA's governance, and to make ASHA more aware and sensitive to the needs of its public school members. PSC has established direct and active communication with ASHA and has developed a supportive, informative, and visible networking system for school issues. PSC publishes a newsletter, *Practically Speaking*, which provides articles on current school-based issues, discusses ASHA's direction in school concerns, and announces workshops, seminars, and conferences that are related to the practice of speech-language pathology and audiology in the schools.

To become a PSC member, you must be an ASHA member or a journal group participant who is employed in a private or public school at the elementary or secondary level. The journal group consists of persons employed in the field but not eligible for ASHA membership. Other interested ASHA members not eligible for PSC membership can become contributors. Contributors receive publications but cannot vote or hold office (Public School Caucus, 1993).

American Speech-Language-Hearing Foundation

The American Speech-Language-Hearing Foundation is a private, nonprofit foundation that was established in 1946. It is dedicated to innovation in communication sciences and disorders. Specifically, the foundation identifies and facilitates new directions through the promotion of publications and conferences. It supports research and recognizes the clinical excellence of professionals in the field, as well as scholars, through research grants, graduate scholarships, and other awards. School-based practitioners are recognized annually by the foundation with the presentation of the Rolland J. Van Hattum Award at ASHA's national convention (ASHA, 1995d).

National Student Speech-Language-Hearing Association

The National Student Speech-Language-Hearing Association (NSSLHA) is an organization that is available for students majoring in the field of speech-language and audiology, with chapters at many universities and colleges. It supports students, promotes the professions, and disseminates information. Although housed at ASHA headquarters, NSSLHA has its own structure and governance. It is recognized by ASHA, and the two organizations work closely together. NSSLHA has representatives on various ASHA boards and committees. To become a member of NSSLHA, a student must have declared speech-language pathology or audiology as a major and must pay the membership fee. As a member of NSSLHA, you receive the NSSLHA and ASHA's journals. The membership also permits registration at ASHA's conventions at a reduced rate. For students, membership in NSSLHA is an excellent first step toward participation in a professional association (ASHA, 1995d).

SUMMARY

ASHA is a national, professional organization that promotes the interests of the professions, the consumers, and its members. As the organization pursues its purposes and goals, the membership is an active part of the governance process. Members participate in policy

and decision making by volunteering to serve on committees, boards, councils, and task forces and by electing the executive board and legislative council. Several benefits and services accompany ASHA membership. Position statements, guidelines, reports, and other relevant papers are created by the membership to assist in the provision of services to persons with communication disorders. In the standards program, ASHA sets and implements standards for clinical certification and accreditation for graduate educational programs and agencies that provide services. This certification and accreditation process assures the public that the agency and the persons providing the services in that agency have adequate knowledge and skills.

The integrity and ethics of the professions are paramount. The Code of Ethics of ASHA provides the framework and guidelines for maintaining these standards. Issues in ethics are supplied to assist the membership in their ethical decision making.

ASHA educates its members, the public, and the consumer through publications, conventions, workshops, teleconferences, seminars, and other media avenues. It represents the professions and the consumers at various governmental levels and makes major contributions to legislation concerning speech-language pathology and audiology. It provides forms for debate and networking with other colleagues and professionals. ASHA works in partnership with numerous organizations in its pursuit of quality service for the public.

A large number of ASHA members work in school settings, and ASHA is extremely supportive of these practitioners. A special national office division has been established to address school-based concerns, and a journal is specifically dedicated to clinical, professional, and academic issues in the schools.

Committees, task forces, and other publications also address these needs.

For students majoring in the professions, a student organization is available to address student-related issues. The ASHA foundation is supportive of both students and practitioners through the awarding of scholarships, clinical recognition and research grants.

For the practitioner, ASHA offers an opportunity to meet with other colleagues, be on the cutting edge of professional knowledge and techniques, and be actively involved in the evolution of the professions locally, statewide, and nationally. Prospective clinicians in the professions of speech-language pathology and audiology should consider membership in the organization as soon as they are eligible.

STUDY QUESTIONS

1. What does *ASHA* stand for?

2. What are the purposes of ASHA?

3. Why should a practitioner in the field of speech-language pathology or audiology become a member of ASHA?

4. If you are a member of ASHA, what should you do to be considered for appointment to a committee/board/council?

5. As a member of ASHA, how could you introduce a new policy or change an existing one?

6. Why is ASHA's Code of Ethics important?

7. What are the four basic principles of ethics in ASHA's code?

8. What should you do if you feel someone has committed an alleged violation?

9. How do the Scope of Practice and the practice patterns assist you in the practice of speech-language pathology and audiology?

10. What can you as a student do now to become involved in a professional organization?

11. What is the SSD? What does it do for the school practitioner?

12. What is the PSC? Why is it a valuable organization to join?

13. What are CEUs? What is an ACE? Why would they be important for a school practitioner?

14. Which ASHA committees would you join? Why?

15. The minimum level of preparation needed for entry into speech-language pathology and audiology is _____.

REFERENCES

American Speech-Language-Hearing Association. (1996a). New on the website: http://www.asha.org. *ASHA Leader*, 1 (13), 2.

American Speech-Language-Hearing Association. (1996b). Contact ASHA over the Internet. *ASHA Leader*, 1 (12), 6.

American Speech-Language-Hearing Association. (1996c). New committee will address needs of school-based SLPs. *ASHA Leader*, 1 (12), 6.

American Speech-Language-Hearing Association. (1970). News and comments. *Speech and Hearing Services in Schools*, 3, 3–7.

American Speech-Language-Hearing Association. (1974). *The Public School Caucus: A progress report.* Unpublished report, Rockville, MD.

American Speech-Language-Hearing Association. (1990). Scope of practice, speech-language pathology and audiology. *Asha*, 32 (Suppl. 2), 1–2.

American Speech-Language-Hearing Association. (1992). *ASHA desk reference: Guidelines, position statements, definitions, and relevant papers.* Rockville, MD: Author.

American Speech-Language-Hearing Association. (1993a). *Ethics: Resources for professional preparation and practice.* Rockville, MD: Author.

American Speech-Language-Hearing Association. (1993b). Preferred practice patterns for the professions of speech-language pathology and audiology. *Asha, 35* (Suppl. 11), 1–97.

American Speech-Language-Hearing Association. (1994a, March). Issues in ethics. *Asha, 36* (Suppl. 13), 7–27.

American Speech-Language-Hearing Association. (1994b). *School Services Division: 1994 convention highlights, Fall.* Rockville, MD: Author.

American Speech-Language-Hearing Association. (1994c, March). Statement of practices and procedures. *Asha, 36* (Suppl. 13), 3–5.

American Speech-Language-Hearing Association. (1995a). ASHA 1994 annual report. *Asha, 37* (3), 18–26.

American Speech-Language-Hearing Association. (1995b). ASHA reports. *Asha, 37* (2), 12, 17.

American Speech-Language-Hearing Association. (1995c). ASHA reports. *Asha, 37* (4), 23, 29–30, 47.

American Speech-Language-Hearing Association. (1995d). ASHA reports. *Asha, 37* (5), 14–18, 26, 28, 37.

American Speech-Language-Hearing Association. (1995e). ASHA reports. *Asha, 37* (6/7), 18–19, 24–25, 29, 57.

American Speech-Language-Hearing Association. (1995f). At press time. *Asha, 37* (6/7), 7–8.

American Speech-Language-Hearing Association. (1995g). Boards, committees, councils, and task forces. *Asha, 37* (3), 61–73.

American Speech-Language-Hearing Association. (1995h). Code of ethics 1995. *Asha, 37* (3), 74–75.

American Speech-Language-Hearing Association. (1995i). Legislative Council report. *Asha, 37* (Suppl. 14), 1–9.

American Speech-Language-Hearing Association. (1995j). *Membership and certification handbook speech language pathology.* Rockville, MD: Author.

American Speech-Language-Hearing Association. (1995k). Model Bill of Rights. *Asha, 37* (3), 37.

American Speech-Language-Hearing Association. (1995l). Position statements, guidelines, definitions, and relevant papers. *Asha, 37* (Suppl. 14), 36–37.

Kuster, J.M., & Kuster, T.A. (1995). Finding treasures on the Internet: Gopher the gold. *Asha, 37* (2), 43–47.

Lubinski, R., & Frattali, C. (Eds.). (1994). *Professional issues in speech-language pathology and audiology: A textbook.* San Diego, CA: Singular.

Paden, E.P. (1970). *A history of the American Speech and Hearing Association, 1925–1958.* Washington, DC: American Speech-Language-Hearing Association.

Peters-Johnson, C. (1995). Action: School services. *Language, Speech and Hearing Services in Schools, 26,* 295–297.

Public School Caucus. (1993, Fall). *Practically Speaking, 12.* Marietta, GA: Public School Caucus.

Sharp, H., & Genesen, L. (1996). Ethical decision-making in dysphagia management. *American Journal of Speech-Language Pathology, 5,* 15–22.

Uffen, E. (1995). Ideas into print: ASHA's scholarly journals. *Asha, 37* (4), 35–38.

Appendix 3–A

Position Statement on Facilitated Communication

American Speech-Language-Hearing Association

This position statement is an official policy of the American Speech-Language-Hearing Association (ASHA). It was developed after select and widespread peer review by ASHA's Speech-Language Pathology Division: Diane Paul-Brown, division director; Louise Zingeser, branch director; Crystal S. Cooper, 1994–1996 vice president for professional practices in speech-language pathology, served as monitoring vice president. The contributions of Stan Dublinske, director, Professional Practices Department, and Kelley Turnbull, departmental assistant, Professional Practices Department, are gratefully acknowledged. The Legislative Council adopted this statement in November 1994 (LC 51-94). For additional information, please refer to the Technical Report on Facilitated Communication (Facilitated Communication Subcommittee of the Ad Hoc Committee on Auditory Integration Training and Facilitated Communication, 1994, October).

Facilitated Communication is a technique by which a "facilitator" provides physical and other supports in an attempt to assist a person with a significant communication disability to point to pictures, objects, printed letters and words, or to a keyboard. Personal accounts and qualitative descriptions suggest that messages produced using this technique may reveal previously undetected literacy and communication skills in people with autism and other disabilities. When information available to facilitators is controlled and objective evaluation methods are used, peer-reviewed studies and clinical assessments find no conclusive evidence that facilitated messages can be reliably attributed to people with disabilities. Rather, most messages originate with the facilitator. Moreover, Facilitated Communication may have negative consequences if it precludes the use of effective and appropriate treatment, supplants other forms of communication, and/or leads to false or unsubstantiated allegations of abuse or mistreatment.

It is the position of the American Speech-Language-Hearing Association (ASHA) that the scientific validity and reliability of Facilitated Communication have not been demonstrated to date. Information obtained through or based on Facilitated Communication should not form the sole basis for making any diagnostic or treatment decisions.

Source: Reprinted with permission from Position Statement Facilitated Communication, *Asha*, Vol. 37, Suppl. 14, p. 22, © 1995, the American Speech-Language-Hearing Association.

ASHA strongly supports continued research and clinical efforts to develop scientifically valid methods for developing or enhancing the independent communication and literacy skills of people with disabilities.

Speech-language pathologists are autonomous professionals who are responsible for critically evaluating all treatment techniques in order to hold paramount the welfare of persons served in accordance with the ASHA Code of Ethics. Speech-language pathologists should inform prospective clients and their families or guardians that currently the scientific validity and reliability of Facilitated Communication have not been established, and should obtain their informed consent before using the technique.

Appendix 3–B

Scope of Practice, Speech-Language Pathology and Audiology

Committee on Interprofessional Relationships, American Speech-Language-Hearing Association

The following document, prepared by the American Speech-Language-Hearing Association (ASHA) Committee on Interprofessional Relationships, was adopted as an official statement by the ASHA Legislative Council (LC 6-89) in November 1989. Current and past members of the committee responsible for the development of the document include Crystal S. Cooper, 1988–1990 chair; John L. Peterson, 1988 chair; Rachel E. Stark, 1986–1987 chair; Brenda L.B. Adamovich; Katharine G. Butler; Janina K. Casper; Becky S. Cornett; Ted A. Culler; Frank DeRuyter; Elaine S. Dunn; Anita S. Halper; Anne E. Seltz; Rosalind R. Scudder; Barbara Shadden; and Brenda Y. Terrell, Michelle M. Ferketic, 1988–1989 ex officio; Lynette R. Goldberg, 1989–1990 ex officio; Carol Kamara, 1986–1987 ex officio; Patricia G. Larkins, 1988 ex officio. Ann L. Carey, current vice president for professional and governmental affairs, and Nancy Becker, vice president for professional and governmental affairs, were monitoring vice presidents.

Preamble

The purpose of this statement is to define the scope of practice of speech-language pathology and audiology in order to: (1) inform members of ASHA and certificate holders of the activities for which certification in the appropriate area is required in accordance with the ASHA Code of Ethics; and (2) educate health-care and education professionals, consumers, and members of the general public of the services offered by speech-language pathologists and audiologists as qualified providers.

The scope of practice defined here, and the areas specifically set forth, are part of an effort to establish the broad range of services offered within the profession. It is recognized, however, that levels of experience, skill, and proficiency with respect to the activities identified within the scope of practice will vary among the individual providers. Similarly, it is recognized that related fields and professions may have knowledge, skills, and experience which may be applied to some areas within the scope of practice. By defining the scope of practice of speech-language pathologists and audiologists, there is no intention to exclude members of other professions or related fields from rendering services in common practice areas for which they are competent by virtue of their respective disciplines.

Nothing in the scope of practice statement is intended to affect the licensure laws of the various states or the implementation or interpretation of such laws.

Finally, it is recognized that speech-language pathology and audiology are dynamic and continuously developing practice areas. In setting forth some specific areas as included within the scope of practice, there is no intention that the list be exhaustive or that other, new, or emerging areas be precluded from being considered as within the scope of practice.

Statement

Speech-language pathologists and audiologists hold either the master's or doctoral degree, the Certificate of Clinical Competence of the American Speech-Language-Hearing Association, and state license where applicable. These professionals identify, assess, and provide treatment for individuals of all ages with communication disorders. They manage and supervise programs and services related to human communication and its disorders. Speech-language pathologists and audiologists counsel individuals with disorders of communication, their families, caregivers, and other service providers relative to the disability present and its management. They provide consultation and make referrals. Facilitating the development and maintenance of human communication is the common goal of speech-language pathologists and audiologists.

The practice of speech-language pathology includes:

- screening, identifying, assessing and interpreting, diagnosing, rehabilitating, and preventing disorders of speech (e.g., articulation, fluency, voice) and language (ASHA, 1983, 1989);

- screening, identifying, assessing and interpreting, diagnosing, and rehabilitating disorders of oral-pharyngeal function (e.g., dysphagia) and related disorders;

- screening, identifying, assessing and interpreting, diagnosing, and rehabilitating cognitive/communication disorders;

- assessing, selecting, and developing augmentative and alternative communication systems and providing training in their use;

- providing aural rehabilitation and related counseling services to hearing impaired individuals and their families;

- enhancing speech-language proficiency and communication effectiveness (e.g., accent reduction); and

- screening of hearing and other factors for the purpose of speech-language evaluation and/or the initial identification of individuals with other communication disorders.

The practice of audiology includes:

- facilitating the conservation of auditory system function; developing and implementing environmental and occupational hearing conservation programs;

- screening, identifying, assessing and interpreting, diagnosing, preventing, and rehabilitating peripheral and central auditory system dysfunctions;

- providing and interpreting behavioral and (electro) physiological measurements of auditory and vestibular functions;

- selecting, fitting, and dispensing of amplification, assistive listening, and alerting devices and other systems (e.g., implantable devices) and providing training in their use;

- providing aural rehabilitation and related counseling services to hearing impaired individuals and their families; and

- screening of speech-language and other factors affecting communication function for the purposes of an audiologic evaluation and/or initial identification of individuals with other communication disorders.

REFERENCES

American Speech-Language-Hearing Association. (1983). Definition of language. *Asha, 25* (6), 44.

American Speech-Language-Hearing Association. (1987a). Ad Hoc Committee on Dysphagia report. *Asha, 29* (4), 57–58.

American Speech-Language-Hearing Association. (1987b). The role of speech-language pathologists in the habilitation and rehabilitation of cognitively impaired individuals: A report of the Subcommittee on Language and Cognition. *Asha, 29* (6), 53–55.

American Speech-Language-Hearing Association. (1988). The role of speech-language pathologists in the identification, diagnosis, and treatment of individuals with cognitive-communication impairments. *Asha, 30* (3), 79.

American Speech-Language-Hearing Association. (1989). Standards for the certificates of clinical competence. *Asha, 31* (3), 70–71.

Appendix 3–C

Preferred Practice Patterns for Articulation/Phonology Assessment and Speech-Language Pathology Treatment

ARTICULATION/PHONOLOGY ASSESSMENT

Procedures to assess speech articulation/phonology, delineating strengths, deficits, contributing factors, and implications for functional communication.

Articulation/phonology assessment is conducted according to the Fundamental Components of Preferred Practice Patterns, p. 1

Professionals Who Perform the Procedure(s)

Speech language pathologists.

Expected Outcome(s)

- Assessment is conducted to describe characteristics of speech-sound production and to diagnose a communication disorder.

- Assessment may result in recommendations for treatment or follow-up, or in referral for other examinations or services.

Source: Reprinted with permission from Preferred Practice Patterns for the Professions of Speech-Language Pathology and Audiology, *Asha, Vol. 35,* Suppl. 11, pp. 1–97, © 1993, the American Speech-Language-Hearing Association.

Clinical Indications

- Individuals of all ages are assessed as needed, requested, or mandated, or when they have educational, vocational, social, and health needs caused by impaired communication.

- Assessment is prompted by referral, by the patient's/client's medical status, or by failure of a speech screening (see Statement 02.0).

Clinical Process

- Assessment includes:
  - —Case history
  - —Standardized and/or nonstandardized measures to assess developmental and acquired articulation disorders, oral motor skills, segmental and suprasegmental data, phonological processes, and motor speech control
  - —Observation of interaction between parent and child or adult and significant other
  - —Hearing screening
  - —Observation or review of voice, fluency, cognition, language, and vision
- Patients/clients with identified articula-

tion/phonology disorders receive follow-up services to monitor status and to ensure appropriate treatment.

Setting/Equipment Specifications

- Assessment is conducted in a clinical or natural environment conducive to eliciting a representative sample of the patient's/client's articulation/phonology.

Documentation

- Documentation includes pertinent background information, results and interpretation, prognosis, and recommendations. Recommendations may include the need for further assessment, follow-up, or referral. When treatment is recommended, information is provided concerning frequency, estimated duration, and type of service (e.g., individual, group, home program) required.

ASHA Policy and Related References

In addition to the references listed on p. iv, the following references apply specifically to these procedures:

Source: Reprinted with permission from Definitions of communication disorders and variations, *Asha*, Vol. 35, Suppl. 10, pp. 40–41, © 1993, the American Speech-Language-Hearing Association.

SPEECH-LANGUAGE PATHOLOGY TREATMENT

Procedures to apply strategies that improve, alter, augment, or compensate for comprehension, speech, voice, spoken and written language, and cognitive-communication impairments.

Speech-language pathology treatment is conducted according to the Fundamental Components of Preferred Practice Patterns, p. 1.

Professionals Who Perform the Procedure(s)

Speech-language pathologists.

Expected Outcome(s)

- Treatment is conducted to achieve improved, altered, augmented, or compensated speech, language, and cognitive-communication behaviors and/or processes.
- Treatment may result in recommendations for reassessment or follow-up, or in referral for other examinations or services.

Clinical Indications

- Individuals of all ages receive treatment when their ability to communicate effectively is impaired and there is reason to believe that treatment will reduce the degree of impairment or disability or lead to improved communication behaviors.

Clinical Process

- Short- and long-term functional communication goals and specific objectives are determined from assessment and represent the framework for treatment. They are reviewed periodically to determine appropriateness.
- All individuals involved in the implementation of the treatment plan (e.g.,

patient/client, family, staff) are instructed by the speech-language pathologist regarding the components of the plan and their role(s) in its implementation.

- Patients/clients and families are provided informative and supportive counseling regarding the nature of the communication disorder, the impact of the disorder upon the patient/client and family, and other likely outcomes of treatment.

- Dismissal/discharge planning occurs continually throughout treatment.

- Follow-up services may include reevaluation of the patient's/client's status, referrals, and provision for continuing treatment.

- Speech-language pathologists may be part of an interdisciplinary team.

- The quality of care and utilization of services are assessed.

Setting/Equipment Specifications

- Treatment is conducted in a clinical or natural environment conducive to observing, modifying, and monitoring the patient's/client's communication behavior.

Documentation

- Documentation includes pertinent background information, treatment goals, results, prognosis, and specific recommendations. Recommendations may include the need for further treatment, follow-up, or referral. When further treatment is recommended, information is provided concerning the frequency, estimated duration, and type of service (e.g., individual, group, home program) required.

ASHA Policy and Related References

In addition to the references listed on p. iv, the following references apply specifically to these procedures:

American Speech-Language-Hearing Association. (1987). American Speech-Language-Hearing Association classification of speech-language pathology and audiology procedures and communication disorders (ASHACS). *Asha, 29* (12), 49–53.

American Speech-Language-Hearing Association. (1987). *Quality assurance process indicators.* Rockville, MD: Author.

American Speech-Language-Hearing Association. (1990). Report update. AIDS/HIV: Implications for speech-language pathologists and audiologists. *Asha, 32* (12), 46–48.

American Speech-Language-Hearing Association. (1991). Chronic communicable diseases and risk management in the schools. *Language, Speech and Hearing Services in the Schools, 22* (1), 345–352.

Appendix 3-D

List of Position Statements, Guidelines, Definitions, Reports, and Other Relevant Papers

As directed by an Executive Board resolution of 1979, *Asha* publishes a listing of all current Association Position Statements, Guidelines, and Definitions. The following listing is current through March 1995.

Preferred Practice Patterns

Preferred Practice Patterns for the Professions of Speech-Language Pathology and Audiology, *Asha*, March 1993, Suppl. 1, pp. 1–110

Statements

*Acoustics in Educational Settings, *Asha*, March 1995, Suppl. 14, p. 15

Adults With Learning Disabilities: A Call to Action, *Asha*, December 1995, pp. 39–41

The Audiologist's Role in Occupational Hearing Conservation, *Asha*, April 1985, pp. 41–45

Augmentative and Alternative Communication, *Asha*, March 1991, Suppl. 5, p. 8

*Balance System Assessment, *Asha*, March 1992, Suppl. 7, pp. 9–12

Clinical Management of Communicatively Handicapped Minority Language Populations, *Asha*, June 1985, pp. 29–32

Clinical Supervision in Speech-Language Pathology and Audiology, *Asha*, June 1985, pp. 57–60

Competencies for Aural Rehabilitation, *Asha*, May 1984, pp. 37–41

*Delivery of Speech-Language Pathology Services in Home Care, *Asha*, March 1988, pp. 77–79

*Electrical Stimulation for Cochlear Implant Selection and Rehabilitation, *Asha*, March 1992, Suppl. 7, pp. 13–16

*Evaluation and Treatment for Tracheoesophageal Fistulization/Puncture, *Asha*, March 1992, Suppl. 7, pp. 17–21

*External Auditory Canal Examination and Cerumen Management, *Asha*, March 1992, Suppl. 7, pp. 22–24

Facilitated Communication, *Asha*, March 1995, Suppl. 14, p. 22

In-Service Programs in Learning Disabilities, *Asha*, November 1983, pp. 47–49

*Instrumental Diagnostic Procedures for Swallowing, *Asha*, March 1992, Suppl. 7, pp. 25–33

Interdisciplinary Approaches to Brain Damage, *Asha*, April 1990, Suppl. 2, p. 3

Issues in the Delivery of Service to Individuals With Learning Disabilities, *Asha*, November 1983, pp. 43–45

Issues in Learning Disabilities: Assessment and Diagnosis, *Asha*, March 1989, pp. 111–112

Source: Reprinted with permission from Position Statements, Guideline Definitions, and Relevant Papers, *Asha*, Vol. 37, Suppl. 14, pp. 36–37, ©1995, the American Speech-Language-Hearing Association.

Joint Committee on Infant Hearing 1994 Position Statement, *Asha*, December 1994, pp. 38–41

Learning Disabilities and the Preschool Child, *Asha*, May 1987, pp. 35–38

Learning Disabilities: Issues in the Preparation of Professional Personnel, *Asha*, September 1985, pp. 49–51

Learning Disabilities: Issues on Definition, *Asha*, March 1991, Suppl. 5, pp. 18–20

Learning Disabilities, *Asha*, May 1976, pp. 282–290

Language Learning Disorders, *Asha*, November 1982, pp. 937–944

Language Learning Disorders Statement of ASHA and National Association of School Psychologists, *Asha*, March 1987, pp. 55–56

National Health Care Proposals, *Asha*, November 1971, pp. 683–684

National Health Policy, *Asha*, March 1993, Suppl. 10, p. 1

*Neurophysiologic Intraoperative Monitoring, *Asha*, March 1992, Suppl. 7, pp. 34–36

Position Statement and Guidelines for Oral and Oropharyngeal Prostheses, *Asha*, March 1993, Suppl. 10, pp. 14–16

Position Statement and Guidelines for the Use of Voice Prostheses in Tracheotomized Persons With or Without Ventilatory Dependence, *Asha*, March 1993, Suppl. 10, pp. 17–20

Prevention of Communication Disorders, *Asha*, March 1988, p. 90

Professional Performance Appraisal by Individuals Outside the Professions of Speech-Language Pathology and Audiology, *Asha*, March 1993, Suppl. 10, pp. 11–13

Providing Appropriate Education for Students With Learning Disabilities in Regular Education Classrooms, *Asha*, March 1991, Suppl. 5, pp. 15–17

The Need for Subject Descriptors in Learning Disabilities Research: Preschool Through High School Years, *Asha*, March 1991, Suppl. 5, pp. 13–14

The Role of Speech-Language Pathologists in the Identification, Diagnosis, and Treatment of Individuals With Cognitive-Communicative Impairments, *Asha*, March 1988, p. 79

The Roles of Speech-Language Pathologists in Service Delivery to Infants, Toddlers, and Their Families, *Asha*, April 1990, Suppl. 2, p. 4

The Roles of the Speech-Language Pathologist and Audiologist in Learning Disabilities, *Asha*, December 1979, p. 1015

The Role of Speech-Language Pathologists and Audiologists in Service Delivery for Persons With Mental Retardation and Developmental Disabilities in Community Settings, *Asha*, April 1990, Suppl. 2, pp. 5–6

The Roles of Speech-Language Pathologists and Audiologists in Working With Older Persons, *Asha*, March 1988, pp. 80–83

Serving the Communicatively Handicapped Mentally Retarded Individual, *Asha*, August 1982, pp. 547–553

The Role of the Speech-Language Pathologist in Assessment and Management of Oral Myofunctional Disorders, *Asha*, March 1991, Suppl. 5, p. 7

Scope of Practice, Speech-Language Pathology and Audiology, *Asha*, April 1990, Suppl. 2, pp. 1–2

Social Dialects (and Implications), *Asha*, September 1983, pp. 23–27

The Use of FM Amplification Instruments for Infants and Preschool Children with Hearing Impairment, *Asha*, March 1991, Suppl. 5, pp. 1–2

Training, Credentialing, Use, and Supervision of Support Personnel in Speech-Language Pathology, *Asha*, March 1995, Suppl. 14, p. 21

*Vocal Tract Visualization and Imaging, *Asha*, March 1992, Suppl. 7, pp. 31–40

Guidelines

Competencies in Auditory Evoked Potential Measurement and Clinical Application, *Asha*, April 1990, Suppl. 2, pp. 13–16

Competencies for Speech-Language Pathologists Providing Services in Augmentative Communication, *Asha*, March 1989, pp. 107–110

Determining the Threshold Level for Speech, *Asha*, May 1979, pp. 353–356

Employment and Utilization of Supportive Personnel in Audiology and Speech-Language Pathology, *Asha*, March 1981, pp. 165–169

Guidelines for Audiologic Assessment of Children from Birth–36 Months of Age, *Asha*, March 1991. Suppl. 5, pp. 37–43

Guidelines for Audiologic Screening of Newborn Infants Who Are at Risk for Hearing Impairment, *Asha*, March 1989, pp. 89–92

Guidelines for Audiology Services in the Schools, *Asha*, March 1993, Suppl. 10, pp. 24–32

Guidelines for Audiometric Symbols, *Asha*, April 1990, Suppl. 2, pp. 25–30

Guidelines for Caseload Size and Speech-Language Service Delivery in the Schools, *Asha*, March 1993, Suppl. 10, pp. 33–39

Guidelines for the Delivery of Speech-Language Pathology and Audiology Services in Home Care, *Asha*, March 1991, Suppl. 5, pp. 29–34

Guidelines for Determining Threshold Level for Speech, *Asha*, March 1988, pp. 85–89

Guidelines for Education in Audiology Practice Management, *Asha*, March 1995, Suppl. 14, p. 20

Guidelines for Fitting and Monitoring FM Systems, *Asha*, March 1994, Suppl. 12, pp. 1–9

Guidelines for Gender Equality in Language Use, *Asha*, March 1993, Suppl. 10, pp. 42–46

Guidelines for Graduate Education in Amplification, *Asha*, March 1991, Suppl. 5, pp. 35–36

Guidelines for Meeting the Communicative Needs of Persons With Severe Disabilities, *Asha*, March 1992, Suppl. 7, pp. 1–8

Guidelines for Practice in Stuttering Treatment, *Asha*, March 1995, Suppl. 14, p. 26

Guidelines for Screening for Hearing Impairments and Middle Ear Disorders, *Asha*, April 1990, Suppl. 2, pp. 17–24

Guidelines for Speech-Language Pathologists Serving Persons With Language, Socio-Communicative, and/or Cognitive-Communicative Impairments, *Asha*, March 1991, Suppl. 5, pp. 21–28

Guidelines for the Audiologic Management of Individuals Receiving Cochleotoxic Drug Therapy, *Asha*, March 1994, Suppl. 12, pp. 11–19

Guidelines for the Structure and Function of an Interdisciplinary Team for Persons With Brain Injury, *Asha*, March 1995, Suppl. 14, p. 23

Identification Audiometry, *Asha*, May 1985, pp. 49–52

Knowledge and Skills Needed by Speech-Language Pathologists Providing Services to Dysphagic Patients/Clients, *Asha*, April 1990, Suppl. 2, pp. 7–12

Manual Pure-Tone Threshold Audiometry, *Asha*, April 1978, pp. 297–301

Mental Retardation and Developmental Disabilities Curriculum Guide, *Asha*, March 1989, pp. 94–96

Nonsexist Language in the Journals of ASHA, *Asha*, November 1979, pp. 973–978

Orofacial Myofunctional Disorders: Knowledge and Skills, *Asha*, March 1993, Suppl. 10, pp. 21–23

Suggested Competencies for Effective Clinical Supervision, *Asha*, December 1982, pp. 1021–1023

Definitions

Bilingual Speech-Language Pathologists and Audiologists, March 1989, p. 93

Communicative Disorders and Variations, *Asha*, November 1982, pp. 949–950

Definitions of Communication Disorders and Variations, *Asha*, March 1993, Suppl. 10, pp. 40–41

Definition of Language, *Asha*, June 1983, p. 44

Definition of Private Practice, *Asha*, March 1987 p. 35

Learning Disabilities: Issues on Definition, *Asha*, November 1982, pp. 945–947

Prevention of Speech, Language and Hearing Problems, *Asha*, June 1982, pp. 425, 431

Severely Hearing Handicapped (Effective November 1978), *Asha*, March 1979, p. 191

Bibliographies

Acoustic-Immittance Measures: An Annotated Bibliography, *Asha*, March 1991, Suppl. 4, pp. 1–44

Audiological Assessment of Central Auditory Processing: An Annotated Bibliography, *Asha*, February 1990, Suppl. 1, pp. 45–62

Aural Rehabilitation: An Annotated Bibliography, *Asha*, February 1990, Suppl. 1, pp. 1–2

Business, Marketing, Ethics, and Professionalism in Audiology: An Updated Annotated Bibliography (1986–1989), *Asha*, January 1991, Suppl. 3, pp. 39–45

Reports

Ad Hoc Committee on Dysphagia Report, *Asha*, March 1989, pp. 63–67

Ad Hoc Committee on Labial-Lingual Posturing Function, *Asha*, November 1989, pp. 92–94

AIDS/HIV: Implications for Speech-Language Pathologists and Audiologists, *Asha*, December 1990, pp. 46–48

A Model for Collaborative Service Delivery for Students With Language Learning Disorders in the Public Schools, *Asha*, March 1991, Suppl. 5, pp. 44–50

Amplification as a Remediation Technique for Children with Normal Peripheral Hearing, *Asha*, January 1991, Suppl. 3, pp. 22–24

Augmentative and Alternative Communication, *Asha*, March 1991, Suppl. 5, pp. 9–12

Autonomy of Speech-Language Pathology and Audiology, *Asha*, May 1986, pp. 73–77

Committee on Personnel and Service Needs in Communication Disorders, *Asha*, November 1988, pp. 59–60

Communication-Based Services for Infants, Toddlers, and Their Families, *Asha*, May 1989, pp. 32-34

Considerations for Establishing a Private Practice in Audiology and/or Speech-Language Pathology, *Asha*, January 1991, Suppl. 3, pp. 39–45

Considerations in Screening Adults/Older Persons for Handicapping Hearing Impairment, *Asha*, August 1992, pp. 81–87

Deinstitutionalization: Its Effects on the Delivery of Speech-Language-Hearing Services for Persons With Mental Retardation and Developmental Disabilities, *Asha*, March 1989, pp. 84–87

Issues in Determining Eligibility for Language Intervention, *Asha*, March 1989, pp. 113–118

Major Issues Affecting the Delivery of Speech-Language Pathology and Audiology Services in Hospital Settings: Recommendations and Strategies, *Asha*, April 1990, pp. 67–70

Professional Liability and Risk Management for the Audiology and Speech-Language Pathology Professions, *Asha*, March 1994, Suppl. 12, pp. 25–38

Provision of Audiology and Speech-Language Pathology Services to Older Persons in Nursing Homes, *Asha*, March 1988, pp. 72–74

Report of the Ad Hoc Committee on Cochlear Implants, *Asha*, April 1986, pp. 29–52

Report of the Ad Hoc Committee on Instrument Evaluation, *Asha*, March 1988, pp. 75–76

Report of the Task Force on Audiology II, *Asha*, November 1988, pp. 41–45

Report on Doctoral Education, *Asha*, January 1991, Suppl. 3, pp. 1–9

Report on Private Practice, *Asha*, September 1991, Suppl. 6, pp. 1–4

Role of the Speech-Language Pathologist and Teacher of Singing in Remediation of Singers With Voice Disorders, *Asha*, January 1993, p. 63

Sedation and Topical Anesthetics in Audiology and Speech-Language Pathology, *Asha*, March 1992, Suppl. 7, pp. 41–46

Survey of States' Workers' Compensation Practices for Occupational Hearing Loss, *Asha*, March 1992, Suppl. 8, pp. 1–8

Telephone Hearing Screening, *Asha*, November 1988, p. 53

The Protection of Rights of People Receiving Audiology or Speech-Language Pathology Services, *Asha*, January 1994, pp. 60–63

The Role of Research and the State of Research Training Within Communication Sciences and Disorders, *Asha*, March 1994, Suppl. 12, pp. 21–23

Utilization and Employment of Speech-Language Pathology Supportive Personnel With Underserved Populations, *Asha*, November 1988, pp. 55–56

Utilization of Medicaid and Other Third Party Funds for "Covered Services" in the Schools, *Asha*, March 1991, Suppl. 5, pp. 51–58

Tutorial Papers

Calibration of Speech Signals Delivered Via Earphones, *Asha*, June 1987, pp. 41–48

Prevention of Communication Disorders Tutorial, *Asha*, September 1991, Suppl. 6, pp. 15–42

Short Latency Auditory Evoked Potentials, June 1987

Sound Field Measurement Tutorial, *Asha*, January 1991, Suppl. 3, pp. 25–37

Tympanometry, *JSHD*, November 1988, pp. 354–377

REACH: A Model for Service Delivery and Professional Development Within Remote/Rural Regions of the United States and U.S. Territories, *Asha*, September 1991 Suppl. 6, pp. 5–14

Other Relevant Papers

A Plan for Special Interest Divisions and Study Sections, *Asha*, February 1990, pp. 59–61

Classification of Speech-Language Pathology and Audiology Procedures and Communication Disorders, *Asha*, December 1987, pp. 49–50

Code of Ethics, *Asha*, March 1994, Suppl. 13, pp. 1–2

Standards for Professional Service Programs in Audiology and Speech Language Pathology, *Asha*, September 1992, pp. 63–70

ASHA Work Force Study, *Asha*, March 1989, pp. 63–67

Evaluation of the Requirements for the Certificate of Clinical Competence in Speech-Language Pathology and Audiology, *Asha*, September 1988, pp. 75–78

Preparation Models for the Supervisory Process in Speech-Language Pathology and Audiology, *Asha*, March 1989, pp. 97–106

These documents are available in the ASHA Desk Reference. To order, contact Fulfillment Operations. (301) 897-5700 ext. 218.

Appendix 3–E

Code of Ethics and Partial List of Issues in Ethics Statements

Last Revised January 1, 1994

Preamble

The preservation of the highest standards of integrity and ethical principles is vital to the responsible discharge of obligations in the professions of speech-language pathology and audiology. This Code of Ethics sets forth the fundamental principles and rules considered essential to this purpose.

Every individual who is (a) a member of the American Speech-Language-Hearing Association, whether certified or not, (b) a non-member holding the Certificate of Clinical Competence from the Association, (c) an applicant for membership or certification, or (d) a Clinical Fellow seeking to fulfill standards for certification shall abide by this Code of Ethics.

Any action that violates the spirit and purpose of this Code shall be considered unethical. Failure to specify any particular responsibility or practice in this Code of Ethics shall not be construed as denial of the existence of such responsibilities or practices.

The fundamentals of ethical conduct are described by Principles of Ethics and by Rules of Ethics as they relate to responsibility to

Source: Reprinted with permission from Code of Ethics 1995, *Asha,* Vol. 37, No. 3, pp. 74–75, © 1995, the American Speech-Language-Hearing Association.

persons served, to the public, and to the professions of speech-language pathology and audiology.

Principles of Ethics, aspirational and inspirational in nature, form the underlying moral basis for the Code of Ethics. Individuals shall observe these principles as affirmative obligations under all conditions of professional activity.

Rules of Ethics are specific statements of minimally acceptable professional conduct or prohibitions and are applicable to all individuals.

Principle of Ethics I

Individuals shall honor their responsibility to hold paramount the welfare of persons they serve professionally.

Rules of Ethics

A. Individuals shall provide all services competently.

B. Individuals shall use every resource, including referral when appropriate, to ensure that high-quality service is provided.

C. Individuals shall not discriminate in the delivery of professional services on the basis of race or ethnicity, gender, age, religion, national origin, sexual orientation, or disability.

D. Individuals shall fully inform the persons they serve of the nature and possible effects of services rendered and products dispensed.

E. Individuals shall evaluate the effectiveness of services rendered and of products dispensed and shall provide services or dispense products only when benefit can reasonably be expected.

F. Individuals shall not guarantee the results of any treatment or procedure, directly or by implication; however, they may make a reasonable statement of prognosis.

G. Individuals shall not evaluate or treat speech, language, or hearing disorders solely by correspondence.

H. Individuals shall maintain adequate records of professional services rendered and products dispensed and shall allow access to these records when appropriately authorized.

I. Individuals shall not reveal, without authorization, any professional or personal information about the person served professionally, unless required by law to do so, or unless doing so is necessary to protect the welfare of the person or of the community.

J. Individuals shall not charge for services not rendered, nor shall they misrepresent,[1] in any fashion, services rendered or products dispensed.

K. Individuals shall use persons in research or as subjects of teaching demonstrations only with their informed consent.

L. Individuals whose professional services are adversely affected by substance abuse or other health-related conditions shall seek professional assistance and, where appropriate, withdraw from the affected areas of practice.

Principle of Ethics II

Individuals shall honor their responsibility to achieve and maintain the highest level of professional competence.

Rules of Ethics

A. Individuals shall engage in the provision of clinical services only when they hold the appropriate Certificate of Clinical Competence or when they are in the certification process and are supervised by an individual who holds the appropriate Certificate of Clinical Competence.

B. Individuals shall engage in only those aspects of the professions that are within the scope of their competence, considering their level of education, training, and experience.

C. Individuals shall continue their professional development throughout their careers.

D. Individuals shall delegate the provision of clinical services only to persons who are certified or to persons in the education or certification process who are appropriately supervised. The provision of support services may be delegated to persons who are neither certified nor in the certification process only when a certificate holder provides appropriate supervision.

---

[1]For purposes of this Code of Ethics, misrepresentation includes any untrue statements or statements that are likely to mislead. Misrepresentation also includes the failure to state any information that is material and that ought, in fairness, to be considered.

E. Individuals shall prohibit any of their professional staff from providing services that exceed the staff member's competence, considering the staff member's level of education, training, and experience.

F. Individuals shall ensure that all equipment used in the provision of services is in proper working order and is properly calibrated.

Principle of Ethics III

Individuals shall honor their responsibility to the public by promoting public understanding of the professions, by supporting the development of services designed to fulfill the unmet needs of the public, and by providing accurate information in all communications involving any aspect of the professions.

Rules of Ethics

A. Individuals shall not misrepresent their credentials, competence, education, training, or experience.

B. Individuals shall not participate in professional activities that constitute a conflict of interest.

C. Individuals shall not misrepresent diagnostic information, services rendered, or products dispensed or engage in any scheme or artifice to defraud in connection with obtaining payment or reimbursement for such services or products.

D. Individuals' statements to the public shall provide accurate information about the nature and management of communication disorders, about the professions, and about professional services.

E. Individuals' statements to the public—advertising, announcing, and marketing their professional services, reporting re-search results, and promoting products—shall adhere to prevailing professional standards and shall not contain misrepresentations.

Principle of Ethics IV

Individuals shall honor their responsibilities to the professions and their relationships with colleagues, students, and members of allied professions. Individuals shall uphold the dignity and autonomy of the professions, maintain harmonious interprofessional and intraprofessional relationships, and accept the professions' self-imposed standards.

Rules of Ethics

A. Individuals shall prohibit anyone under their supervision from engaging in any prac\ fraud, deceit, misrepresentation, or any form of conduct that adversely reflects on the professions or on the individual's fitness to serve persons professionally.

C. Individuals shall assign credit only to those who have contributed to a publication, presentation, or product. Credit shall be assigned in proportion to the contribution and only with the contributor's consent.

D. Individuals' statements to colleagues about professional services, research results, and products shall adhere to prevailing professional standards and shall contain no misrepresentations.

E. Individuals shall not provide professional services without exercising independent professional judgment, regardless of referral source or prescription.

F. Individuals shall not discriminate in their relationships with colleagues, students, and members of allied professions on the basis of race or ethnicity, gender, age, religion, national origin, sexual orientation, or disability.

G. Individuals who have reason to believe that the Code of Ethics has been violated shall inform the Ethical Practice Board.

H. Individuals shall cooperate fully with the Ethical Practice Board in its investigation and adjudication of matters related to this Code of Ethics.

ISSUES IN ETHICS

Conflicts of Professional Interest

Representation of Services for Insurance Reimbursement or Funding

Clinical Practice by Certificate Holders in the Profession in Which They Are Not Certified

Supervision of Student Clinicians

Competition

Prescription

Use of Graduate Degrees by Members and Certificate Holders

Ethics in Research and Professional Practice

Public Announcements and Public Statements

Drawing Cases for Private Practice from Primary Place of Employment

Clinical Fellowship Supervisor's Responsibilities

ASHA Policy Regarding Support Personnel

Ethical Practice Inquiries: State Versus ASHA Jurisdictions

Fees for Clinical Service Provided by Students

Identification of Members Engaged in Clinical Practice Without Certification

For the complete Issues in Ethics statements, see March 1994 *Asha*, Suppl. 13.

Appendix 3–F

Model Bill of Rights

Model Bill of Rights for People Receiving Audiology or Speech-Language Pathology Services

Clients as consumers receiving audiology or speech-language pathology services have:

The Right to be treated with dignity and respect

The Right that services be provided without regard to race or ethnicity, gender, age, religion, national origin, sexual orientation, or disability

The Right to know the name and professional qualifications of the person or persons providing services

The Right to personal privacy and confidentiality of information to the extent permitted by law

The Right to know, in advance, the fees for services, regardless of the method of payment

The Right to receive a clear explanation of evaluation results; to be informed of potential or lack of potential for improvement; and to express their choices of goals and methods of service delivery

The Right to accept or reject services to the extent permitted by law

The Right that services be provided in a timely and competent manner, which includes referral to other appropriate professionals when necessary

The Right to present concerns about services and to be informed of procedures for seeking their resolution

The Right to accept or reject participation in teaching, research, or promotional activities

The Right to the extent permitted by law, to review information contained in their records, to receive explanation of record entries upon request, and to request correction of inaccurate records

The Right to adequate notice of and reasons for discontinuation of services; an explanation of these reasons, in person, upon request; and referral to other providers if so requested

These rights belong to the person or persons needing services. For sound legal or medical reasons, a family member, guardian, or legal representative may exercise these rights on the person's behalf.

This document is available in a two-color, suitable-for-framing version. For details, contact Actionline 1-800-638-6868.

Source: Reprinted with permission from Model Bill of Rights for People Receiving Audiology, *Asha*, Vol. 36, No. 3, p. 75, © 1994, the American Speech-Language-Hearing Association.

Appendix 3–G

Related Professional Organizations

Academy of Dispensing Audiologists

Kenneth E. Smith
8901 West 74th Street
Suite 150
Shawnee Mission, KS 66204
    (913) 384-5880
FAX: (913) 384-9612

Academy of Neurologic Communication Disorders and Sciences

Kathryn A. Bayles
University of Arizona
Dept. of Speech and Hearing
Building #71
Tucson, AZ 85721
    (602) 621-1819
FAX: (602) 621-2226

Academy of Rehabilitative Audiology

Judy Abrahamson
Audiology/Speech Pathology Services
Olin E. Teague Veterans Center
Temple, TX 76504
    (817) 778-4811, ext. 4901
FAX: (817) 771-4563

Source: Reprinted with permission from Presidents/ Chairs, Allied and Related Professional Organizations, *Asha,* Vol. 37, No. 3, pp. 82–83. © 1995 the American Speech-Language-Hearing Association.

Air Force Audiology Association

Lt. Colonel Ben Sierra
Consultant USAF Surgeon General for Audiology and Speech Language Pathology
AI.\XPTT
2509 Kennedy Circle
Brooks Air Force Base, TX 78235-5118
    (210) 536-2661
FAX: (210) 536-2810

American Academy of Audiology

Robert W. Keith
Division of Audiology
University of Cincinnati Med. Center
Cincinnati, OH 45267
    (513) 558-9728
FAX: (513) 558-5203

American Academy of Private Practice in Speech-Language Pathology and Audiology

Barbara Samuels
7349 Topanga Canyon Boulevard
Canoga Park, CA 91303
    (818) 883-1381
FAX: (818) 883-3583

American Auditory Society

Deborah Hayes
Children's Hospital
Dept. of Audiology, Speech Pathology
and Learning Services
1056 East 19th Avenue
Mail Station B030
Denver, CO 80218-1088
(303) 861-6800
FAX: (303) 861-3992

Audiology Foundation of America

David P. Goldstein
2100 N. Salisbury
W. Lafayette, IN 47906
(317) 463-5446
FAX: (317) 494-0771

Communication Disorders Prevention and Epidemiology Study Group

Bobbie B. Lubker
University of North Carolina
CB 3500 014 Peabody Hall
Chapel Hill, NC 27599
(919) 962-5579
FAX: (919) 962-1533

Computer Users in Speech and Hearing

Art Schwartz
Hearing and Speech Sciences
Cleveland State University
Cleveland, OH 44115
(216) 687-6990
FAX: (216) 687-9366

Council of AuD Programs

James Lynn
University of Akron

School of Communication Disorders
Akron, OH 44325
(216) 972-6803
FAX: (216) 972-7884

Council of Graduate Programs in Communication Sciences and Disorders

John Ferraro
Department of Speech and Hearing
University of Kansas
Medical Center
Kansas City, KS 66160-7650
(913) 588-5937
FAX: (913) 588-5923

Council of Language, Speech and Hearing Consultants in State Education Agencies

Carolyn Weiner Isakson
212 Mohawk Drive
West Hartford, CT 06117
(203) 638-4260
FAX: (203) 638-4231

Council of School Supervisors

Carolyn S. Zeller
1331 Frankfort Street
New Orleans, LA 70122-2121
(504) 830-4437

Council of State Association Presidents

Herease Frazier
1204 East 85th Street
Chicago, IL 60619
(312) 978-6428

Council of Supervisors in Speech-Language Pathology and Audiology

Sally Jones-McNamara
5501 Seminary Road, Rt. 106 South

Falls Church, VA 22041
 (800) 477-4002, ext. 4031
FAX: (703) 820-2798

Directors of Speech and Hearing Programs in State Health and Welfare Agencies

Lorraine Michel
Bureau of Family Health & Environment
Maternal & Child Health
900 S.W. Jackson, 10th Floor
Topeka, KS 66612-1290
 (913) 296-6134
FAX: (913) 296-8626

Educational Audiology Association

Laurie Allen
99 Cambridge Court
Dubuque, IA 52001
 (319) 556-3310
FAX: (319) 556-3310

Hispanic Caucus

Luis F. Riquelme
167 Park Place
Brooklyn, NY 11238
 (718) 783-0760
FAX: Same, press * after beep

Alexandra Heinsen-Combs
86-48 111th Street
Richmond Hill, NY 11418
 (718) 250-8431
FAX: (718) 250-8669

Infant and Family Special Interest Group

Debra Reichert Hoge
Box 1776 SIUE
Edwardsville, IL 62026
 (618) 692-3662
FAX: (618) 692-3307

International Affairs Association

Margo Wilson
8039 Cholla Street
Scottsdale, AZ 85260
H: (602) 483-6572
W: (602) 965-2373
FAX: (602) 965-8516
(Dept. Speech and Hearing Sciences)

Lesbian, Gay, and Bisexual Audiologists and Speech-Language Pathologists

Richard K. Adler
1169 Conway Road
Decatur, GA 30030
 (404) 370-1394
FAX: (404) 933-4135

Ellen Fye
239 Dale Drive
Silver Spring, MD 20910
 (301) 589-3063

Military Audiology Association

LTC Nancy Vause
Vanderbilt University
ATTN: Audiology
Station B
PO Box 6141
Nashville, TN 37235
 (615) 320-5353
FAX: (615) 343-7705

National Academy of Preprofessional Programs in Communication Sciences and Disorders

Sandra Salisch, M.S.
Pace University
Speech Communication Studies
Pace Plaza

New York, NY 10038
 (212) 346-1204
FAX: (212) 346-1933

National Black Association for Speech, Language and Hearing

Eugene Wiggins, Executive Director
3542 Gentry Ridge Court
Silver Spring, MD 20904
 (202) 727-2608

National Council of State Boards of Examiners for Speech-Language Pathology and Audiology

Virginia G. Walker
3220 Robinhood Road
Tallahassee, FL 32312
W: (904) 644-8460
H: (904) 385-0290
FAX: (904) 644-8994

National Hearing Conservation Association

Barbara Garrett
St. Luke's Hospital
Occupational Health Care Center
PO Box 3026
Cedar Rapids, IA 52406-3026
 (319) 369-7569
FAX: (319) 369-8119

Navy Audiology Society

Leslie Sims
2262 Evergreen Avenue, SE
Port Orchard, WA
 (206) 895-3462
FAX: (206) 476-3744
ATTN: Lt. Sims CODE 061.1A

Public School Caucus

Monica Ferguson
PO Box 74608
Fairbanks, AK 99707
H: (907) 479-0028
W: (907) 452-2000
FAX: (907) 451-6160

Society of Hospital Directors of Communicative Disorders Programs

Alex Johnson
Henry Ford Hospital–Neurology
2921 West Grand Boulevard
Detroit, MI 48202
 (313) 874-7170
FAX: (313) 874-7168

Treatment Research in Communication Disorders—Special Interest Group

Nancy Scherer
Department of Communication Disorders
Box 70643
East Tennessee State University
Johnson City, TN 37614
 (615) 929-5254
FAX: (615) 929-5238

United States Society for Augmentative and Alternative Communication

Mary Blake Huer
Dept. of Speech Communication
California State University–Fullerton
Fullerton, CA 92634
 (714) 773-3617
FAX: (714) 773-3142

Speech-Language Pathology and Audiology in the Educational Setting: Professional Qualifications, Roles, and Services

Nancy H. Huffman and Pamelia F. O'Connell

This chapter has two major divisions. Qualifications, roles, and services in speech-language pathology and audiology are examined separately by different authors who have different professional backgrounds. Because most of this book has a speech-language pathology focus, the two sections do not share an identical format. Many aspects of the services of speech-language pathologists in schools are given extensive discussion in the chapters that follow; audiological services receive in-depth coverage in this chapter.

SPEECH-LANGUAGE PATHOLOGY SERVICES IN THE EDUCATIONAL SETTING

Pamelia F. O'Connell

Chapter 1 documented the beginnings of speech services in school settings in the early decades of this century and traced the subsequent changes in the nature of the services and the kinds of students receiving them. Chapter 3 introduced the national organization, the American Speech-Language-Hearing Association (ASHA), and provided a discussion of professional standards set by the association. What standards are currently required of the speech-language pathologists who serve in the nation's schools? What changes from the early days of "additional course work" have taken place? Are requirements congruent with the roles assumed by the speech-language specialist? The answers to these important questions will not be either simple or clear, for the situation regarding professional standards in schools is complex.

CREDENTIALS IN SPEECH-LANGUAGE PATHOLOGY: PROFESSIONAL REGULATION

There are three types of regulation; registration, certification and licensure. The term "regulation" refers to any of the three but the term "licensure" is generally reserved to describe the process which restricts the use of certain titles and prohibits certain acts to those holding the license. Certification and registration are lesser forms of regulation and are voluntary. Although certification generally refers to the credential bestowed by private associations, like ASHA, states may also use certification to regulate a profession. (S. Larson, personal communication, 1996).

There are three major types of professional credentials that an individual speech-language pathologist may hold. Many school speech-language pathologists hold all three of them; many do not. These credentials are: (a) the Certificate of Clinical Competence, or CCC-SLP, issued by ASHA; (b) the professional license, issued by a state licensure board; and (c) the school credential, issued by a state education agency, enabling the holder to provide speech and language services in schools in a certain state.

Certificate of Clinical Competence

The CCC-SLP, as granted by ASHA, "allows the holder to provide independent clinical services and to supervise the clinical practice of student trainees, clinicians who do not hold certification, and support personnel" (ASHA, 1995a, p. 2).

Individuals who have the CCC-SLP must have a graduate degree in speech-language pathology or speech-language and hearing science or an allied field. They must abide by ASHA's Code of Ethics. The CCC-SLP is awarded through ASHA's Clinical Certification Board, whose members are appointed by ASHA's Executive Board.

Effective on January 1, 1994, all graduate course work and graduate clinical practicum required in the professional area for which the certificate is sought must have been completed at an institution whose program was accredited by the Educational Standards Board of ASHA (ASHA, 1995a).

The applicant must meet academic requirements that include course work in the basic sciences and professional areas and supervised clinical observation and clinical practicum. Supervised clinical experience must be obtained in eight specific areas. Applicants must pass the national examination in the area for which the certificate is sought. After completion of academic course work and clinical practicum, the applicant must successfully complete a clinical fellowship year. The fellowship must consist of at least 36 weeks of full-time professional experience or its part-time equivalent and must be completed under the supervision of an individual holding the CCC in the area for which certification is sought. ASHA's requirements for the CCC change periodically. More current and or more complete information may be obtained from ASHA.

Although ASHA has provided the profession with a nationally recognized set of standards for professional practice, it lacks enforcement power. That is, like other professional and scientific organizations such as the American Psychological Association and the American Medical Association, ASHA has no method of ensuring that all service providers meet this standard. A movement began, therefore, in the late 1960s, toward professional regulation through state licensure boards. In this regard, speech-language pathology and audiology followed other professional groups such as physicians, dentists, psychologists, and many more, in seeking to ensure professional competence and consumer protection via a state license to practice.

The State License

In 1969, the state of Florida became the first to require a license to practice for speech-language pathologists and audiologists. Other states followed, and by January 1996, all but five states and the District of Columbia required a license or its equivalent through a registration process. Two other states regulate audiology but not speech-language pathology, and one state, New Hampshire, does not license audiologists but does license speech-language pathologists. Though states vary somewhat in their regulatory requirements, there are several common elements. All states except Georgia require a master's degree or its equivalent; most have a supervised clinical clock-hour requirement. Almost all states accept the ASHA credential as proof of meeting some requirements or waive their examination for holders of the CCC-SLP. This suggests a fairly uniform standard for practice throughout the United States, with one major and very relevant exception. Of the 45 states that regulate one or both of the professions, 36 of them exempt school speech-language pathologists from licensure requirements, according to 1995 figures (ASHA, 1995b). Several states, however, have since raised their standards, and many more will do so sometime in the next century. If licensure is not required for so many school-based professionals, what is the standard?

State Educational Agency Requirements

Although there are minor differences between the states in regulatory requirements, differences at the state education agency level are more significant, and these requirements also are subject to change. The best source of current information for any given state is that state's education department. Though 36 states require a master's degree or its equivalent, most states have no supervised clock-hour requirement. Thirty-four states do require a school-based practicum, frequently referred to as "student teaching." At least one state, New York, which requires a master's degree for permanent certification, does not require that the degree be in speech-language pathology. Eight states require a bachelor's degree only, and seven others grant entry-level or provisional certification to bachelor's degree holders. Five states have policies to upgrade certification requirements by a "date-certain" before 2000. It should be noted that almost every state has a system for awarding emergency certificates to people who do not meet the qualifications. The criteria for awarding these certificates vary from state to state.

Clearly, a double standard exists, one that is confusing to professionals and the public. Though the situation is improving, an implication exists that school speech-language pathologists do not necessarily meet the highest professional standards, those required of speech-language pathologists in other settings. Yet the services they provide depend upon high levels of education and supervised experience for their adequate execution.

The reasons for this discrepancy are doubtless as varied as the states themselves. Some common contributing factors lie in the nature of early services provided (only services to speech-impaired students from regular classrooms) and in political considerations that made state licensure obtainable only if school exemptions were granted. Shortages of master's-level personnel are often cited to support continuation of bachelor-level service providers.

At present, the nature of the services and the population served point toward adherence to the highest of professional standards. The vast majority of children and adolescents who receive speech-language pathology services receive them in schools. They deserve the best that the profession has to offer.

ROLES AND SERVICES: SPEECH-LANGUAGE PATHOLOGY

The ASHA Scope of Practice statement is found in Appendix 3–B. The preferred practice patterns included in Appendix 3–C enlarge upon the statement by describing some of the activities that make up the practice of the profession. These provide a brief introduction to the roles and services of speech-language pathologists in schools.

It is somewhat difficult to differentiate between roles and services because the role assumed by any individual is at least partially defined by the activities or services performed. If there in an overarching role for the school speech-language pathologist, it seems to be that of expert in communication disorders. That is, the school speech-language pathologist is presumed to be the most knowledgeable school professional in the areas of speech and language difficulties or differences. This role alone calls for a high level of professional competence. Other roles more clearly defined by the services that the speech-language pathologist provides are discussed below.

Management

A school speech-language pathologist may find him- or herself in complete charge of a small school program, may function as a part of a large department in a large school district, or may be one of several within a single school. In any event, the individual will be responsible for organizing and managing at least a part of the program. Management of time is an important function (Neidecker & Blosser, 1993), one that can be divided into several sections.

Managing the School Year

Certain activities traditionally take place in the beginning of the school year, such as screening, assessments, case selection, Individual Educational Plan (IEP) preparation, scheduling of students for direct services, and scheduling of time to be spent in classrooms or in consultation with other school personnel. There may be midyear and end-of-school-year activities as well that involve additional screening, assessments, documentation, and planning for the year to come.

Managing the School Week

The speech-language pathology schedule is usually planned by the week. Blocks of time are set aside on certain days for certain activities to be performed. Some speech-language pathologists serve more than one school. In these cases, travel time must be built into the schedule, and differences in starting and ending the school day, lunch periods, and so on must be taken into account. Building an effective and manageable weekly schedule may prove a difficult task because so many factors, including the needs and wishes of others, as well as optimum programming for individual students and classrooms, must be considered. The weekly schedule should include time for such activities as telephone calls, report writing and other documentation activities, and conferences with parents, teachers, administrators, and other school personnel. Smith, Carter, and Gilder (1988) conducted a study involving 57 school speech-language pathologists that examined the amount of time spent on activities other than direct student services. They found that the range of activities was large as was the amount of time consumed. For example, an average of 57 IEPs were written over the course of the school year, consuming 29 hours; 40 hours were required for 80 parent conferences; and another 27 hours were spent in additional conferences. The authors concluded that these activities, termed "coordination time," though necessary for effective programming, were frequently inadequately provided for within the schedule.

Managing the School Day

Weeks, of course, take place day by day, and each day must be carefully managed to achieve the maximum benefit from the relatively small number of hours that make up the school day. The length of each session must be planned effectively, the time between sessions must be scheduled, the best days for the scheduling of extra activities must be chosen, and so on. The school speech-language pathologist must be familiar with the individual school's daily routines. Gaining that familiarity must be accorded a high priority.

Identification, Case Finding, and Assessment

Activities associated with the selection of students to receive services have always formed a prominent portion of the job of the speech-language pathologist. This continues to be true; the major changes in this regard lie in the increasing complexity of the case-finding process because the scope of services has broadened over time to include many students not previously served. The assessment process has also become more complex because new assessment instruments appear constantly. Assessment of the more seriously handicapped student may be a difficult and lengthy process.

The numbers of students who may be effectively served will vary according to types of disabilities and levels of performance (Shewan, 1988). Issues involved in setting appropriate caseload figures and a detailed discussion of assessment methods may be found in Chapter 6.

Providing Direct and Indirect Services

The provision of direct student services, frequently termed *therapy*, has always been the hallmark of the school speech-language pathologist. Typically, children have been removed from their classrooms to work in small groups on skills to improve their communicative effectiveness. This model, called the "pull-out" model, is still found today. It is, however, increasingly being supplemented by collaboration and consultation. Chapter 8 provides an in-depth analysis of current models of service delivery.

Documentation

Screening, assessment, and reassessment results; IEPs; progress reports; reports to parents; and reports to other professionals all are necessary. All require attention to detail and the ability to write clearly. Most students in speech-language and audiology programs receive training on report writing; probably few realize how important this will prove in the practice of a career in speech-language pathology, whatever the setting. Chapter 7 details IEP creation, demonstrating how assessment results are translated into programs of service. As the IEP is the heart of any school intervention program, this emphasis is warranted. It should be stressed, however, that all significant professional activities must be adequately documented.

Counseling

The word *counseling* may be used to denote a variety of activities and approaches. In a narrow sense, counseling is a psychological term referring to professional guidance in resolving personal problems or conflicts. In a broader perspective, to counsel is to offer advice and information. Thus we have debt counselors, substance abuse counselors, academic guidance counselors, and the like. In this broader sense, the speech-language pathologist is a counselor in the area of communication disorders, and this constitutes a significant portion of the services provided.

Effective counseling of whatever type takes place within a relationship that seeks to promote knowledge, growth, and change (Taylor, 1992). Speech-language pathologists in school settings usually engage in parent counseling, student counseling, or both. Through the relationships established, the speech-language pathologist may discover the need for additional counseling and may make referrals to other professionals. Parent counseling was addressed a generation ago by Webster (1966, 1968). Much of what she stated then still has relevance for those who work with children. She stressed that parental anxiety and guilt are frequently present and may make obstacles to the child's progress. She also emphasized respect for parents as individuals who have their own needs and responsibilities. Parents usually need information regarding their children's speech, language, or hearing problems, and they may also need guidance in improving their communicative interactions with their children. These ideas have increased relevance today as speech-language pathologists work with infant and toddler populations in which child–parent interaction may constitute the major part of an intervention program (Fitzgerald & Fischer, 1987). Both Luterman (1991) and Rollins (1987) have provided books devoted to counseling in communication disorders. Many professionals have recommended that students in training receive a graduate-level course in counseling. The beginning speech-language pathologist, who may enter school service without such a course, should seek information in this crucial area through course enrollment, continuing education programs, and reading.

Team Membership

The speech-language pathologists of earlier times were frequently professional isolates, working alone in small rooms on skills unrelated to the curriculum. This may be partially true today, but more commonly the speech-language pathologist will function as a member of a team devoted to ensuring an optimum program for each student. The exact manner in which teams operate and their composition will vary from one school setting to another. The speech-language pathologist will always be expected to interact with classroom teachers, in either regular or special education, and building administrators; other educational specialists may be involved as well. These may include physical therapists, occupational therapists, educational audiologists, and other hearing specialists (see the second division of this chapter), learning disability specialists, and reading specialists. Chapter 8 provides detailed discussions of various service delivery models that further elaborate upon the role of the speech-language pathologist as a team member.

Advocacy

The speech-language pathologist, whatever the work setting, should view him- or herself as an advocate for the communicatively impaired. The needs and potential of the communicatively handicapped student may not be fully understood by others. Lack of understanding may be compounded by competition for scarce resources among a variety of contenders. That is, budgetary constraints may limit the availability of special equipment and individual instruction time.

Difficult choices must at times be made. The speech-language pathologist should not shrink from stating the needs of the individual student and making the strongest possible case for meeting these needs. For example, alternate and augmentative communication (see Chapter 9) devices may be costly but crucial for a child's academic success and communication development. Another example lies in unrealistic caseload expectations. The speech-language pathologist should not be expected to serve an excessive number of children. It is not only a question of overwork for the professional but of inevitable underservice for the students involved. Self-advocacy may also be required to obtain, for example, time off for professional meetings, expenses for professional obligations, resources for supplies and equipment, and adequate space and furnishings. For the novice, the advocacy role may be especially difficult because it involves asserting oneself and may involve challenging authority. Membership in local professional organizations such as regional or state Speech-Language Hearing Associations may be very helpful. Of course, membership in ASHA is highly recommended.

Dysphagia Management

The inclusion of the more severely handicapped students within our schools has made many additional demands on speech-language pathologists. One of these involves dysphagia management, or the feeding of neurologically impaired students who experience difficulty in swallowing. Although dysphagia management is within the scope of practice, many speech-language specialists in schools lack training and experience in this area. If the beginning school speech-language pathologist has not had direct, supervised ex-

perience in feeding the neurologically impaired, it is strongly recommended that this practice be avoided until the necessary skills are obtained. Works by Alexander (1987a, 1987b, 1987c), Langley & Lombardini (1991), Morris (1985, 1987), and Morris & Klein (1987) may serve to familiarize the reader with some of the issues involved.

KNOWLEDGE AND SKILLS

To accomplish the roles and services discussed above and throughout this volume, an extensive knowledge base in communication disorders is obviously required. The need for an extensive educational background is also obvious. The qualified and effective speech-language pathologist will have a master's degree from an ASHA-approved institution, will have completed a clinical fellowship year, will have passed the national examination, and will be eligible for both the CCC-SLP and a state license, as well as school certification. A more programmatic listing of knowledge and skills in speech-language pathology, created by Monroe # 1 Board of Cooperative Educational Services in New York State, may be found in the attachments at the end of Chapter 10.

Almost equal to professional knowledge in importance are good communication skills. Effective communication depends upon a host of interlocking abilities and attitudes. Perhaps the first requisite of effective communication is active listening. Also of prime importance is the ability to adjust communication style and vocabulary to meet the needs of others. Clarity, brevity, and truthfulness characterize good communication skills. Written communications share these parameters and are especially demanding.

Interpersonal skills probably determine professional success or failure to a great extent. A recent article by Kahmi (1995) stressed the importance of personal attributes for clinical success in any setting. He reported on a series of studies aimed at illuminating the development and maintenance of clinical expertise. His data indicated that clinicians rated interpersonal/attitudinal factors as much more important than technical skills. The attitudes receiving the highest ratings were interest and adaptability. The profession of speech-language pathology makes great interpersonal demands. The students, parents, other professionals, and paraprofessionals must be considered as individuals and collectively. Although these abilities are not easily taught, they may be acquired or improved over time with a combination of observation of others and self-awareness. Chapter 10's treatment of supervision includes a section on mentoring, which is a means of refining interpersonal skills, among other professional attributes, within the context of a nurturing relationship.

Employment in a setting that offers the new professional a mentor is highly desirable. Kahmi (1995) noted that clinical excellence seems to involve a process of continual growth and change.

CONCLUSION

In sum, the school speech-language pathologist is, ideally, a highly qualified, flexible, and enthusiastic professional, committed to continuing growth and equipped with excellent oral and written communication skills and strong abilities in the area of interpersonal relationships.

AUDIOLOGY SERVICES IN THE EDUCATIONAL SETTING

Nancy P. Huffman

Prior to 1975, children with disabilities were not routinely visible in public school classrooms. In many instances, the identified "disability" created the educational program, placement, technique, and personnel. There was minimal attention given to continuum of service. Local school districts had little involvement with or ownership of the identification and placement of students with disabilities. Children went to schools for "the blind," "the deaf," "the physically handicapped," or "the retarded." They were taught solely by teachers of the deaf, teachers of the blind, or teachers of the mentally retarded. Large school districts may have had buildings dedicated to "exceptional children" or special programs for "the trainable" or "the educable retarded." Preschool programs for children with disabilities, if they existed at all, were privately funded and certainly not accessible through publicly supported systems.

Where were the children with hearing loss going to school? Children regarded as "deaf" may have attended a school for the deaf. In fact, for many children with hearing loss, a school for the deaf was the only option so it is probable too that the definition of *deaf* was broad. Many students who today might not be regarded as "deaf" received their education in schools for "the deaf." Children with milder hearing problems went to public schools, but they may not even have been identified as having a "hearing problem." The "hearing problem" was invisible. They may have been treated as they were perceived by the current teacher—strange? unable to speak clearly? retarded? a behavior problem?

Prior to 1975, the audiology profession was growing and changing as well. For many years, audiologists were only the prescribers of hearing aids. They tested hearing, determined hearing aid candidacy, and made recommendations for the type of hearing aid, which was then fit and managed by someone else. The idea of an audiologist's dispensing hearing aids was "unthinkable" in terms of professional ethics. With regard to children, hearing aid use and technology was in its infancy compared to the amplification and sensory options available today for virtually every kind of hearing loss. Body-type hearing aids were the norm, over-the-ear hearing aids were improving, and in-the-ear hearing aids were being developed. In fact it was not uncommon for "experts" to suggest waiting before considering the fitting of amplification to see if the child was "ready."

DOORS OPENED: ENABLING LEGISLATION AND REGULATION

The Education for All Handicapped Children Act of 1975, which later became the Individuals with Disabilities Education Act of 1990 (IDEA), had significant impact on the audiology profession and the services that were and are now provided in schools. The legislation gave birth to the expansion of audiology services in schools, defined the practice of "educational audiology," and placed school audiology services in the public sector.

Prior to the opportunity created by the act, children with hearing loss and hearing disorders in schools had access to audiology services primarily through clinics, community agencies, university facilities, physicians, and some private practices. Unfortunately, the providers were "off site" and had little familiarity with the educational setting issues. Ex-

cept for schools for the deaf and some forward thinking school systems, audiology services in public school agencies were rare.

The Education of the Handicapped Amendments of 1986 created new opportunity for infants, toddlers (Part H) and preschoolers (Part B) with disabilities to access service and education. The legislation created additional responsibilities and involvement for audiologists, speech-language pathologists, and other related service providers in all kinds of educational and early intervention programs for children ages birth through 5 and their families.

In 1990, the Education for All Handicapped Children Act and its 1986 amendments were again reauthorized and amended as the Individuals with Disabilities Education Act (IDEA). In sum, the legislation created accessibility to education for disabled children at no cost to their parents—a presumed and operational given for nondisabled children. We now have in place regulations, policies, procedures, programs, facilities, and a myriad of professional services related to early intervention and special education to fulfill the goal of access to public education. IDEA was reauthorized in 1996. It faced a number of challenges related to funding, regulatory issues, outcome data, professional personnel, and service delivery.

The IDEA regulations define *audiology* as a related service.

Audiology includes:

(i) Identification of children with impairments using at risk criteria and appropriate screening techniques;

(ii) Determination of the range, nature, and degree of hearing loss and communication functions, by use of audiologic evaluation procedures;

(iii) Referral for medical and other services necessary for the habilitation or rehabilitation of children with auditory impairment;

(iv) Provision of auditory training, aural rehabilitation, speech reading and listening device orientation and training, and other services;

(v) Provision of services for prevention of hearing loss; and

(vi) Determination of the child's need for individual amplification, including selecting, fitting, and dispensing of appropriate listening and vibrotactile devices, and evaluating the effectiveness of those devices. (34 CFR 303.12 [d])

IDEA's regulations also provide definitions for the disability categories of "deaf" and "hard of hearing" as follows:

"Deaf" means a hearing impairment which is so severe that the child is impaired in processing linguistic information through hearing, with or without amplification, which adversely affects educational performance. (34 CFR 300.5)

"Hard of Hearing" means a hearing impairment, whether permanent or fluctuating, which adversely affects a child's educational performance but which is not included under the definition of deaf in this section. (34 CFR 300.5)

The significant role of the audiologist is implicit in these definitions in terms of the need to determine the presence of hearing loss, whether it is permanent or fluctuating, the effect of hearing loss on the processing of spoken language, the effectiveness of amplification, and the need for specialized equipment to access the learning environment. Further, regulations state that "each public agency shall insure that hearing aids worn by deaf and hard of hearing children in school are functioning properly" (34 CFR 300.303), which again acknowledges and reinforces the role of the audiologist.

TURNING REGULATION INTO REALITY

Although federal regulations establish parameters, as in defining *audiology services*, states have the responsibility to develop their own regulations to comply with federal mandates. Many states do not have requirements for credentials to be held by audiologists who practice in schools, nor do they define roles. Only a few states have guidelines for audiology services in the schools. Many have licensure requirements for audiologists, but often public schools are exempt from those requirements. Audiology services, then, are sometimes defined and delivered by individuals who are not audiologists. DeConde Johnson (1991) in a survey conducted for the Educational Audiology Association, found that licensure and/or ASHA certification (CCC-A) were required in all but 14 states for individuals who provided audiology services in schools. Of those 14 states, 12 had no requirements, or schools were exempt from their licensure requirements; 2 specified ASHA certification (CCC-A). Only 13 states reported that they had written guidelines for school audiology services. Four years later, English (1995) reported that still "most states do not have established guidelines for providing audiology services in schools" (p. 216). Further, she stated that "many school professionals do not have basic information regarding the impact of hearing impairment on learning, nor are they aware of the contributions and expertise of the educational audiologist" (p. 216).

PROFESSIONAL QUALIFICATIONS AND COMPETENCIES FOR AUDIOLOGISTS WHO WORK IN SCHOOLS

Most states require audiologists who work in schools to hold the Certificate of Clinical

Competence in Audiology (CCC-A) from ASHA and/or to be licensed as an audiologist in the state in which they are practicing. Licensure requirements differ from state to state, and some states have separate credentialing/certification requirements for audiologists who work in schools (DeConde Johnson, 1991). The Educational Audiology Association (1994) in June 1994 approved a statement entitled "Minimum Competencies for Educational Audiologists" (Exhibit 4–1).

AUDIOLOGY RESOURCES

There are now a wide variety of professional and grassroots organizations for the deaf and hearing impaired, their families, and the professionals who work with them. A list of these organizations is provided in Appendix 4–A. ASHA has published numerous position papers, guidelines, policy statements, and reports for the professional audiologist; these are listed in Appendix 4–B.

WHAT ARE THE HEARING NEEDS OF STUDENTS IN EDUCATIONAL SETTINGS?

Although IDEA focuses on students with disabilities, it is important to understand that audiology services in schools are not focused solely on students with hearing loss and/or other disabilities. Audiology services touch and benefit all students in a variety of ways.

Identification and Screening

Prior to entering school (formal education), most, if not all, children experience some kind of screening that may place them on a high-risk register for hearing loss, or rule out hearing loss, or identify them as having a hearing loss. A child may have been identified at birth or as an infant as being at risk for hearing loss and involved in periodic audiologic evaluation and monitoring. As a toddler or preschooler, a child may have been involved in a number of health-related screening programs that typically include hearing screening.

Screening and early identification are so important because it is now widely understood and accepted that hearing is a critical factor for the development of speech and language, communication skills, and learning. The presence of hearing loss of any kind, including minimal or fluctuating loss, is a form of sensory deprivation. It is also widely recognized that the most common etiology of hearing loss in young children is otitis media causing a conductive type of loss that is usually fluctuant. Otitis media most frequently occurs during the first 3 years of life (Klein, 1986) yet can continue through ages 8 to 10 (Davis, Shepard, Stelmachowicz, & Gorga, 1981). It is critical that any hearing loss be identified early and appropriately managed.

Many, if not all states, require schools to carry out hearing screening on a periodic basis as students begin, move through, and complete their formal education. All states do not, however, follow the same guidelines. Speech-language pathologists and audiologists working in schools should familiarize themselves with their state's requirements for hearing screening.

Typically, it is required that all children be screened for hearing loss either prior to or upon entry into formal education at age 5 and at regularly defined intervals thereafter. The screening is more frequent in the elementary grades, followed by a screen occurring at least once during high school. In New York State, for example, hearing screening must be administered at least annually to students in Grades K through 7 and Grade 10 and to all new entrants into the school district (NYS Ed, 1992). In California, hearing screening occurs in kindergarten, Grades 2, 5, 8 and 10

Exhibit 4–1 Minimum Competencies for Educational Audiologists

---

I. The educational audiologist should demonstrate competency for providing services to individuals birth through 21 years of age and their families in the following areas:

A. Identification audiometry, including pure tone audiometric screening, immittance measures, and newborn screening criteria.

B. Threshold audiometric evaluation for pure tone air and bone conduction, speech reception and word recognition testing, immittance measurements, otoscopy, special tests including interpretation of electrophysiological measures, differential diagnosis of auditory disorders, and diagnosis of central auditory processing disorders.

C. Medical and educational referral and follow-up procedures and criteria.

D. Audiological assessment of individuals using procedures appropriate to their receptive and expressive language skills, cognitive abilities, and behavioral functioning.

E. Evaluation of the need for and selection of hearing aids, FM systems, cochlear implants, vibrotactile devices, and other hearing assistance technology. This includes making earmold impressions and modifications.

F. The structure of the learning environment, including classroom acoustics and implications for learning.

G. General child development and management.

H. Written and verbal interpretation of auditory assessment results and implications appropriate for the intended audience, such as parents, teachers, physicians, and other professionals.

I. IFSP/IEP planning process and procedures:

1. Interpretation of auditory assessment results and their implications on psychosocial, communicative, cognitive, physical, academic, and vocational development.

2. Educational options for individuals who are deaf or hard of hearing including appropriate intensity of services and vocational and work–study programming as part of a multidisciplinary team process.

3. Legal issues and procedures, especially the legal rights of and due process for students, parents, teachers, administrators, and school boards, including the implications of the Americans with Disabilities Act, the Individuals with Disabilities Education Act, and Section 504 of the Vocational Rehabilitation Act of 1974.

J. Consultation and collaboration with classroom teachers and other professionals regarding the relationship of hearing and hearing loss to the development of academic and psychosocial skills:

1. Ensure support for enhancing the development of auditory functioning and communication skills.

2. Recommend appropriate modifications of instructional curricula and academic methods, materials, and facilities.

K. Participation in team management of communication treatment for individuals who are deaf or hard of hearing or who have difficulties processing speech/language through the auditory system. These procedures should integrate the following:

1. Orientation to, and the use and maintenance of, appropriate amplification instrumentation and other hearing assistance technologies.

2. Auditory skills development.

3. Speech skills development including phonology, voice, and rhythm.

4. Visual communication including speechreading and manual communication.

5. Language development (expressive and receptive oral, signed, and/or written language).

6. Selection and use of appropriate instructional materials and media.

7. Structure of learning environments including acoustic modifications.

continues

Exhibit 4–1 continued

> 8. Case management/care coordination with family, school, medical, and community services.
> 9. Facilitation of transitions between levels, schools, programs, agencies, etc.
> L. Knowledge of communication systems and language used by individuals who are deaf and hard of hearing.
> M. Counseling for the family and individual who is deaf or hard of hearing, including emotional support, information about hearing loss and its implications, and interaction strategies to maximize communication and psychosocial development.
> N. Selection and maintenance of audiological equipment.
> O. Maintenance of records including screening, referral, follow-up, assessment, IFSP/IEP planning, and services.
> P. Implementation of a hearing conservation program.
> Q. Awareness of cerumen management concerns and techniques.
> R. Implementation of inservice training for staff and support personnel.
> S. Train and supervise paraprofessionals.
> T. Sensitivity to family systems, diversity, and cultures, including Deaf culture.
> U. Knowledge of school systems, multidisciplinary teams, and community and professional resources.
> V. Effective interpersonal and communication skills.
> II. The educational audiologist should have an internship/practicum in a school setting under the supervision of an educational audiologist. A preferred internship would be a full-time experience lasting approximately six weeks.
>
> *Source:* Reprinted with permission from Minimum competencies for educational audiologists, *Educational Audiology Association Newsletter*, Vol. 11, No. 4, p.7, © 1994, Educational Audiology Association.

or 11. (California State Department of Education, 1986).

It is not commonly required by states that all children be screened for middle-ear disorders, although some states, such as New York, suggest it can be done on an optional basis or "if available." Immittance measures identify individuals with potentially medically significant ear disorders who may or may not have accompanying hearing loss.

It should be noted that screening programs may or may not specify who performs the hearing screening. In fact, in most cases, screening procedures themselves are performed by nonaudiologist personnel, such as nurses, speech-language pathologists, or technicians. Best practice would warrant that any program conducting screening for hearing loss or middle-ear dysfunction be supervised and managed by a licensed and certified audiologist. All identification/screening programs require systematic procedures for protocol, interpretation, referral, follow-up, and management. ASHA has published guidelines for identification audiometry (ASHA, 1985) and guidelines for screening for hearing impairment and middle-ear disorders (ASHA, 1990) that are a valuable reference for speech-language pathologists in school practice.

Assessment

Audiologists in educational practice are involved in assessment and evaluation of students for a number of reasons.

Assessment as a Result of Failing a Hearing Screen

Hearing screening programs operate according to pass–fail criteria. They simply separate individuals into two groups; those who passed (and are therefore presumed to have no hearing loss) and those who failed (and are presumed to have hearing loss).

Children who fail hearing screening must have audiological assessment performed by a licensed and certified audiologist to determine the degree, nature, and extent of the suspected hearing loss. The evaluation results may also document that no hearing loss exists and the screen failure was a false positive.

The evaluation will yield data that allow the audiologist to describe the degree, nature, and extent of the hearing loss. With regard to *degree of hearing loss*, the audiologist is looking for quantitative information. Hearing levels are expressed in decibels based on pure tone average for the frequencies 500 to 4000 Hz and discussed using descriptors related to severity: normal hearing (–10 to +15 dB HL), borderline hearing loss (16–25 dB HL), mild hearing loss (26–40 dB HL), moderate hearing loss (41–55 dB HL), moderate to severe hearing loss (56–70 dB HL), severe hearing loss (71–90 dB HL), and profound hearing loss (91 dB HL or greater).

With regard to the *nature of hearing loss*, the audiologist is looking for the type of hearing impairment and information suggesting the site of lesion. The loss may be conductive (a temporary or permanent hearing loss typically due to abnormal conditions of the outer and/or middle ear), sensorineural (typically a permanent hearing loss due to disease, trauma, or inherited conditions affecting the sensory and/or nerve cells in the cochlea or inner ear or conditions affecting the eighth cranial nerve), mixed (a combination of conductive and sensorineural components), or

due to a central auditory processing disorder (a condition that is found in the presence of normal hearing but may occur in combination with conductive, sensorineural, and mixed hearing loss such that there is difficulty processing audible signals).

With regard to *extent of hearing loss*, the audiologist is looking at qualitative attributes such as bilateral versus unilateral hearing loss; symmetrical versus asymmetrical hearing loss; high-frequency versus low frequency hearing loss; and flat versus sloping versus precipitous hearing loss.

Assessment for the Purpose of Monitoring a Condition

Once a particular hearing loss has been identified, a treatment and management plan is put into place. The plan may include medical intervention, prescription of personal hearing aids, prescription/provision of assistive listening devices, habilitative skills development, or simply monitoring of the condition through periodic assessment. It is important, however, for a student's hearing loss to be checked periodically to determine its stability: Is it fluctuating? Has it improved as a result of medical intervention? Is it progressing? Have new conditions come into play that have affected the original condition? It is also important that a student's ability to hear using amplification (i.e., personal hearing aids and any assistive listening devices that are used in place of, or in conjunction with, personal amplification) be monitored and documented. This monitoring would include functional gain assessment, real ear measurement, electroacoustic analysis, listening check, and informal "functional" assessment in the listening environment in which the student operates (i.e., the classroom, the work–study placement, the home).

Assessment because of Suspected Hearing Loss

Although students may have successfully passed periodic school hearing screenings, they may have experienced a change in hearing as a result of an event or a particular condition that causes concern for a change or loss in hearing.

Assessment to Determine Eligibility for Various Programs

As students move through their school careers, they are often required to have reports of hearing testing before they can participate in some contact sports (some state laws and regulations may require this as a part of a health examination), as part of application for certain vocational and postsecondary programs, as part of applications to qualify for SSI, or to demonstrate eligibility for 504 and IDEA programs.

Assessment as Part of a Multidisciplinary Team Evaluation

Audiologists are a frequent resource for school placement teams as part of the evaluation process for students who are suspected of having a disability. Sometimes the purpose of the audiological assessment is to confirm the presence of normal hearing. Sometimes the purpose is to conduct tests of central auditory processing and to work with teams of professionals in analyzing listening and auditory processing behaviors of a particular student and the impact on learning. Sometimes as part of early intervention (birth to age 5) and early childhood (ages 3–5) assessment teams, the purpose is to determine eligibility for service and a description of services needed.

Prevention

The educational setting is the ideal and natural forum to introduce values and practices relative to hearing hygiene and prevention of hearing loss. It is interesting to note that although schools typically have health education curricula and provide health education, health educators, when surveyed (Lass et al., 1990), were shown to have deficiencies in knowledge of hearing, hearing loss, hearing health practices, and, in particular, the effect of noise on hearing. There is no question that information about methods of prevention, as well as causes and effects, of hearing loss need to be provided not only to students but also to teachers and administrators.

Hearing hygiene and hearing preservation require education not only on diseases and medical conditions that place one at risk for hearing loss but also on the effects of drugs and over-the-counter medications on hearing. Approximately 200 drugs have been identified as being ototoxic; that is, having the potential to cause toxic reactions to structures of the inner ear, including the cochlea, vestibule, semicircular canals, and otoliths (ASHA, 1994; Miller, 1985). Audiologists are prepared to develop curricula or assist in the development of curricula pertaining to hearing, hearing health, and hearing hygiene as part of school health education programs.

There is ongoing concern about the high prevalence of high-frequency sensorineural hearing loss in school-age students, particularly older students (Anderson, 1967; Woodford, 1973, 1980, 1981; Woodford & O'Farrell, 1983). Researchers have concluded that exposure to excessive noise levels occurring in the educational setting and during recreational activities such as listening to music, riding snowmobiles and motorcycles, and using power tools appears to be the primary etiology of high frequency hearing loss in older school-age students (Clark, 1991; Katz,

Gertsman, Sanderson & Buchanan, 1982; Woodford & O'Farrell, 1983). The educational setting as an environment for hazardous noise exposure might come as a surprise to many, yet the demonstration of noxious noise levels in vocational and industrial arts classes led the state of Iowa to adopt a law requiring that hearing protection be worn in all educational classes in which noise levels exceed Occupational Safety and Health Administration (OSHA) guidelines for excessive noise (Plakke, 1985, 1991). Audiologists in the educational setting are equipped to determine noise levels, recommend and provide ear protection for both students and staff, and carry out education programs with regard to noise.

Treatment and Management

The Audiologist as a Team Member and Team Player

The educational audiologist, traditionally linked with providing services to students with hearing loss, is an increasingly visible member of school district teams involved in educational programs and placement planning for all students, disabled and nondisabled. The use of the plural *teams* is deliberate because often there are a number of teams on which an audiologist might participate. They may have differing composition, and they may operate in sequence, at different points in time, or simultaneously. The audiologist's and speech-language pathologist's need to participate productively on school teams cannot be overstated.

Let us look at this complex and dynamic team process. In a school setting, when a child's needs become apparent or a concern emerges, there is usually a resource team within the building to address concerns, solve problems, and identify areas in which testing

is necessary. The building resource team typically includes the school psychologist, the speech-language pathologist, a teacher, a school nurse, a social worker, a reading/curriculum specialist, and a school administrator. They are responsible for a student's initial testing and for referral, perhaps to an intermediate unit or an evaluation center familiar with educational contexts, for testing to be done in specific areas addressing the suspected disability, such as audiology, occupational therapy, or others. In addition to a building resource team, there is also the school district's placement team. In some states, such as New York, this is called the "Committee on Special Education," consisting of mandated members and others selected by the district, who work with the family and the building resource team in developing a child's IEP, determining related services, and making placement decisions. Finally, regardless of whether the student is disabled or nondisabled, there is the team of educators, related services providers, and school administrators who, with the support of the parents, work together to implement the student's education program wherever it is located.

It is critical that a team work together under administrative leadership to create goals and objectives for a particular student or to implement the goals and objectives that have been created by someone else. This is a dynamic process because when team members come to the table, they bring their various perspectives (Hearing Instruments, 1994). Each team member may have identified different goals and objectives. Perhaps members agree on the goals and objectives, but each member may rank them differently in terms of priority. Team members may each have differing perceptions of time frames in which goals can be achieved. They may have differing perceptions as to who is responsible for a particular goal or objective. And, they may have different ideas for methods and techniques to use to achieve the goal or objective. The team members around the table are at the same time experts (in their particular field) and novices (in the fields of the other team members). Further, they may not know each other. And finally, they must work together!

In looking at the needs of students with hearing and listening problems, the audiologist's priority may not be the same as that of the teacher of the deaf, which may be different still from the priority of the speech-language pathologist, which may not satisfy the goal of the parents. Each sees him- or herself as a key stakeholder. Goals and objectives for a particular student must be a common focus, and the roles of the audiologist, speech-language pathologist, teacher of the deaf and hearing impaired, interpreter, note taker, classroom teacher, parent, and any others involved in program implementation must be clearly defined and understood by all.

Team members must recognize and acquire the necessary skills that allow them to work as a team to identify, work toward, or achieve the student's outcome. These skills include collaboration, consensus building or whole-group support, collaborative problem solving, conflict resolution, capitalizing on divergent thinking, collecting and analyzing data, nonjudgmental information sharing, and finally, understanding what is and what is not under the control of the team or an individual member of the team (Katzenbach & Smith, 1994; Kayser, 1994). It is critical that the educational audiologist be seen not only as a team member but also as a team player in this process.

The Role of the Audiologist in Educational Management and Treatment Plans for Students with Hearing Loss. As they participate on teams developing and carrying out treatment and management plans for students with hearing loss, audiologists and speech-language pathologists know that hearing loss negatively affects the development of receptive and expressive language skills, which in turn causes learning problems, which then jeopardizes and often lowers academic achievement. In fact, the relationship between hearing loss and poor academic performance has been documented over the years (Bess, 1985; Brackett & Maxon, 1986; Davis, 1977). Further, Bess (1985) has shown that even a mild hearing loss or a unilateral hearing loss can result in academic failure. The student's communication difficulties frequently lead to social isolation and poor self-esteem. Often the student's vocational choice and vocational success are affected.

As a first step, the audiologist may have a lead role in determining candidacy for and prescribing personal amplification (i.e., hearing aids). When possible, the audiologist prescribes hearing aids that can easily connect to assistive listening device fittings, using audio input and telecoil options. The hearing aid/assistive device combination should also allow for various listening options, such as (a) listening only through the hearing aid microphone, (b) listening only to the signal coming in via audio input or through the telecoil (e.g., the teacher's voice being transmitted), and (c) listening to the signals coming from both the hearing aid microphone and the signal from the telecoil or audio input together. As a team member, the audiologist is also prepared to design and carry out programs to assist students in developing listening skills, managing their hearing aids, and managing various listening situations and environments. The audiologist, in partnership with parents, speech-language pathologists, and others working with the student, is prepared to assist those partners in recognizing when amplification may not be working, to perform listening checks, and to do basic trouble-shooting. This is consistent with the federal regulation cited earlier that requires school districts to ensure that hearing aids worn by hearing-impaired and deaf students are working properly.

The audiologist is also a key player in determining candidacy for sensory aids such as vibrotactile devices or cochlear implants.

> A cochlear implant is an electronic prosthetic device that is surgically placed in the inner ear and under the skin behind the ear for the purpose of providing useful sound perception via electrical stimulation of the auditory nerve. Cochlear implants are intended to provide prelingually or postlingually deafened children, who obtain limited functional benefit from conventional amplification, improved sound and speech detection and improved auditory perception of speech. (American Academy of Audiology, 1995, p. 14).

Cochlear implantation program teams depend upon the on-site school audiologist as the connection between the implant center and the school team implementing training to maximize benefit that is expected from the device. Implant programs want school personnel to have a thorough understanding of how the device functions and how to maintain it. They also want school site staff to work to have the child acquire new listening skills within meaningful communicative contexts.

For students who are deaf, it is necessary for the team to have particular sensitivity to issues pertaining to educational placement, amplification, communication methods, the cultural aspects of deafness, and the deaf community. The *deaf community* has been defined as "the community of people whose primary mode of communication is signed language and who share a common identity, a common culture and a common way of interacting with each other and the hearing community" (National Association of State Directors of Special Education [NASDE], 1994, p. 78). It is again crucial that the team work together to identify needs and resources consistent with the family's expectation of outcome. Team members such as the audiologist, the teacher of the deaf and hearing impaired, and the speech-language pathologist are valuable resources for further understanding of philosophies of education of the deaf, communication modes (American Sign Language [ASL], Cued Speech, Signed English, Signing Exact English, fingerspelling, the Rochester Method, Total Communication), and, depending on the placement and communication system used, the need for educational interpreters/transliterators, note takers, and other supports required to achieve outcomes identified for the student. These specialists have unique preparation, certification, and roles. Teachers of the deaf and hard of hearing have preparation in general education and additional special education preparation and expertise in the learning needs of children who are deaf. They should be able to communicate proficiently in the primary language and preferred mode of communication of their students. They are skilled in using technology that is known to enhance instruction for students who have hearing loss, they can modify curriculum and apply instructional techniques for clearer presentation and ease of comprehension of information in specific content areas, they carry out appropriate test modification, and they are frequently the coordinators of educational programs for students in mainstreamed settings. The note taker is trained to take notes for a student who has hearing loss (and, more recently, students with other disabilities) and is unable to receive instruction and take notes simultaneously. (If a student with hearing loss is trying to listen, follow a visual media presentation, read lips, or attend to an interpreter, taking notes becomes virtually impossible!) The note taker attends classes with the student, takes notes, and provides copies of the notes to the student, the classroom teacher, and the teacher of the deaf who may be providing support. Educational interpreters/transliterators facilitate communication exchange between students and others, including teachers, service providers, and peers within the educational environment (NASDE, 1994, p. 66). They interpret for the student the spoken communication of the teacher, using the student's preferred communication mode. For the teacher and others who are not fluent in the student's preferred communication mode, they interpret into spoken English the student's communication. Educational interpreters are trained and must meet competencies. The Registry of Interpreters for the Deaf, the Council of Education of the Deaf, and the National Cued Speech Association have standards and ethics codes that all interpreters must meet.

The Role of the Audiologist in Educational Management and Treatment Plans for Students Whose Primary Disability is Not Hearing Loss. Audiologists are involved in teams developing treatment and management plans for students whose primary disability is not hearing loss. Students with learning disabilities, for example, may have central auditory processing disorders that cause them to have difficulty paying attention (particularly in the presence of background noise), following spoken directions, remembering heard information, and performing fine sound analyses

and discrimination. In an attempt to overcome listening problems associated with background noise and poor attending, audiologists are prepared to explore amplification systems that improve signal-to-noise ratio, such as sound field classroom amplification systems, or to prescribe individually fitted assistive listening systems. Audiologists can also assist teachers and staff in modifying their presentation and instructional style so the student can more easily process spoken information. Audiologists can assist in making environmental modifications to improve the listening situation. They can also provide instruction to the student in managing his or her listening habits and skills. Students with attention-deficit disorder (ADD) or attention-deficit disorder with hyperactivity (ADHD) can often benefit from the same intervention and management. It must be reinforced that any amplification device used with children with normal hearing should be prescribed and managed by an audiologist.

Students with mental retardation and other developmental disabilities have a higher incidence of hearing loss than the general pediatric population (ASHA, 1983; Fulton & Lloyd, 1969). There is a particularly high incidence of conductive hearing loss (occurring, for example, as a result of craniofacial anomalies and other medical conditions), which requires management and monitoring. The audiologist is prepared to explore a number of strategies in addition to personal amplification and/or assistive listening systems to make the listening environment more accessible to students with mental retardation and developmental disabilities.

Audiologists are involved on teams designing services for students with vision impairments. Hearing loss and impairments of vision and blindness frequently have a common etiology—as, for example, in the cases of Usher's syndrome and maternal rubella. It is important that a student with vision disabilities have audiologic evaluation that includes a detailed case history. Monitoring and documentation of vision and hearing status on a periodic basis are necessary. Students with dual-sensory disabilities of vision and hearing (deaf–blindness or visual impairment–hearing impairment) require joint, collaborative management between the audiologist, the vision specialist, and the speech-language pathologist, particularly in the prescription and management of assistive technology for learning and for environmental control.

In the early 1990s, students with autism became the focus of a novel listening treatment program called *auditory integration training* (AIT), and audiologists became a visible member of the team of professionals providing services to these students. AIT was developed in the 1960s in France by a physician, Guy Berard. He used the program with individuals having a number of disabling conditions, such as dyslexia, depression, learning problems, and autism (Veale, 1994a, b). AIT became associated with autism in the United States when Annabel Stehli (1991) wrote a book entitled *The Sound of a Miracle*, in which she described her daughter's recovery from autism following auditory integration training.

AIT is administered by trained practitioners, not necessarily audiologists, using specific instrumentation. The technique is controversial (Friel-Patti, 1994; Gravel, 1994; Madell, 1994; Rimland & Edelson, 1994a, b). Those who see it as successful report that individuals with autism have improved language development and reduced irritability, echolalic speech, and distractibility (Madell, 1994; Monville & Nelson, 1994). Research and clinical data collection are ongoing.

Meanwhile, however, the American Academy of Audiology (1993) and some state licensing boards in speech-language pathology and audiology caution that the technique is experimental and that potential candidates and their parents or caregivers should be so informed. Audiologists in educational settings would be prepared to advise about and perhaps, if trained themselves, to administer the technique.

WHEN A STUDENT IN SCHOOL HAS HEARING LOSS, WHAT NEEDS TO BE DONE TO PROMOTE LEARNING ACCESS AND LEARNING SUCCESS?

Consider the Hearing Loss

Although the statement may be simplistic (and may risk being too simplistic), the primary difficulty of students with hearing loss is that they cannot hear in their instructional settings! They are unable to access spoken and other acoustic information to benefit from instruction because they cannot hear it. Let us now look at some examples of hearing loss and the problems they pose in "hearing" and ability to benefit from instruction. Recall that earlier in this chapter, hearing loss was discussed with regard to its degree, nature, and extent. The examples here are discussed in terms of these attributes.

Degree of Hearing Loss

Mild Hearing Loss. A student whose average hearing, between 500 and 2,000 HZ on the audiogram, lies in the mild loss range (26–40 dB hearing level) will probably not hear 25% to 40% of speech signals under ideal conditions (Anderson & Matkin, 1991). Successful "hearing" is dependent upon the level of noise present, the distance from the speaker, and the specific configuration (across all frequencies) of the hearing loss. In instructional settings, the student may miss up to 50% of class discussions because (a) distances vary between the classmates and teachers who are speaking to the student who is trying to hear, (b) communication exchanges and contributions occur and shift rapidly, (c) speakers have different volumes and rates of speaking, and (d) background noise is usually present. Because hearing ability is inconsistent based on specific conditions of communication experience, a mild hearing loss may go undetected. Instead, the student is seen as not paying attention, having selective hearing, or daydreaming.

Moderate Hearing Loss. A student whose average hearing (between 500 and 2,000 Hz) lies between 41 and 55 dB HL may understand conversation (a) within a distance of 3 to 5 feet, (b) when it is face to face, and (c) when it occurs with carefully controlled speaking and vocabulary (Anderson & Matkin, 1991). Those around the child would most likely suspect hearing loss because inability to "hear" would demonstrate itself in most situations. The child would be expected to have speech-language problems involving articulation, sentence structure, use of syntax, limited vocabulary both receptively and expressively, and self-monitoring of voice loudness and quality.

Nature or Type of Hearing Loss

Fluctuating Hearing Loss. Fluctuating hearing loss commonly occurs in young children secondary to otitis media with effusion, which is the accumulation of fluid into the middle ear. If hearing is typically within normal range without fluid, the presence of fluid may create a conductive hearing loss of mild or moderate degree. When the fluid dissipates, hearing returns to previously normal

levels. Hearing loss that fluctuates causes the student to have inconsistent ability to "hear." The student on some days may perform consistently in terms of response to instructional expectations. Yet at other times, the student will simply not hear or will respond inappropriately in comparison to previously demonstrated behaviors and responses in similar situations.

Unilateral hearing loss. Unilateral hearing loss is a situation in which hearing levels in one ear are within normal range, while in the other ear there is a hearing loss of mild or greater severity. Individuals with unilateral hearing loss cannot "hear" conversation or sounds originating on the "bad" side. They have the greatest difficulty locating and localizing sound source and direction. They have difficulty in noisy situations, particularly when the noise source is on the "good" side. Because one ear is normal, this type of loss may go undetected for quite some time or, if detected, may be regarded as insignificant. The child might be viewed as having selective hearing or poor attention or as hearing only what he or she wants to hear.

Extent of Hearing Loss

High-Frequency Hearing Loss. High-frequency hearing loss refers to a situation in which hearing levels in the low to middle frequencies (250–1,000 Hz) lie within normal limits but then hearing drops off to mild and greater loss levels in the higher frequencies (1,500–8,000 Hz). There are variations on the theme, but the essence is that lower pitches (frequencies) are easily heard, and high pitches (frequencies) are not heard. This causes distortion in hearing because the student hears the vowel and some voiced consonant portions of what is said but does not hear the unvoiced consonants in the spoken message. The unvoiced consonants are markers of verb tense, possession, gender, plurality, and so on, and, if not heard, serve to confuse or misconstrue the intended message. For example, "What *time* is it?" might be heard as "What *kind* is it?" or "I passed the test" might be heard as "I packed the rest." Words like *paint, painting,* and *painted* might all sound like *aint.* The end result is miscommunication, a response that to the listener, is way "off base." Depending on the degree and configuration of the high-frequency loss, the student will demonstrate articulation errors, poor receptive and expressive language development and skills, and inappropriate responses in instructional and social contexts.

These are but a few arbitrary examples of various kinds and types of hearing loss that are managed in educational settings. As stated earlier, there are variations on the theme. Of course, the attributes of degree, nature, and extent or configuration of hearing loss, though separated here for purpose of example, become extricably intertwined as we study a particular student's individual situation. In addition to these attributes, other important features of the hearing loss, such as age of onset, age of discovery, etiology, and age at which intervention was introduced, all influence decision making regarding instruction and access to instruction. Mark Ross, an audiologist who himself has a severe to profound hearing loss, suggested that the problem with having a hearing loss is that (a) you hear what you thought you heard, (b) you don't know what you didn't hear, and (c) you don't know what you misheard because you didn't hear it correctly in the first place (Ross, Brackett, & Maxon, 1991). Any student with hearing loss requires a carefully designed and monitored management program based on the attributes of the hearing loss unique to that individual student and on the demands of the instructional program.

Consider the Setting and Context of Instruction

Access to spoken and other acoustic information that enhances instruction is influenced by the setting and context of instruction—that is, where it occurs. Instruction today occurs in a multitude of places. For most, the traditional school classroom immediately comes to mind—the kind that houses 20 to 25 desks and chairs, a few small tables, and a teacher's desk. Those classrooms exist in buildings that could be as old as 70 years or brand new. The buildings exist in urban, suburban, and rural areas. They are subject to air, ground, and underground traffic noise and other external factors that are completely out of our control. Unfortunately, even the most recently constructed buildings have not been designed with acoustics necessary for learning in mind. Classrooms vary in function and therefore may be large, with specialized equipment and workstations, as in the case of a shop, a kitchen, or a gymnasium. Or they may be rather small, as in the case of a room in which small-group instruction or therapy occurs.

Instruction today also occurs in naturalistic and/or functional settings. These include the student's home, day care centers, nursery schools, work–study placements, and field placements. Some unique, forward-thinking special education programs provide full-time instruction in settings such as farms, greenhouses, and carpentry shops, where the setting is the "classroom" and academics are integrated into the functional instructional activity. Instruction occurs in hospitals, jails, and other specialized settings. For some, the "classroom" might be "home," where a student engaged in distance learning receives instruction via computer and telephones. The list is endless, as are the acoustic challenges posed by each setting. The point is that the physical setting and context of instruction today extend far beyond our traditional paradigm and perception of the "classroom" with walls as boundaries. For a student with hearing loss, the setting and context of instruction pose access challenges that must be recognized and addressed in educational planning.

Consider the Instructional Dynamics

Our discussion of instructional dynamics focuses on (a) instructional staff (teachers, related service providers, support staff) and their interaction as an instructional team, (b) instructional models and strategies or the techniques of instruction, and (c) the tools used as part of instruction. The dynamics of instruction vary widely and change constantly as a function of the contexts and settings described above. Hence the emphasis on *dynamics*.

Instructional Staff

Instructional staff may operate in instructional contexts in a variety of ways, a few of which are described here:

- Single teacher with a class of 25 students in a "traditional" classroom.
- Co-teacher, in a situation in which two teachers *together* provide instruction.
- Teacher with classroom aide or aides. Some regulated special education classroom ratios provide for an aide or even an aide for every 4 students in a classroom that has a maximum size of 12. It is therefore possible for a teacher and up to four paraeducators to be providing and carrying out an instructional program.

- Teacher with one or more students in a class who have an assigned one-to-one aide.
- Teacher and related service providers participating in integrated instruction in which therapies and related services such as occupational therapy, physical therapy, and speech-language pathology occur within the context of the classroom for extended periods of time.
- Related or special instructional services delivered by providers outside of the classroom context (as when the student leaves the classroom instructional staff for resource room service, instruction from a teacher of the deaf, speech-language services, occupational therapy, physical therapy, tutoring, or audiology services). The classroom instruction continues while the student is out of the class receiving related or special instructional services. These service providers and the classroom instructional staff are expected to keep in touch with each other to coordinate services that are relevant to the student's educational program.
- Single teacher who instructs students who cannot be seen (as in a distance-learning instructional context, in which the "class" may include many, many students from a wide geographical area).

Models and Strategies of Instruction

Staff who provide instruction use a number of models and strategies. Again, the "traditional" model comes to mind of a teacher instructing from the front of the room, a class of 25 students sitting at desks in rows. Instruction today, however is highly interactive and may include

- cooperative learning strategies, in which small groups of students work with each other under the guidance of a teacher who may be cruising, monitoring, and prompting
- blended classrooms, in which teachers and aides are instructing simultaneously and moving among students to monitor and target and assist
- instruction that combines lecture with periodic small-group interaction and reporting
- instruction that is highly interactive, such as large-group discussion, debate, questioning, and clarifying

In any model or strategy that involves more than one adult, an additional dynamic of adult interaction or "adult talk" becomes a factor. Adult talk means the communication between and among instructional staff to manage and coordinate the instruction as it is occurring. Adult talk may come from a teacher who advises an aide to change technique, a one-to-one aide who is providing feedback to the teacher, or an interpreter who is working with a student who is deaf, or, unfortunately, it may be irrelevant social talk that distracts from instruction.

Instructional Tools

Finally, the tools and technology used in instruction are extensive, expanding in scope, and constantly changing. Instructional tools include computers (with and without speakers), televisions and VCRs, film projectors, overhead projectors, tape recorders, compact disc players, and telephones. We use these tools to enhance an instructor's presentation as it is happening, to "substitute" for the in-person instructor, and to offer optional enrichment programs for self-study.

Contexts, settings, and instructional dynamics present significant access issues for students who have hearing loss or listening disorders (hearing problems occurring in the absence of hearing loss, such as central auditory processing disorders). According to Berg (1987), students spend at least 45% of the school day engaged in listening activities. That is confirmed by teachers, who, when asked to name a crucial skill necessary for classroom success, usually resoundingly reply—listening! Yet we as an educational team of speech-language pathologists, audiologists, teachers of the deaf, and classroom teachers often fail to recognize the importance of structuring and enhancing the listening environment within the instructional setting. Often, in the midst of instruction, we ask the student with limited hearing, "Can you hear me?" And what does the student automatically reply? "Yes." As Flexer, Wray, and Ireland (1989) pointed out, one would not expect the student to state the real answer: "I hear your voice, but I can't hear the unstressed linguistic markers of plurality and tense; nor can I hear articles, voiceless consonants or new vocabulary words clearly enough to distinguish them from other known words" (p. 77). Because instruction today is so dynamic, access considerations must be included in planning for a student with hearing loss.

Questions of management that need to be planned for include the following:

- What is the student's primary communication mode? How does the student receive information? Through hearing? a manual language system? a total communication system? a vibrotactile system? Is communication mediated through an interpreter or a transliterator?

- How will multitalker instruction be handled so the student can "hear" or receive the information from each talker when the talker speaks? How will the student know to whom (which talker) he or she should attend?

- How will "adult talk" (noninstructional talk among adults in the classroom) be managed?

- How will assistive listening devices be used in each of the instructional models in which the student participates? How will interpreters, note takers, and so forth be used within instructional models?

- Can the tools used in instruction be accessed by the student with hearing loss? What will the plan be for each of the tools typically used in the student's particular instructional context?

Facilitating Listening in Instructional Settings

Typically, the effort to facilitate listening focuses first on assistive listening devices. The availability of assistive listening systems as an easy and accessible tool to overcome poor listening/instructional environments has increased the value of educational audiologists because many well-intended school districts, in seeking to provide listening accessibility for their students with hearing loss, made purchases of equipment without the advice of an audiologist. Many found that they had invested in equipment that they came to perceive as nonfunctional, with no one on site who understood its fitting or its operation. Although the number of educational audiologists and/or audiologists practicing in educational settings is growing, it is the exception rather than the rule for a school district to have its own audiologist. The audiologist who is familiar with instructional settings, instructional models, and instructional tools is increasingly seen as a valuable and cost-effective resource to a school district in the prescribing, procuring, fitting, troubleshooting, and managing of assistive listening systems programs in educational settings.

The educational audiologist is the architect and overall manager of a school assistive listening device program. All assistive listening systems attempt to eliminate the listening problems created by poor acoustics: noise, distance, and reverberation. Although there are several kinds of assistive listening systems, frequency modulation (FM) systems are most commonly used. The FM system operates like a miniature radio station. A transmitter/microphone is placed at the sound source (the teacher wears a small microphone). The signal is transmitted to a receiver worn by the student; then it is changed back to an audio signal and routed to the ear through the student's hearing aid or through a receiver (speaker/earphone).

Some still believe that a hearing aid performs the same function as an assistive listening system, but it does not. Students who use only hearing aids are still subject to listening problems created by distance, noise, and reverberation. Assistive listening systems must fulfill the following requirements (Fettinger & Huffman, 1994; Huffman, 1982, 1985):

- The system must allow the student to receive the teacher's voice at a *constant intensity level, regardless of the distance* between the student and the teacher (FM—Yes; HA [Hearing Aid]—No).

- The system must allow the teacher's voice to be *heard more prominently* than background noise (such as papers rustling, chairs scraping, whispering, footsteps, outside noises), *even when the background noise is closer to the student* than the teacher's voice (FM—Yes; HA—No).

- The system must allow the student to *hear his or her own voice* and the voices of other students who are close by in small-group discussion (FM—Yes; HA—Yes).

- The system must be easily wearable and must allow the student and teacher to *move about freely.* (FM—Yes; HA—Yes).

- The system must be adjustable in frequency response and maximum power output to suit the individual student's hearing loss (FM—Yes; HA—Yes).

- The system must be sturdy and convenient to use (FM—Yes; HA—Yes).

The application and use of assistive listening systems in the instructional setting is an art and a science! See Appendix 4–C for instructional applications of FM systems.

Communication Management

Whereas the educational audiologist is the architect and manager of an assistive listening device program, the speech-language pathologist is the architect of the communication management program. More often than not, there is a strong joint partnership between the specialists because one management program cannot happen without the other. In designing programs for students with hearing loss, it is important pragmatically to think in terms of "listening" and "communication" instead of "hearing" and "speaking." By adopting this frame of reference, we broaden our own thinking to tie listening into the receiving of information, and speaking into the sending of information. This creates roles and responsibilities for all members of the team who may be involved in

instruction—the teacher, the aide, related services therapists, speech-language pathologists, teachers of the deaf, interpreters—to craft a learning environment in which the student can successfully receive and send information as part of instruction regardless of the mode he or she uses.

In working to design a communication management program, the speech-language pathologist's goal is for the student to engage successfully in academic conversation and social conversation. If speaking is an element of that "conversation," then intervention must include helping the student to receive speech. This involves working with the audiologist to make sure the student has appropriate hearing aids and assistive listening devices. It also involves learning how to determine if hearing aids and listening devices are working. Speech-language pathologists have indicated that they have little or no experience in inspecting hearing aids (Lass et al., 1989). This is not necessarily surprising because for many this is a low-incidence population. But this documented information is a signal to both speech-language pathologists and audiologists that they together must ensure that the speech-language pathologist, and ideally others on site, will have the demonstrated capability to carry out listening checks and basic troubleshooting of the student's amplification devices. In addition to carrying out listening checks, the "Five-Sound Test," attributed to Daniel Ling and described by Frederick Berg (1987), is a highly functional tool that can be easily employed by the speech-language pathologist in a variety of listening settings. Speech sounds representing energy in low, middle, and high frequencies are used. They are /u/, /a/, /i/, /2/, and /s/. If the student can hear these five sounds, it can be assumed that all 40 speech sounds in the English language can be heard. The test can first be administered in a quiet setting. The speaker should be within 3 feet and behind the student or seated so that the student cannot see the speaker's face. The student is instructed to raise his or her hand when he or she hears the sound. The speaker proceeds to present the sounds in the order presented above. Raising the hand upon hearing the sound is a "detection" response. If the student can repeat the sound, the student is demonstrating "recognition." The task can be altered to provide additional information. For example, speaker distances can be varied, the order of sounds can be changed, and the test can be administered in different types of listening environments. Information provided by this test helps the teacher determine optimum speaking distances in different listening settings. It can also be a way to help the student to begin to learn how to position him- or herself in different settings. If he or she knows that he or she cannot hear when the speaker is beyond 5 feet, then she can begin self-advocacy by requesting optimal seating.

Along with working to have the student receive speech optimally, the speech-language pathologist designs programs to ensure that the student is understanding the speech that has been received (i.e., the focus is on receptive language development, vocabulary skills, and processing of conversation that occurs in the context of instruction). Representative examples of activities addressing understanding of speech might include training the student to recognize his or her name when called upon during play; word and phrase recognition and understanding; training the student in listening for and identifying tense markers (/t/ and /d/) in sentences; preteaching of vocabulary words; vocabulary expansion; use of context clues to anticipate the outcome of a story; awareness of conversational rules (recognizing that someone is talking, waiting one's turn to speak); training

the student to recognize and understand routine, "unique to the teacher" phrases/directions that the teacher uses as part of instruction; recognizing and applying contextual clues; and helping the student to understand his or her hearing loss and what he or she is unable to hear because of it. The speech-language pathologist also designs programs to help the student generate messages that express the intended idea (i.e., with a focus on expressive language): use of correct vocabulary, form, and sentence structure within the pragmatic context. Representative examples of activities focusing on generating messages might include paraphrasing sentences, requesting clarification, providing more than one meaning for common words, generating sentences, object identification, action-agent activities, noun-verb agreement, topic maintenance, and successfully negotiating problem solving with peers. Finally, the speech-language pathologist designs programs to ensure that the student can produce speech that is intelligible to others. Hence the focus on articulation, phonological development, rate, prosody, and temporal aspects of speaking. Representative activities might include teaching sound production, drill and practice activities, transfer of skills into context, identifying feedback mechanisms, developing an oral report, and application of pronunciation rules for letter combinations.

Lasting Partnerships

As educational audiology services continue to grow and become more visible in schools, the speech-language pathologist continues to be the advocate and often the first to be involved in dealing with issues of hearing. It is important for both professionals to recognize and use each other as resources in planning and implementing programs for the hearing needs of all children in school. From the points made in this chapter, some guidelines for speech-language pathologists in school practice emerge:

1. Determine the requirements in your state for audiologists who work in schools.

2. Determine if your state has requirements for the kinds of audiology services to be provided by school districts.

3. Determine your state's hearing screening requirements and who is responsible for screening.

4. If there is any question whatsoever about a student's hearing (even if the student has passed a school screening), advocate for an evaluation to be done by an audiologist.

5. Determine your audiology resources, and develop a strong working partnership with an audiologist.

6. Make sure that any assistive listening system provided to a student is prescribed, fitted, and managed by a licensed audiologist.

7. Make it your priority to be able to perform a listening check on the hearing aids and assistive listening devices that your students use.

8. Work with your audiologist to develop student education programs on hearing, hearing loss, hearing hygiene, the protection of hearing, and the prevention of hearing loss.

9. Develop your teamwork skills so that all on the instructional team will be working toward common outcomes.

10. Broaden your thinking to include the concepts of listening and communication.

CONCLUSION

This discussion of audiology services in educational settings focused on the needs of children with hearing loss and/or listening disorders who spend major portions of their day in instructional experiences and settings. Some children are in these instructional programs for as long as 21 years. They enter the system as infants and age out at the end of their 21st year. In schools, the instructional milieu is highly linguistic, and student success is highly dependent upon a student's ability to hear and process spoken information. Audiologists are key players and a critical resource for ensuring optimum listening environments conducive to learning, ensuring optimum hearing among children who must function in those environments, and ensuring that the professionals who work in these environments understand the listening needs of their students.

STUDY QUESTIONS

1. What are the purposes of audiological assessment and the rationale for each?

2. IDEA defines the disability categories of "deaf" and "hard of hearing." Some think the definitions lack guidelines. How would you expand upon the definitions to add greater clarity? What would be indicators that a child's disability would be deafness? What would be indicators that a child's disability would be classified under "hard of hearing"? What would be indicators that a child's educational performance was being adversely affected by hearing loss?

3. How, in your state, would you find out what the guidelines were for audiology services delivered in schools?

4. As a communication specialist, what strategies would you provide a teacher to use to determine if a child needed hearing instruction?

5. How would you go about setting up a system in your school for daily checks of

hearing aids and assistive listening systems?

6. What are potential issues for a student with hearing loss in each of the instruction models and staff combinations discussed in this chapter?

REFERENCES

Alexander, R. (1987a). Developing prespeech and feeding abilities in children. In S. Shanks (Ed.), *Nursing and the management of pediatric communication disorders* San Diego, CA: College Hill.

Alexander, R. (1987b). Oral-motor treatment for infants and young children. *Seminars in Speech and Language, 8,* 87–100.

Alexander, R. (1987c). Prespeech and feeding development. In E. McDonald (Ed.), *Treating cerebral palsy.* Austin, TX. Pro-Ed.

American Academy of Audiology. (1993). Position statement: Auditory integration training. *Audiology Today, 5,* 21.

American Academy of Audiology. (1995). Position statement: Cochlear implants in children. *Audiology Today, 7,* 14–15.

American Speech-Language-Hearing Association. (1983). *The hearing impaired mentally retarded: Recommendations for action.* Washington, DC: Department of Health, Education and Welfare, Social and Rehabilitative Services.

American Speech-Language-Hearing Association. (1985). Guidelines for identification audiometry. *Asha, 27,* 49–52.

American Speech-Language-Hearing Association. (1990). Guidelines for screening for hearing impairments and middle ear disorders. *Asha, 32* (Suppl. 2), 17–24.

American Speech-Language-Hearing Association. (1994). Clinical practice by certificate holders in the profession in which they are certified. *Asha, 36* (Suppl. 13), 11–12.

American Speech-Language-Hearing Association. (1994a). Guidelines for fitting and monitoring FM systems. *Asha, 36* (Suppl. 12), 1–9.

American Speech-Language-Hearing Association. (1994b). Guidelines for the audiological management of individuals receiving cochleotoxic drug therapy. *Asha, 36* (Suppl. 12), 11–19.

American Speech-Language-Hearing Association. (1994c). Minimum competencies for educational audiologists. *Educational Audiology Association Newsletter, 11*(4), 7.

American Speech-Language-Hearing Association. (1995a). *Membership and certification handbook speech-language pathology.* Rockville, MD: Author.

American Speech-Language-Hearing Association. (1995b). *State education agency requirements for certification of speech-language pathologists.* Rockville, MD: Author.

Anderson, K., & Matkin, N. (1991). Relationship of degree of loss to psychosocial and educational needs. *Educational Audiology Newsletter, 8*(2), 11–12.

Anderson, U. M. (1967). The incidence and significance of high-frequency deafness in children. *American Journal of Diseases in Children, 113,* 560–565.

Berg, F. S. (1987). *Facilitating classroom listening.* Boston: College Hill.

Bess, F. H. (1985). The minimally hearing-impaired child. *Ear and Hearing, 6,* 43–47.

Brackett, D., & Maxon, A. B. (1986). Service delivery alternatives for the mainstreamed hearing-impaired child. *Language, Speech and Hearing Services in Schools, 17,* 115-125.

California State Department of Education. (1986). *Program guidelines for hearing impaired students.* Sacramento, CA: Author.

Clark, W. (1991). Noise exposure from leisure activities: A review. *Journal of the Acoustical Society of America, 90,* 175–181.

Davis, J. (Ed.). (1977). *Our forgotten children: Hard-of-hearing pupils in the schools.* Minneapolis, MN: Department of Health, Education and Welfare, Bureau of Education of the Handicapped, National Support Systems Project and Division of Personnel Preparation.

Davis, J., Shepard, N., Stelmachowicz, P., & Gorga, M. (1981). Characteristics of hearing impaired children in the schools: Part I—Demographic data. *Journal of Speech and Hearing Disorders, 46,* 123–129.

DeConde Johnson, C. (1991). The "state" of educational audiology: Survey results and goals for the future. *Educational Audiology Monograph, 2,* 74–84.

Education for All Handicapped Children Act of 1975, Pub. L No. 94-142, 89 Stat. 773 (1975).

Education of the Handicapped Amendments of 1986, Pub. L. No. 99-457, xx, 100 Stat. 1145 (1986).

Educational Audiology Association. (1994 Fall). Minimum competencies for educational audiologists. *Educational Audiology Association Newsletter*, 11, 4, 7.

English, K. M. (1995). *Educational audiology across the lifespan: Serving all learners with hearing impairment.* Baltimore: Paul H. Brookes.

Fettinger, M., & Huffman, N. P. (1994). *A teacher's guide to FM assistive devices, revised.* Unpublished manuscript.

Fitzgerald, M. T. & Fischer, R. M. (1987). A family involvement model for hearing impaired infants. *Topics in Language Disorders*, 7(3), 1–8.

Flexer, C., Wray, D., & Ireland, J. (1989). Preferential seating is not enough. *Language, Speech, and Hearing Services in Schools*, 20, 11–21.

Friel-Patti, S. (1994). Commitment to theory. *American Journal of Speech-Language Pathology*, 3, 30–34.

Fulton, R. T., & Lloyd, L. L., Eds. (1969). *Audiometry for the retarded: With implications for the difficult-to-test.* Baltimore: Williams & Wilkins.

Gravel, J. S. (1994). Auditory integration training: Placing the burden of proof. *American Journal of Speech-Language Pathology*, 3, 25–29.

Hearing Instruments Editors. (1994). A special editorial supplement to *Hearing Instruments*. Children and hearing: Strategies for successful teamwork. *Hearing Instruments*, 45 (Suppl. 2).

Huffman, N. P. (1982). *A teacher's guide to educational amplification.* Unpublished manuscript.

Huffman, N. P. (1985). *A teacher's guide to assistive devices.* Unpublished manuscript.

Individuals with Disabilities Education Act of 1990, Pub. L. No. 101–407, (1990).

Kahmi, A. C. (1995). Defining, developing, and maintaining clinical expertise. *Language, Speech, and Hearing Services in Schools*, 26, 353–356.

Katz, A., Gertsman, H., Sanderson, H., & Buchanan, R. (1982). Stereo headphones and hearing loss. *New England Journal of Medicine*, 307, 1460–1461.

Katzenbach, J. R., & Smith, D. K. (1994). *The wisdom of teams: Creating the high-performance organization.* New York: HarperCollins.

Kayser, T. A. (1994). *Building team power: How to unleash the collaborative genius of work teams.* Blue Ridge, IL: Irwin.

Klein, J. (1986). Risk factors for otitis media in children. In J. Kavanaugh (Ed.), *Otitis media and child development* (pp. 45–51). Parkton, MD: York.

Lass, N. J., Woodford, C. M., Pannbacker, M., Carlin, M., Saniga, R., Schmitt, J., & Everly-Myers, D. (1989). Speech-language pathologists' knowledge of exposure to, and attitude toward hearing aids and hearing aid wearers. *Language, Speech, and Hearing Services in Schools*, 20, 115–132.

Lass, N. J., Woodford, C. M., Schmidt, J. F., Pannbacker, M., Lundeen, C., & English, P. J. (1990). Health educators' knowledge of hearing, hearing loss, and hearing health practices. *Language, Speech, and Hearing Services in Schools*, 21, 85–90.

Luterman, D. M. (1991). *Counseling the communicatively disordered and their families.* Austin TX: Pro-Ed.

Madell, J. (1994). Auditory integration training. *American Journal of Audiology*, 3, 14–18.

Miller, J. J. (1985). *Handbook of ototoxicity.* Boca Raton, FL: CRC.

Monville, D. K., & Nelson, N. W. (1994). Parental viewpoints on change following auditory integration training for autism. *American Journal of Speech-Language Pathology*, 3, 41–51.

Morris, S. (1985). Developmental implications for the management of feeding problems in neurologically impaired children. *Seminars in Speech and Language*, 6, 293–315.

Morris, S., (1987). Therapy for the child with cerebral palsy: Interacting frameworks. *Seminars in Speech and Language*, 8, 71–86.

Morris, S. & Klein, M. (1987). *Prefeeding skills.* Tucson, AZ: Therapy Skill Builders.

National Association of State Directors of Special Education. (1994). *Deaf and hard of hearing students: Educational service guidelines.* Alexandria, VA: Author.

Neidecker, E. A., & Blosser, J. L. (1993). *School programs in speech-language organization and management.* (3rd ed.). Englewood Cliffs, NJ: Prentice-Hall.

New York State Education Department. (1992). *School hearing screening guidelines.* Albany, NY: Author.

Plakke, B. L. (1985). Hearing conservation in secondary industrial arts classes: A challenge for audiologists. *Language, Speech, and Hearing Services in Schools*, 16, 75–79.

Plakke, B. L. (1991). Hearing conservation training of industrial technology teachers. *Language, Speech, and Hearing Services in Schools*, 22, 134–138.

Rimland, B., & Edelson, S. M. (1994a). The effects of auditory integration training on autism. *American Journal of Speech-Language Pathology*, 3, 16–24.

Rimland, B. & Edelson, S.M. (1994b) Is theory better than chicken soup? *American Journal of Speech-Language Pathology*, 3, 38–40.

Rollins. W. J. (1987). *The psychology of communication disorders in individuals and their families.* Englewood Cliffs, NJ: Prentice-Hall.

Ross, M., Brackett, D., & Maxon, A. (1991). *Assessment and management of mainstreamed hearing impaired children.* Austin, TX: Pro-Ed.

Shewan, C. (1988). 1988 Omnibus Survey: Adaptation and progress in times of change. *Asha, 30*(8), 27–30.

Smith, J., Carter, M., & Gilder, G. (1988). Trends in time allocation for the school speech-language pathologist: A need for change. *HEARSAY: Journal of the Ohio Speech and Hearing Association*, pp. 45–48.

Stehli, A. (1991). *The sound of a miracle*. New York: Doubleday.

Taylor, J. S. (1992). Speech-language pathology services in the schools (2nd ed.). Boston: Allyn & Bacon.

Veale, T. K. (1994a). Auditory integration training: The use of a new listening treatment within our profession. *American Journal of Speech-Language Pathology, 3*, 12–15.

Veale, T. K. (1994b). Weighing the promises and the problems: AIT may be a risk worth taking. *American Journal of Speech-Language Pathology, 3*, 35–37.

Webster, E. J. (1966). Parent counseling by speech pathologists and audiologists. *Journal of Speech and Hearing Disorders, 31*, 331–340.

Webster, E. J. (1968). Procedures for group parent counseling in speech pathology and audiology. *Journal of Speech and Hearing Disorders, 33*, 127–131.

Woodford, C. M. (1973). A perspective on hearing loss and hearing assessment in school children. *Journal of School Health, 43*, 572–576.

Woodford, C. M. (1980). Notes on audiology in the public schools. *Hearing Aid Journal*, pp. 5–9.

Woodford, C. M. (1981). Hearing protection in the shop. *School Shop*, pp. 17–18.

Woodford, C. M., & O'Farrell, M. L. (1983). High frequency loss of hearing in secondary school students: An investigation of possible etiological factors. *Language, Speech, and Hearing Services in Schools, 14*, 22–28.

Audiology Organizations and Resources

Academy of Rehabilitative Audiology
P.O. Box 26532
Minneapolis, MN 55426

Alexander Graham Bell Association for the
   Deaf
3417 Volta Place NW
Washington, DC 20007

American Society for Deaf Children
814 Thayer Avenue
Silver Spring, MD 20910

American Speech-Language-Hearing Association
School Services Division
10801 Rockville Pike
Rockville, MD 20852

American Speech-Language-Hearing Association
Special Interest Division—Hearing Disorders
   in Children
Special Interest Division—Aural Rehabilitation
10801 Rockville Pike
Rockville, MD 20852

Cochlear Implant Club International
P.O. Box 464
Buffalo, NY 14223

Educational Audiology Association
1000 Carrington Place
Manassas, VA 22110

National Association for the Deaf
814 Thayer Avenue
Silver Spring, MD 20910

National Cued Speech Association
P.O. Box 3145
Raleigh, NC 27622

Network of Educators of Children With Co-
   chlear Implants
Cochlear Implant Center Manhattan Eye,
   Ear & Throat Hospital
210 E. 64th St., 4th Floor
New York, NY 10021

Self Help for Hearing Impaired People
   (SHHH)
7800 Wisconsin Avenue
Bethesda, MD 20814

Appendix 4–B

American Speech-Language-Hearing Association Position Statements, Guidelines, and Reports Pertinent to Audiology Practice in Educational Settings

- Position Statements

  1991. The use of FM amplification instruments for infants and preschool children with hearing impairment. *Asha, 33,* (Suppl. 5), 1-2.

- Guidelines

  1985. Guidelines for identification audiometry. *Asha, 27,* 49–52.

  1990. Guidelines for screening hearing impairments and middle ear disorders. *Asha, 32* (Suppl. 2), 17–24.

  1991. Guidelines for audiologic assessment of children from birth–36 months of age. *Asha, 33* (Suppl. 5), 37–43.

  1993. Guidelines for audiology services in the schools. *Asha, 35* (Suppl. 10), 24–32.

  1994. Guidelines for fitting and monitoring FM systems. *Asha, 36* (Suppl. 12), 1–9.

  1994. Guidelines for the audiological management of individuals receiving cochleotoxic drug therapy. *Asha, 36* (Suppl. 12), 11–19.

- Policy Statements

  1992. External auditory canal examination and cerumen management. *Asha, 34* (Suppl. 7), 22–24.

- Reports

  1990. Audiological assessment of central auditory processing: An annotated bibliography. *Asha, 32* (Suppl. 1), 13–30.

  1990. Aural rehabilitation: An annotated bibliography. *Asha, 32,* (Suppl. 1), 1–12.

  1991. Amplification as a remediation technique for children with normal peripheral hearing. *Asha, 33* (Suppl. 3), 22–24.

FM Assistive Listening Systems: Teaching Applications

TEACHING APPLICATIONS

Below are illustrations of incorrect usage of FM assistive devices and the solution to each problem. T = Teacher; X = Hearing-impaired student; 1, 2, 3, 4 = Other normal-hearing students.

PROBLEM A.

T has transmitter on. X is receiving both the FM and environmental signals. T asks student 2 to read and student 3 is asked to read next. T asks X a question on reading. X does not know answer. 1 answers very softly. T says "correct." X is asked some questions and still does not know answer.

SOLUTION: Cue hearing-impaired student as to who is speaking. Allow students to wear transmitter while reading. Change seating of hearing-impaired student. Teacher should repeat answers.

PROBLEM B.

T has transmitter on. X is receiving both FM and environmental signals. T is conducting reading group, asks (1) to read out loud. X is asked to continue where (1) has left off and starts at wrong spot.

SOLUTION: Student who is reading should use the microphone. Cue X that he or she will be called on next and where to begin reading.

PROBLEM C.

T has FM microphone on. X is receiving both FM and environmental signals. T is conducting reading group. X is doing seat work.

SOLUTION: Teacher should turn off transmitter.

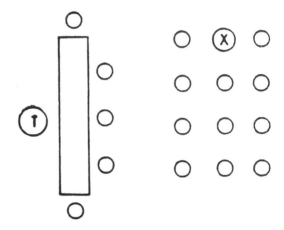

PROBLEM D.

T has FM microphone on. X is receiving both FM and environmental signals. T is helping (3) and (4) with alphabet. X is *not* responding verbally to (1) and (2).

SOLUTION: Teacher should turn off transmitter.

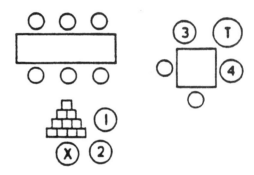

PROBLEM E.

T has FM microphone on while teaching her table numbers. X is receiving both FM and environmental signals. An aide (A) is also teaching numbers concepts.

SOLUTION: Aide should be using transmitter/microphone.

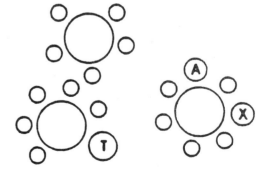

PROBLEM F.

T has FM microphone on. X is receiving both FM and environmental signals. T has been teaching group. Principal (P) visits to talk to teacher about a child. X is listening in on conversation.

SOLUTION: Teacher should turn off transmitter. Student should be trained to re-mind teacher to turn off transmitter should teacher forget.

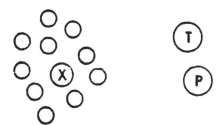

PROBLEM G.

T has FM microphone on. X is receiving both FM and environmental signals. (1) is giving oral book report. T makes comment and asks questions. X unable to answer.

SOLUTION: Student giving oral report should wear transmitter. Teacher should stand near hearing-impaired student while making comments and asking questions.

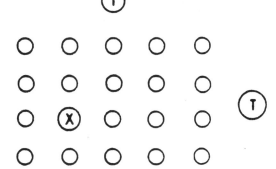

PROBLEM H.

T has FM microphone on. X is receiving both FM and environmental signals. T is showing videotape. X is expected to follow content presented on the videotape.

SOLUTION: Use audio-input capabilities of transmitter. See section in this guide under Transmitter on how to do this. If audio-input cord is not available, place transmitter near television (less desirable).

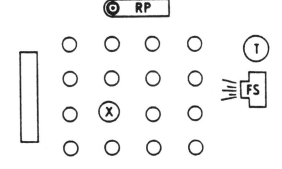

PROBLEM I.

T is talking with FM microphone on. X is listening in classroom noise with a less than optimal signal-to-noise ratio. Both FM and environmental mics are on.

SOLUTION: Student should turn off environmental mic. Teacher could also consider moving student closer to teacher.

PROBLEM J.

T has transmitter on and asks student a question. X has receiver turned on. (1) child responds. X cannot hear (1).

SOLUTION: Teacher should cue hearing-impaired student as to who is answering. Teacher should repeat answer. Hearing-impaired student should be trained to cue teacher if he is missing other students' answer.

PROBLEM K.

Film is being shown to class; sound source is projector (SP). X is sitting too far from projector. Motor noise from projector interferes if student moves closer to it.

SOLUTION: Use the audio input connection from the FM transmitter to the projector. Or, place transmitter near speaker of projector with student advising as to distance.

PROBLEM L.

T is conducting group work, with questions and answers around the table. T has FM transmitter on. X has receiver on with both FM and EM mics turned up. The rest of the class is at free play and circulating, making some noise. X is having difficulty hearing.

SOLUTION: Hearing/impaired student should turn off environmental mic on FM receiver.

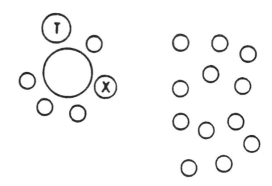

Chapter 5

Language-Impaired Students in Today's Schools

Pamelia F. O'Connell

Children who "stammered" were the initial focus of speech-language pathology professional involvement in our nation's schools. They were quickly joined by other students who exhibited difficulty in speech sound production. Today, children and adolescents with fluency disorders are still seen for speech-language pathology services, as are students with articulatory/phonological disorders. Students with voice disorders are also seen within our schools. Increasingly, however, the caseloads of school professionals have been dominated by students whose deficits in language negatively affect academic achievement.

Because every communication disorder that can be found among the young may now be encountered in our schools, a single chapter in a book of this type cannot possibly provide meaningful material on all of them. Even a comprehensive listing would run to multiple pages without offering any useful information.

This chapter will attempt only to remind the reader, once again, of the tremendous diversity among school-aged children who receive speech and language services and the need for high standards of qualification for those who provide them.

Some of the groups of students who are currently served in schools are discussed in other chapters. Part II of this book, "Program Implementation," includes case histories, one of them concerning a phonologically impaired first grader. Nonspeaking students receive emphasis in Chapter 9, and those from culturally and linguistically diverse backgrounds are featured in Chapter 11. The remainder of this chapter is devoted to four groups of language-impaired students who have been relatively recent entrants into the caseloads of school professionals: the learning disabled, pre-kindergarten children, students with autism, and the traumatically brain injured.

LEARNING DISABILITY

Learning disability has grown to be the largest category of students receiving special services in our schools. There has also been a continuing trend toward classification of language-impaired students as "LD." Because learning-disabled students form such a significant population, issues concerning them need to be addressed.

No attempt, however, will be made to summarize the vast and ever-growing literature on LD. Rather, two issues that seem to be key concerns for the school speech-language pathologist will be discussed. They are: (a) the heterogeneous nature of the group; and (b) the language connection.

The Nature of the Group

The learning disabled, as a group, show more variability than many others. This partially accounts for the large size of the group. Other factors, however, have influenced the rapid growth of the learning disability category.

From 1977 to 1980, that growth was quite dramatic. Whereas in 1977, 782,055 were receiving special education services, almost 2 million were receiving services in 1990. The rate of growth has slowed in the past decade as some states have begun to change eligibility criteria to limit the numbers of children receiving services (U.S. Department of Education, 1990). These changes do not suggest that an epidemic of disability has occurred but that many children experiencing school difficulties have been labeled LD to receive special help. Some of these children might have been labeled "slow learners" in the past. Many would agree that LD is less pejorative and therefore a preferred term. Others might argue that "learning disabled" and "slow learner" are separate categories, not to be confused with each other. In many of our schools, however, the line has been blurred. Thus one may find students bearing a label of *LD* whose overall cognitive abilities, though in the normal range, may be considered somewhat low.

Students with a diagnosis of attention-deficit hyperactivity disorder (ADHD) or undifferentiated attention deficit disorder (ADD) usually display learning problems in the classroom as well as unwelcome behavioral characteristics. Such students are increasingly identified, with some authorities stating that as many as 20% of school-aged children are affected (Shaywitz, Fletcher, & Shaywitz, 1994). Some authorities feel that such disorders are perhaps being overidentified. Nevertheless, many of these children are being added to the learning disability category. In some school districts, they carry the label "other health impaired."

As the research findings on attentional disorders have accumulated, there have been numerous conceptual and definitional shifts. The latest view of the symptoms of inattention, impulsivity, and hyperactivity proposes four subtypes (Shelton & Barkeley, 1994):

1. attention-deficit hyperactivity disorder, predominantly inattentive type
2. attention-deficit hyperactivity disorder, predominantly hyperactivity type
3. attention-deficit hyperactivity disorder, combined type
4. attention-deficit hyperactivity disorder, not otherwise specified

These four subtypes assume two distinct mechanisms of disorder, one involving difficulty in the focus and sustaining of attention and one reflecting difficulty in inhibition or self-regulation. There is some evidence that early ADHD may be symptomatic of risk for later reading problems (Ferguson & Horwood, 1992).

As previously noted, there is an increasing tendency for children with specific language impairment to be characterized as LD, especially as they grow older. These students are usually identified through the presence of oral language deficits during the preschool years. It is well to recognize that these early manifestations of language disability may change as the child matures; oral language skills may improve considerably, but the child may be vulnerable to reading failure and other academic difficulties (Scarborough & Dobrich, 1990).

There will be many more students who were not identified as being at risk for learning failure in the early years. The increased

complexity of school language and the demands made by the need for literacy cause
school failure to begin to occur. That is, more
covert and subtle language weaknesses characterize the majority of LD students. The
school-based speech-language pathologist
needs to be aware of the great variability
within the LD group and the concomitant
need to tailor services to individual needs and
demands of the curriculum.

Learning Disability and the Language Connection

It may seem unnecessary to stress the connection between language and learning. It
has become an educational "given" in the
1990s—one that has grown out of several decades of research findings, all underscoring
the primary importance of such a connection.
Wallach and Butler (1994) provided a comprehensive and thoughtful discussion of
much of this research. If language and learning are so closely associated, the relationship
between language deficits and learning problems seems obvious. There are several reasons, however, to emphasize the language
connection. One is that this linkage has not
always been recognized, at least not explic-
itly. Many LD children have difficulty with
reading, and reading failures were often, in
the past, attributed to sensory perception
deficits (Vellutino, 1979). Not until the relatively recent past have we witnessed explicit
and research-supported linkages between oral
and written language (Blachman, 1991;
Kahmi & Catts, 1991; Kahmi & Koenig,
1985; Wallach, 1990). Reading failure or dyslexia is increasingly seen as a developmental
language disorder. Yet the reading specialist
and the speech-language pathologist are
separate professional specialists within our
schools, and they often approach the LD stu-

dent from different perspectives. This is not
necessarily negative, yet the language connection should be recognized by both so that
a meaningful and genuinely helpful collaboration may take place.

The second reason for the need for emphasis here lies in the complex, multifaceted nature of language itself. I am reminded of a
conversation held about 10 years ago with an
educational psychologist. "When you say *language* you mean syntax, right?" she asked con-
fidently, surprised when I replied "Well, not
entirely."

The following is a listing, accompanied by
brief discussions, of some of the areas of language that the school speech-language pathologist must consider when planning services for a learning-disabled student.

Metalinguistic skill or *language awareness* "refers to ability to reflect consciously on the
nature and properties of language" (Van
Kleek, 1994, p. 53). Van Kleek (1994) further stated that metalinguistic skills fall into
two categories: (a) those reflecting awareness
of language as an arbitrary code and (b) those
reflecting awareness of language as a system
of elements that may be combined in certain
ways. Examples of the first category include
word awareness, such as differentiation between a word and its referents, between words
and nonwords, and among multiple meanings, as well as humor. Examples of the second category include segmentation, as well as
rules or regularities involved in syntax, morphology, and phonology.

Phonological awareness, in the view of
many, plays a crucial role in early reading success, and this is a prime area of investigation
for the reading-disabled student (Vellutino &
Scanlon, 1987). A number of studies, (e.g.,
Ball & Blachman, 1991; Blachman, 1991)
suggest that a combination of instruction in
phoneme awareness and letter-sound knowl-

edge results in superior reading and spelling performance. This research also suggests that phonological awareness can be taught during the preschool years.

Discourse refers to naturally occurring language in which the unit is larger than a sentence. Discourse may be oral or written. There are many types of discourse in both modalities; the major divisions are narration, description, argument, and exposition (Scott, 1994).

Narration has been extensively studied, in both normally developing children and learning-disabled students. For the latter, multiple weaknesses in producing and comprehending oral narratives have been documented. These include (a) shorter and incomplete episodes, (b) shallow characterization, (c) decreased awareness of the needs of listeners, and (d) increased rates of communication breakdowns (Garnett, 1986; Ripich & Griffith, 1988).

Differences between home and school language may constitute a hurdle for younger LD children. Some writers (Creaghead, 1990) refer to these differences as different scripts or generalized representations of the experiences within a given event. School success requires that children learn a large number of scripts regarding classroom behavior and expectations, and these scripts differ considerably from those of the home.

Discourse demands change over time. The older student, from about age 10, must deal increasingly with written texts. Scott (1991) has summarized some of the common difficulties that LD students have in writing: (a) lack of productivity, (b) lack of organization, (c) grammatical errors, (d) spelling errors, (e) restricted lexicon, and (f) handwriting problems.

Nonliteral language is language in which meaning differs from the literal interpretation of the words used. It can take many forms, such as metaphors, similes, allegories, idioms, and irony. In both spoken and written language, nonliteral or figurative usage is quite common in conversation, in the classroom, and in children's literature (Milosky, 1994). Research findings on LD children in this area have been limited and somewhat contradictory, but the pervasiveness of nonliteral language use suggests it is an area requiring the attention of the speech-language pathologist.

Word retrieval has been studied extensively in many different populations, among them children with learning problems. Difficulties in word finding or the inability to "call up a word from the stored lexicon" (Wiig & Becker-Caplan, 1984, p. 1) have been widely documented, but the significance of this deficit is not generally agreed upon. Word-finding problems may be manifested by semantic or phonemic word substitutions, circumlocutions, perseverations, and delays (German, 1994). Poor readers have frequently shown impaired word-finding ability in rapid naming and confrontation naming tasks (Denckla & Rudel, 1976; Wolf & Goodglass, 1986). Some children display word-finding problems in the absence of comprehension problems; for others, comprehension and vocabulary weaknesses may also be found, or as Long and Long (1994) have stated, a generalized semantic deficit may be present.

And then there is *syntax*—still an area of considerable interest, as LD students have frequently been found to have difficulty with the structural properties of language, especially if they have previously been classified as language impaired. Chapters 6, 7, and 8 contain detailed accounts of assessment and management in the area of syntax/morphology.

There has been increasing emphasis, in the recent past, on literacy as a broad concept, cutting across both oral and written modalities (Silliman & Wilkinson, 1994). A growing body of research supports the connection between written and spoken language. As a consequence, the language-learning connection becomes ever stronger, and the speech-language specialist in the schools becomes increasingly drawn into active participation in the language of the classroom.

THE PREKINDERGARTEN CHILD

Recognition of speech and language impairment in preschool children has existed for a long time. It is a fairly recent development, however, for school services to be routinely supplied for prekindergarten children. Federal legislation, the Education of the Handicapped Amendments of 1986, is primarily responsible for the change. Services for infants, toddlers, and children aged 3 to 5 with handicapping conditions or who are considered at risk for developmental delays were encouraged by this legislation. Now a wide variety of youngsters with handicapping conditions of many types receive early intervention services in a variety of settings. Although some services for infants are provided through hospitals or other health care facilities, many services are offered through community public schools. Thus a school-based speech-language pathologist may work exclusively with the very young.

Two principal types of intervention are currently in practice, with the decisive factor usually being the age of the child. Infants and toddlers, from birth to 2 years old, are most frequently served in their homes. The model followed, in most cases, stresses a family systems approach. As Butler (1994) pointed out, "It is impossible to separate consideration of infants and toddlers from consideration of their parents and families" (p. v). To a certain extent, of course, this principle applies to

all children and adolescents. As with many groups, a team approach is most frequently used and is deemed most appropriate by many authorities (Wilcox, 1989).

Within the general model of team-based intervention, there are several varieties: multidisciplinary, transdisciplinary, and interdisciplinary. These differ in the manner in which professionals cooperate in planning and programming. The school-based speech-language pathologist who functions in such a program must be familiar with the model of service in practice and his or her role within the team.

Somewhat older preschoolers often receive services from center-based programs. One of the benefits of center-based programs is the opportunity provided for parents to share with other parents—to explore options and to become mutually supportive. Center-based programs also focus on the child's family to maximize the potential benefits to the child (Prizant & Wetherby, 1990).

Wilcox (1989) stated that three approaches may be applied when dealing with infants and toddlers. They are (a) remedial, used when a specific deficit has been identified; (b) preventive, when, in the absence of a specific deficit, the child is judged to be at risk; and, (c) compensatory, in which aids or devices may be employed to compensate for a disability. These are not mutually exclusive; more than one approach may be used with a given child.

Language development in the infant–toddler group is frequently characterized as delayed. Language milestones are late to occur, and growth of the language system may be slowed. Whether or not such delays constitute actual disorders is subject to controversy (Reed, (1994). The term *slow expressive language development* (SELD) is currently the preferred one. Note that the word *disorder* is avoided; the term is also usually reserved for children who exhibit delayed language development in the absence of such general disabilities as mental retardation or autism.

The 3- to 5-Year-Old Child

Paul (1991) and other writers have suggested that many toddlers who are slow in language development continue to exhibit linguistic deficits at ages 3, 4, and 5. Further, many of these children will have persistent language learning problems. A plethora of terms have been employed over the years to designate this group of children. Currently, the term *specific language impairment* (SLI), is preferred by many. Some authorities, however (Leonard, 1991), have questioned its appropriateness. Other writers, such as Lahey (1988), have stressed our lack of understanding of both typical and atypical language development. Although a search for causative factors and increased understanding of developmental language problems should, and will, continue, the challenge for school practitioners remains. That is, in the absence of complete knowledge, children with slow language development will need to be identified and assisted.

Prekindergarten children with language impairments frequently have phonological problems. Although the exact relationship between difficulty with phonology and problems with other components of the language system is not well understood, there does appear to be a relationship between phonology and the lexicon (Shriberg & Kwiatkowski, 1988). Lexical acquisition appears to be slowed in preschoolers with SLI, leading to restricted vocabulary and over- and undergeneralization of lexical items.

Syntax morphology is considered by many authorities to pose a special challenge for SLI youngsters (Loeb & Leonard, 1991; Watkins

& Rice, 1991). Indeed, difficulty with grammatical morphemes is often viewed as the hallmark of SLI.

Conflicting results have characterized the research on pragmatics in SLI preschoolers. Deficits have been documented in certain areas such as politeness (Prinz & Ferrier, 1983), whereas other investigations of revision behaviors (Fey & Leonard, 1984) have found normal-range abilities.

Although the delay in expressive language appears to be the defining characteristic of the SLI child, research by Thal (1991) and her colleagues suggests that language comprehension deficits are better predictors of persisting language difficulty than the degree of expressive language delay.

Tallal (1988) has suggested that early language disability, frequently relabeled *LD* when reading and writing deficits become apparent in later years, is really a different manifestation of the same problem.

Blank, Marguis, and Kimovitch (1995) suggested that language intervention for the young child should focus on the concept of "text," a basic unit of complex meaning that may exist in oral or written form. They stated that we need to help the young child move from the simpler demands of preschool oral language toward the more abstract and complex requirements of the grade-school curriculum. Whereas Blank and others have emphasized the unity of language, whatever its expression, Van Kleek (1995), suggested teaching form and meaning separately at the beginning, when early reading instruction starts in the first and second grades. The speech-language specialist may play an important role, at the preschool level and at later years, in assisting those young students who appear at risk for not achieving literacy.

The language-delayed preschooler must be considered at serious risk for later school difficulties. Intervention with these children is a process of accelerating development and fostering learning (Blank et al., 1995). It should also take into account the linguistic demands that the child will encounter in the future. The foundations of literacy are constructed long before we expect the child to read and write.

AUTISM

No other children with handicapping conditions have been subject to the degree of controversy and the number of profound shifts in conceptualization as those with autism. Even now, the status of our understanding of the cause or causes and the nature of the disorder itself is far from complete. Certainly, however, we have traveled a long way from the initial view of autism promulgated by Leo Kanner in 1943. Observing a small group of children characterized by aloofness and marked social isolation, Kanner (1943) provided the name *autism* and proposed it as a psychiatric illness similar to childhood schizophrenia. Causation was sought in environmental influences, primarily inadequate parenting (Bettelheim, 1967). In the 1970s, however, scholars and researchers began to shift toward an orientation that placed autism among the developmental disorders of childhood (Rutter, 1978), more akin to mental retardation than mental illness, with a probable but unknown organic etiology.

With this shift in thinking about the nature of the problem came a significant shift in approaches to management. Autism fell increasingly within the province of special education and not psychiatry. Children with symptoms of autism began to be identified at earlier ages and began to receive intervention and educational services within our schools. Today, it is not unusual for school speech-language pathologists to number students

with autism among their caseloads. Amid persisting controversy and continuing lack of complete understanding, intervention is taking place and is making a difference.

Description and Diagnostic Criteria

The term *autism* refers to a syndrome, or co-occurring set of symptoms, with unique characteristics. As a clinical category, it has been revised a number of times, and additional revision is quite likely. At present, there is considerable interest in the subject of subtypes of autism and the relationship between autism and other pervasive developmental disorders.

The *Diagnostic and Statistical Manual (DSM)* of the American Psychiatric Association (APA) serves as the official definitional arbiter. The third, revised edition of the *DSM DSM-III-R*; APA, 1987) lists the following diagnostic criteria for autism:

1. qualitative impairment in reciprocal social interaction, such as marked lack of awareness of the existence or feelings of others

2. qualitative impairment in verbal and nonverbal communication such as absence of a mode of communication, gesture, mime, or speech, and abnormal language form or content

3. restricted repertoire of activities and interests, such as preoccupation with parts of objects and insistence on following routines

Although no single behavior is always present, it is generally agreed that impaired social interaction is the hallmark (Seigel, Vukicevic, Elliott, & Kraemer, 1989).

Pervasive developmental disorder not otherwise specified (PDDNOS) is a related diagnostic category, introduced in the *DSM-III-R*, that is used for children who exhibit some but not all of the criteria for autism. These children usually are less functionally impaired than those with autism. Asperger syndrome is regarded as a pervasive developmental disorder that has recently been accorded a separate diagnostic category. Ghaziuddin, Leininger, and Tsai (1995), however, noted that it is not clear to what extent Asperger syndrome differs from high-functioning autism.

This brings us to a consideration of the topic of types of autism. As research findings have accumulated, it has become increasingly apparent that children with autism form a highly variable group, even when all diagnostic criteria are met. Associated neurological problems and language and cognitive levels can exhibit marked variation. Functional levels at adulthood, including the capacity for independent living, also vary significantly. A recent study by Sevin et al. (1996) employed a cluster-analysis method that yielded four subtypes:

1. high functioning, atypical PDD with good verbal skills and intelligence quotient (IQ) ranges from mild mental retardation (MR) to low normal

2. mild autism with variable verbal skills and IQ ranges from mild to moderate MR

3. moderate autism with delayed language development, some functional speech, and IQ ranges from moderate to severe MR

4. severe autism with little or no functional speech and IQ ranges from moderate to severe MR

Although this study does not report on them, there also seems to be a small group of high-functioning individuals with autism or Asperger syndrome who have IQ ranges from normal to superior (Sacks, 1994).

Older definitional criteria for autism included an age of onset before 30 months. It is now generally agreed that autism is usually present at birth and does not, therefore, have an "onset." Also, there have been rare cases of children who did not exhibit a full range of symptoms until age 5 or 6 (APA, 1987). Although it may be present, autism is not readily identifiable at birth, as there are no characteristic physical signs. With the increasing availability of early intervention services and the widespread belief that early intervention is more effective than later efforts (Prizant & Wetherby, 1988), the primary diagnostic challenge in autism, it would seem, is early identification of the disorder and of other forms of PDD. The reliable diagnosis of young nonverbal children has continued to pose a problem (DiLavore, Lord, & Rutter, 1995).

Because many children with autism have accompanying MR, problems exhibited by nonspeaking toddlers could be due to a variety of causes. DiLavore et al. (1995) have devised a semistructured assessment of play, interaction, and social communication skills appropriate for use with children with developmental ages less than 3 years who are suspected of autism. Lord, Rutter, and LeCouteur (1994) have published a revised version of a diagnostic interview to be used with caregivers of such children. Both are recommended sources for speech-language specialists who perform assessments of prekindergarten children.

The estimated prevalence of autism at present is 4 to 5 children per 10,000 with an additional 4 to 5 per 10,000 with PDDNOS (APA, 1987). All forms of PDD, including autism, occur more frequently in males. Among the problems associated with autism, MR is the most frequently observed, with approximately three quarters of all autistic children showing some degree of MR, based on

IQ (APA, 1987). Seizure disorder is also frequent (Gillberg, 1991). Fragile-X syndrome, a genetic disorder, may also be found in a small number of cases (Piven, Gayle, Wzorek, & Folstein, 1991).

Communication, Language, and Speech

One of the three major categories of impairment in autism involves communication, language, and speech. This is, of course, the area of primary interest and responsibility of the speech-language pathologist. Although the level of language ability and the functional use of speech may vary widely in individuals with autism, some generalizations about the group can be made with some degree of confidence. Concerning the range of impairment, Long (1994) has stated, "The verbal abilities of children with autism range from the total absence of speech to communication that is fully adequate in phonological and grammatical form but is remarkable for its semantic or pragmatic irregularities" (p. 240).

Long (1994) further commented on a profile of language skills that is generally characteristic, a profile of relative strengths and weaknesses. Among the relatively preserved abilities in autistic children who are verbal are segmental phonology and syntax. That is, verbal children with autism do not tend to display the developmental articulatory/phonological and syntactic errors frequently observed in young normally developing children and in children with MR unaccompanied by autism, specific language impairment, or hearing impairment. Speech is usually intelligible, and utterances may be syntactically correct. Similarly, children with autism are able to comprehend vocabulary items and meaning conveyed by word order

at a level consistent with mental age (Beisler, Tsai, & Vonk, 1987; Eskes, Bryson, & McCormick, 1990).

On the other hand, other areas of language show impairment and/or atypical features. Prosodic aspects of spoken language are frequently abnormal, and stereotyped rhythmic patterns, excessive whispering, and inappropriate tonal contrasts have all been noted (Baltaxe & Guthrie, 1987). Pragmatics is another area of difficulty; this is not unexpected, as pragmatics encompasses a wide variety of communication skills that underlie the social uses of language (Prizant & Wetherby, 1988), and reciprocal social interaction is always impaired in autism. The use of idiosyncratic language and neologisms or invented words contributes to difficulty in social interactions (Volden & Lord, 1991). Children with autism are also thought to be delayed in using language to share or direct attention and to tend to initiate communication infrequently (Mundy, Sigman, & Kasari, 1990).

One of the most striking characteristics of the language of children with autism is the frequent repetition of utterances addressed to them. This is called *echolalia*, and it may be either immediate or delayed. Another type is mitigated echolalia, in which some part of the utterance has been changed. Long viewed as uncommunicative imitation, echolalia seems to serve the children who employ it in a variety of ways (Prizant & Duchan, 1981). That is, some echoed utterances may play roles in communication interchanges. The child may be calling attention, answering, or attempting to keep a conversational interchange from ending. Perhaps associated with echolalia is another language characteristic: pronoun reversal, or the confusion of first- and second-person pronouns. Although other language-impaired children may confuse subject and object pronouns, saying "me" for "I" or "him" for "he," the use of "you" for "I" or "me" for "you" appears to be found only in children with autism (Long, 1994). Explanations for this phenomenon, like those for other characteristics of autism, are far from satisfactory.

No discussion of communication in autism can be complete without reference to one of the latest and largest controversies: facilitated communication (FC). This variant of augmented and alternate communication (AAC) appeared in the early 1990s (Biklin, 1990, 1992; Crossley, 1992) and, for a time, appeared to have the promise not only of greatly improving the communication status of individuals with autism but of forcing a complete reevaluation of the nature of the disorder itself. The method involves a "facilitator" who provides physical and emotional support that allows the individual with autism to access a keyboard and produce typed messages. Because many severely impaired individuals have little or no functional speech, nonspeech methods of management, such as signing, have been employed in the past with some success. Initial reports of FC described highly dramatic changes in communication functioning and unexpected levels of literacy.

Individuals with autism, using FC, typed messages with high-level vocabulary, good awareness of the communicative partner, and sophisticated insights. Assumptions about cognitive and social interaction deficits were questioned by these reports, and speculation was offered regarding motor planning deficits as the underlying cause of poor communicative functioning (Biklin, 1990a). Use of the method spread rapidly; perhaps as rapidly, doubts about its validity arose. The primary question about FC concerns message authorship. Is the individual with autism the true author of facilitated messages or is there facilitator influence on content? And if so, what is the extent of such influence? This question arose, in part, from the extreme discrepancy between the level of facilitated messages, and previous estimates of linguistic and cognitive functioning and, in part, from observations that many facilitated students failed to look at the keyboard while typing. It should also be noted that the physical support supplied frequently involved actual control of the individual's hand and fingers by the facilitator.

To date, the overwhelming majority of the evidence points toward an unacceptably high degree of facilitator influence (Bebko, Perry, & Bryson, 1996; Green, 1994; Hudson, Melita, Arnold, & Brey, 1993; Shane & Kearns, 1994; Vasquez, 1994.) Although there has been criticism of the experimental methods used in some FC validation studies (Sonnenmeier & Duchan, 1994), a recent study by Vasquez (1995) addressed some of these concerns and concluded that a generalized language deficit and not word retrieval or perceptual problems is implicated in failures to name pictures without facilitator knowledge of correct answers. That is, this study, among many others, points to the facilitator as the primary author of many FC messages. At present, the American Psychiatric Association, APA, American Association of Pediatrics, American Association of Adolescent and Adult Psychiatry, and the American Speech-Language-Hearing Association (ASHA) have warned of the risks of using FC (Vasquez, 1994). Schopler (1996), in an editorial in the *Journal of Autism and Developmental Disabilities*, made a strong statement against its use. Although a complete resolution of the questions raised by FC eludes us, at present it seems that the method is best avoided, especially by novices.

Issues in Management

In light of the above, we need to address issues in management of autism from somewhat older and more conservative sources. Even so, we find a relatively short history of such approaches and, within this brief span of some 30 years or so, a number of shifts in dominant orientation. Behavior modification (Lovaas, 1977) was the earliest approach, and it has been largely superseded by a social interaction perspective (Duchan, 1984). This is less a method than a belief that adults and peers can interact with children with autism in ways that promote their communicative competence. This philosophy has been joined with early intervention practices that are used with other handicapped children. See the previous section entitled "The Prekindergarten Child" for a brief description of the family systems approach. Preliminary results point toward effectiveness of early intervention (Handleman, Harris, Kristoff, Fuentes, & Alessandri, 1991) for children with autism. Providing the young autistic child with opportunities for group interaction in a supportive environment while providing parents with information, support, and encouragement for meaningful communication with their children seems to produce benefits, whether or not the children are grouped with typically developing peers.

Koegel and Koegel (1995) stressed what they termed as a "natural language paradigm" and stated that it is effective for many autistic children. Their methods are based on the following four principles: (a) language is taught within natural interactions, (b) age-appropriate, child-selected stimuli are employed, (c) language targets result in natural consequences, and (d) all attempts at communication are reinforced. They also emphasized increasing communicative skills in higher functioning autistic children by increasing eye contact and peer involvement and decreasing perseveration.

Difficulty with generalization of new learning is characteristic of many students with handicapping conditions, including those with autism. This has led to an emphasis on communication intervention in natural settings, such as the classroom. Dyer, Williams, and Luce (1991) described a procedure for training special education teachers in the use of communication strategies in the classroom and provided some evidence of its effectiveness.

The search for innovative and effective methods for promoting communication in autism is relatively new and will continue. Although the hopes engendered by FC, that children with autism might possess high levels of cognition, literacy, and interactive capacity, have not materialized, there is ample reason to believe that the condition can be ameliorated. Early and sustained intervention efforts are surely warranted.

TRAUMATIC BRAIN INJURY

Understanding of traumatic brain injury (TBI) in school-aged populations has grown in the recent past. Studies have shown that moderate to severe traumatically brain-injured individuals have persistent academic and social interaction problems. Loss of knowledge and skills acquired prior to the accident, the integration of developmental skills, and difficulty in new learning may all be present.

The Individuals with Disabilities Education Act (IDEA) of 1990, recognized TBI as a distinct educational disability category, and many states have done so as well. The federal law specifies a common etiology, that of an external physical force, resulting in a possibly wide variety of impairments in many processes relevant to academic performance. These include motor, sensory, behavioral, cognitive, and communicative. Traumatic brain injuries are caused by the sudden acceleration or deceleration of the head when the moving head strikes a stationary object or a quickly moving object strikes the head (Brookshire, 1992). There are two principal types: (a) penetrating or open head injuries; and (b) nonpenetrating injuries, in which the meninges remain uninterrupted, or closed head injuries. Unfortunately, these injuries are all too common; many are motor vehicle related. Adolescents and young adults are at greatest risk for sustaining TBI (Ylsivaker, Kolpan, & Rosenthal, 1994). It has been estimated that 150,000 to 200,000 school-aged or younger children are hospitalized each year with TBI. Perhaps as many as 20,000 of these may require extensive hospitalization and sustain permanent deficits of some kind.

The nature of such impairments and the wide variations among them may be accounted for by the injury, in which the brain and/or brain stem may receive significant damage from abrasions, lacerations, contusions, and shearing of brain tissue. This damage is caused by the rapid movement of the brain's relatively soft tissue against the rough, bony interior surfaces of the skull. The resulting damage may be thought of as diffuse or scattered, frequently bilateral or multifocal (Hagen, 1981). The pattern of deficits resulting from such an injury is subject to extensive variation.

The recognition of TBI as a distinct category was welcome, as students with TBI represent a complex educational challenge. Prior to the passage of IDEA in 1990, these students were increasingly seen in community schools. Some of them who had residual physical deficits were often classified as "other health impaired" whereas children who did not display physical problems were frequently labeled as learning disabled. The services these youngsters received may or may not have been sufficient for their needs (Szkeres & Meserve, 1994).

Understanding of the needs of TBI students has grown over the past decade, but a knowledge base regarding this group continues to evolve. Improved medical and rehabilitative care has meant that increasing numbers of TBI survivors return to school settings. For many, school reentry is a difficult process due to problems: communicative, emotional, cognitive, behavioral, or a combination of these (Savage & Carter, 1984). Blosser and de Pompei (1989) stressed that each TBI individual is unique. The combinations of deficits and severity levels will differ across students. Preserved abilities may suggest a higher overall level of functioning than actually exists. Although it is especially difficult to generalize about this population, a number of commonly observed characteristics are listed below:

- a sense of being normal that persists from the premorbid period

- uneven ability levels

- slowed processing and poor memory

- impaired ability for self-management

- disorientation and confusion

- inconsistent performance

- poor judgment and difficulty with emotional control

- combinations of handicapping conditions

- learning style that requires compensation

- previous learning that may facilitate relearning (Rosen & Gerring, 1986;

Szkeres & Meserve, 1994; Ylsivaker, 1985)

Communication problems may include impaired comprehension, word-finding problems, and inappropriate speech. Some TBI students will also display dysarthric speech that may be mild or severe. (dePompei & Blosser, 1987).

Although many of these problems may be found in other groups, it is well to emphasize that head-injured students differ from other handicapped groups in many significant ways. If physical problems do not exist and speech production is "normal," the student may not seem to be impaired. The student him- or herself does not have a history of being a member of an impaired group. And the combination and unevenness of the deficits differ from the patterns seen in other groups.

Many professionals feel that collaboration is the most appropriate model for providing services for TBI students. An excellent discussion of collaboration may be found in Chapter 8 of this book. It means that the speech-language pathologist will work actively with special or regular education teachers, guidance counselors, and other rehabilitative or educational specialists and also with the families of the students. The speech-language pathologist working with a TBI student needs to be aware of the importance of including such factors as attention, memory, organization, and social interactions in the assessment process and in the plans for management. Ongoing assessment is also very important, as these students may show changes over time; educational demands on the student will also change over time. Recovery rates and levels will vary across students.

Fortunately for the school practitioner, the literature on TBI and school reentry continues to grow. Suggestions for further reading may be found in the reference list at the end of this chapter.

CONCLUSION

Although our portrait of the populations served in schools is far from complete, there are some commonalities in the groups we have described. These shared factors, which can be viewed as common needs, can be generalized to other groups not included in this brief discussion. They include (a) the need to view the individual student, whatever the label, within the total school environment, with its increasing cognitive linguistic demands as that student progresses through the system; (b) the need to view the language system in as broad a fashion as possible; (c) the need to foster literacy in developmentally appropriate ways; and (d) the need to provide services to the student that are integrated with and crucial to the entire educational experience.

STUDY QUESTIONS

1. Why have language problems become increasingly the focus of school services for the speech-language pathologist?

2. In what ways might difficulty with nonliteral language affect classroom success?

3. Comment on the relationship between metalinguistic skill and reading ability.

4. What areas of language might form the focus of assessment for a 4-year-old?

5. Prepare a list of activities appropriate for fostering communication in a nonverbal child with autism. What activities might be appropriate for a verbal child?

6. In what ways might a TBI student be similar to an LD student? In what ways might they differ?

REFERENCES

American Psychiatric Association. (1987). *Diagnostic and statistical manual of mental disorders.* (3rd ed., Rev.). Washington, DC: Author.

Ball, E. W., & Blachman, B. A. (1991). Phonological coding, phonological awareness, and reading ability: Evidence from a longitudinal and experimental study. *Merrill-Palmer Quarterly, 26*(1), 49–66.

Baltaxe, C., & Guthrie, D. (1987). The use of primary sentence stress by normal and aphasic autistic children. *Journal of Autism Development Disorders, 17,* 255–271.

Bebko, J., Perry, A., & Bryson, S. (1996). Multiple method validation study of facilitated communication: II. *Journal of Autism and Developmental Disorders, 26,* 19–42.

Beisler, J., Tsai, L., & Vonk, D. (1987). Comparisons between autistic and nonautistic children on the Test for Auditory Comprehension of Language. *Journal of Autism and Developmental Disorders, 17,* 95–102.

Bettelheim, B. (1967). *The empty fortress: Infantile autism and the birth of the self.* New York: Free Press.

Biklin, D. (1990). Communication unbound: Autism and praxis. *Harvard Educational Review, 60,* 291–314.

Biklin, D. (1992). Typing to talk: Facilitated communication. *American Journal of Speech-Language Pathology, 1,* 15–17, 21–22.

Blachman, B. A. (1991). Early intervention for children's reading problems: Clinical applications of the research in phonological awareness. *Topics in Language Disorders, 12*(1), 51–65.

Blank, M., Marguis, M. A., & Kimovitch, M. O. (1995). *Directing early discourse: Making the transition to school language.* Tucson, AZ: Communication Skill Builders.

Blosser, J., & dePompei, R. (1989). The head injured student returns to school. *Topics in Language Disorders, 9*(2), 67–77.

Brookshire, R. (1992). *An introduction to neurogenic communication disorders:* (4th ed.). St. Louis, MO: Mosby Year Book.

Butler, K. G. (1994). *Early intervention I: Working with infants and toddlers.* Gaithersburg, MD: Aspen.

Creaghead, N. A. (1990). Mutual empowerment through collaboration: A new script for an old problem. *Best Practices in School Speech-Language Pathology, 1,* 109–116.

Crossley, R. (1992). Lending a hand: A personal account of the development of facilitated communication training. *American Journal of Speech-Language Pathology, 1,* 15–18.

Denckla, M. B., & Rudel, R. (1976). Naming of objects and drawings by dyslexic and other learning disabled children. *Brain and Language, 3,* 1–16.

dePompei, R. & Blosser, J. (1987). Strategies for helping head injured children successfully return to school. *Language, Speech and Hearing Services in Schools, 18,* 292–300.

DiLavore, D., Lord, C., & Rutter, M. (1995). The prelinguistic autism diagnostic observation schedule. *Journal of Autism and Developmental Disorders, 25,* 355–379.

Duchan, J. (1984). Clinical interactions with autistic children: The role of theory. *Topics in Language Disorders, 4,* 53–71.

Dyer, K., Williams, L., & Luce, S. (1991). Training teachers to use naturalistic communication strategies in classrooms for students with autism and other severe handicaps. *Language, Speech and Hearing Services in Schools, 22,* 313–321.

Eskes, G., Bryson S., & McCormick, T. (1990). Comprehension of concrete and abstract words in autistic children. *Journal of Autism and Developmental Disorders, 20,* 61–73.

Ferguson, D., & Horwood, L. (1992). Attention deficit and reading achievement. *Journal of Child Psychology and Psychiatry, 33,* 375–385

Fey, M., & Leonard, L. (1984). Partner age as a variable in the conversational performance of specifically language-impaired and normal language children. *Journal of Speech and Hearing Research, 27,* 413–423.

Garnett, K. (1986). Telling tales: Narratives and learning disabled children. *Topics in Language Disorders, 6,* 44–56.

German, D. J. (1994). Word finding difficulties in children and adolescents. In G. P. Wallach and K. G. Butler (Eds.), *Language learning disability in school age children and adolescents: Some principles and applications* (pp. 323–347). Needham Heights, MA: Allyn & Bacon.

Ghaziuddin, M., Leininger, L., & Tsai, L. (1995). Brief report. Thought disorder in Asperger syndrome: Comparison with high functioning autism. *Journal of Autism and Developmental Disorders, 25,* 311–317.

Gillberg, C. (1991). Outcome in autism and autistic-like conditions. *Journal of the American Academy of Child and Adolescent Psychiatry, 30,* 375–382.

Green, G. (1994). The quality of the evidence. In H. Shane (Ed.), *Facilitated communication: The clinical and social phenomenon,* (pp. 157–226). San Diego, CA: Singular.

Hagen, C. (1981). Language disorders secondary to closed head injury: diagnosis and treatment. *Topics in Language Disorders, 1*(4), 73–88.

Handleman, J., Harris, S., Kristoff, B., Fuentes, F., & Alessandri, M. (1991). A specialized program for preschool children with autism. *Language, Speech and Hearing Services in Schools, 22,* 107–110.

Hudson, A., Melita, B., & Arnold, N. (1993). Brief report: A case study assessing the validity of facilitated communication. *Journal of Autism and Developmental Disorders, 23,* 165–173.

Individuals with Disabilities Act of 1990, (IDEA) Pub. L. No. 101-407, 20 U.S.C. § 1400 et seq. Formerly titled the Education for All Handicapped Children Act, originally enacted as P.L. 94-142 (1975).

Kahmi, A. G. & Catts, H. W. (1991). *Reading disabilities: A developmental perspective.* Boston: Allyn & Bacon.

Kahmi, A. G., & Koenig, L. (1985). Metalinguistic awareness in normal and language disordered children. *Language, Speech and Hearing Services in Schools, 16,* 199–210.

Kanner, L. (1943). Autistic disturbances of affective contact. *Nervous Child; 2,* 217–250.

Koegel, R. & Koegel, L. (Eds.). (1995). *Teaching children with autism: Strategies for initiating positive interactions and improving learning opportunities.* Baltimore: Paul H. Brookes.

Lahey, M. (1988). *Language disorders and language development.* New York: Merrill/Macmillan.

Leonard, L. (1991). Specific language impairment as a clinical category. *Language, Speech and Hearing Services in Schools, 22,* 66–68.

Loeb, D., & Leonard, L. (1991). Subject case marking and verb morphology in normally developing and specifically language-impaired children. *Journal of Speech and Hearing Research, 34,* 340–346.

Long, S. (1994). Language and children with autism. In V. Reed (Ed.), *An introduction to children with language disorders* (2nd ed., pp 231–256). New York: Merrill.

Long, S. H., & Long, S. T. (1994). Language and children with learning disabilities. In V. Reed (Ed.), *An introduction to children with language disorders* (2nd ed., pp. 193–229). New York: Merrill.

Lord, C., Rutter, M., & LeCouteur, A. (1994). Autism diagnostic interview revised. *Journal of Autism and Developmental Disorders, 24,* 659–686.

Lovaas, O. (1977). The autistic child: *Language development through behavior modification.* New York: Irvington.

Milosky, L. (1994). Nonliteral language abilities: Seeing the forest for the trees. In G. Wallach & K. Butler (Eds.), *Language learning disabilities in school-age children and adolescents: Some principles and applications* (pp. 275–303). Needham Heights, MA: Allyn & Bacon.

Mundy, P., Sigman, M., and Kasari, C. (1990). A longitudinal study of joint attention and language development in autistic children. *Journal of Autism and Developmental Disorders, 20,* 115–128.

Paul, R. (1991). Profiles of toddlers with slow expressive language development. *Topics in Language Disorders, 11*(4), 1–13.

Piven, J., Gayle, J., Landa, R., Wzorek, M., & Folstein, S. (1991). The prevalence of Fragile X in a sample of autistic individuals diagnosed using a standardized interview. *Journal of the American Academy of Child and Adolescent Psychiatry, 30,* 825–830.

Prinz, P., & Ferrier, L. (1983). "Can you give me that one?": The comprehension, production and judgment of directives in language-impaired children. *Journal of Speech and Hearing Disorders, 55,* 179–192.

Prizant, B.M., & Duchan, J. F. (1981). The functions of immediate echolalia in autistic children. *Journal of Speech and Hearing Disorders, 46,* 241–249.

Prizant, B.M. & Wetherby, A.M. (1988). Providing services to children with autism (ages 0 to 2 years) and their families. *Topics in Language Disorders, 9,*1–23.

Prizant, B. M. & Wetherby, A.M. (1990). Toward an integrated view of early language and communication development and socioemotional development. *Topics in Language Disorders. 10*(4), 1–16.

Reed, V. A. (1994). *An introduction to children with language disorders:* (2nd ed). New York: Merrill.

Ripich, D. N. & Griffith, P. L. (1988). Narrative abilities of children with learning disabilities and nondisabled children: Story structure, cohesion, and proposition. *Journal of Learning Disabilities, 21,* 165–173.

Rosen, C. D., CA & Gerring, J. P. (1986). *Head trauma: Educational re-integration.* San Diego, CA: College Hill.

Rutter, M. (1978). Diagnosis and definition of childhood autism. *Journal of Autism and Childhood Schizophrenia, 8,* 139–161.

Sacks, O. (1994). *An anthropologist on Mars.* New York: Random House.

Savage, R. C. & Carter, R. (1984). Re-entry: The head injured student returns to school. *Cognitive Rehabilitation, 2*(6), 28–33.

Scarborough, H., & Dobrick, W. (1990). Development of children with early language delay. *Journal of Speech and Hearing Research, 33,* 70–83.

Schopler, E. (1996). Editorial. *Journal of Autism and Developmental Disorders, 21,* 8.

Scott, C. M. (1989). Problem writers: Nature, assessment and intervention. In A. G. Kahmi & H. W. Catts (Eds.), *Reading disabilities: A developmental language perspective* (pp. 303–344). Boston: Allyn & Bacon.

Scott, C. M. (1994). A discourse continuum for school-age students: Impact of modality and genre. In G. P. Wallach & K. G. Butler (Eds.), *Language learning disability in school age children and adolescents: Some principles and applications* pp. 219–252. Needham Heights, MA: Allyn & Bacon.

Seigel, B., Vukicevic, J., Elliott, G., & Kraemer, H. (1989). The use of signal detection theory to assess DSM III-R criteria for autistic disorder. *Journal of the American Academy of Child and Adolescent Psychiatry, 28,* 542–548.

Sevin, J., Matson, J., Coe, D., Love, S., Matese, M., & Benavidez, D. (1996). Empirically derived subtypes of PDD: A cluster analytic study. *Journal of Autism and Developmental Disorders, 21*, 59–86.

Shane, H., & Kearns, K. (1994). An examination of the role of the facilitator in FC. *American Journal of Speech-Language Pathology, 3*, 48–54.

Shaywitz, S. H., Fletcher, J. M., & Shaywitz, B. A. (1994). Issues in the definition and classification of attention deficit disorder. *Topics in Language Disorders, 14*, 1–25.

Shelton, T. L., & Barkley, R. A. (1994). Critical issues in the assessment of attention deficit disorders in children. *Topics in Language Disorders, 14*(4), 26–41.

Shriberg, L., & Kwiatkowski, J. (1988). A followup study of children with phonological disorders of unknown origin. *Journal of Speech and Hearing Disorders, 53*, 144–155.

Silliman, E. R. & Wilkinson, L. C. (1994). Observing is more than looking. In G. P. Wallach and K. G. Butler (Eds.), *Language and learning disability in school age children and adolescents: Some principles and applications* (pp. 27–52). Needham Heights, MA: Allyn & Bacon.

Sonnenmeier, R., & Duchan, J. (1994). *Issues of validation: A history and review of methods used to validate facilitated communication.* Paper presented at the Facilitated Communication Conference, Syracuse University, Syracuse, NY.

Szkeres, S. F., & Meserve, N. F. (1994). Collaborative intervention in schools after traumatic brain injury. *Topics in Language Disorders, 15*(1), 21–36.

Tallal, P. (1988). Developmental language disorders. In J. Kavanaugh & T. Truss (Eds.) *Learning disabilities: Proceedings of the national conference* (pp. 181–272). Parkton, MD: York.

Thal, D. (1991). Language and cognition in normal and late talking toddlers. *Topics in Language Disorders, 11*(4), 33–42.

U.S. Department of Education (1991). *Thirteenth annual report to Congress on the implementation of the Individuals with Disabilities Education Act.* Washington, D.C.: U.S. Department of Education, Office of Special Education Programs.

Van Kleek, A. (1994). Metalinguistic development. In G. P. Wallach & K. G. Butler (Eds.), *Language and learning disability in school age children and adolescents: Some principles and applications* (pp. 53–98). Needham Heights, MA: Allyn & Bacon.

Van Kleek, A. (1995). Emphasizing form and meaning separately in prereading and early reading instruction. *Topics in Language Disorders, 16*(1), 50–66.

Vasquez, C. (1994). Brief report: Multi-task controlled evaluation of facilitated communication. *Journal of Autism and Developmental Disorders, 24*, 369–376.

Vasquez, C. (1995). Failure to confirm the word retrieval problem hypothesis in facilitated communication. *Journal of Autism and Developmental Disorders, 25*, 597–610.

Vellutino, F. R. (1979). *Dyslexia: Theory and research.* Cambridge, MA: MIT Press.

Vellutino, F. R. & Scanlon, D. M. (1987). Phonological coding, phonological awareness, and reading ability: Evidence from a longitudinal and experimental study. *Merrill-Palmer Quarterly, 33*, 321–363.

Volden, J., & Lord, C. (1991). Neologisms and idiosyncratic language in autistic speakers. *Journal of Autism and Developmental Disorders, 21*, 109–130.

Wallach, G. P. (1990). Magic buries Celtics: Looking for broader interpretations of language, learning and literacy. *Topics in Language Disorders, 10*(2), 62–80.

Wallach, G. P. & Butler, K. G. (1994). (Eds.). *Language and learning disability in school age children and adolescents: Some principles and applications.* Needham Heights, MA: Allyn & Bacon.

Watkins, R. & Rice, M. (1991). Verb particle and proposition acquisition in language-impaired preschoolers. *Journal of Speech and Hearing Research, 34*, 1130–1141.

Wiig, E. H. & Becker-Caplan, L. (1984). Linguistic retrieval strategies and word finding difficulties among children with language disabilities. *Topics in Language Disorders, 4*(3), 1–18.

Wilcox, M. J. (1989). Delivering communication-based services to infants, toddlers and their families: Approaches and models. *Topics in Language Disorders, 10*(1), 68–79.

Wolf, M., & Goodglass, H. (1986). Dyslexia, dysnomia, and lexical retrieval: A longitudinal investigation. *Brain and Language, 28*, 154–168.

Ylsivaker, M. (Ed.) (1985). *Head injury rehabilitation: Children and adolescents.* San Diego, CA: College Hill.

Ylsivaker, M., Kolpan, K., & Rosenthal, M. (1994). Collaboration in preparing for personal injury suits after TBI. *Topics in Language Disorders, 15*(1), 1–20.

Part II

Program Implementation

Chapter 6

Assessment

Jacqueline Meyer

Because this textbook represents many different views, you, as student or instructor, should know where the author of this particular chapter and Chapter 8 is "coming from." As a speech-language professional who has worked in the school environment for many years, and as an instructor in undergraduate and graduate diagnostics, language, and school organization courses, I wanted to develop a chapter that could serve as a practical introduction to assessment in the schools. At different times, I have acted as a "master teacher" or a college supervisor to speech pathology students during their student teaching practicum. Because of this experience, you will find that I often favor lists and examples over an explanation of theory. This is not because theory is not vitally important in assessment and intervention. It is, but although theoretical information may answer the "why," it usually does not answer the "how." As befits a text of this type, I hope these chapters will speak to that ever-present student question, "What should I do tomorrow morning?"

Both chapters will be written as if I were talking to you in class or the "speech" room—that is, in the first and second person, "I" and "you." I loved Rhea Paul's (1995) description of the first person in the preface to her text

Language Disorders From Infancy Through Adolescence as "cranky, preachy, and personal" (p. xi   ). Replacing the third-person point of view serves several purposes. It streamlines sentences, as in "Plan your assessment with great care" versus "Assessment must be planned with great care by the school speech-language professional". It also helps remove infallibility from the statements I make in these two chapters. Part of the reason our field of speech-language pathology is so intellectually exciting is that within it there are so many different ways to accomplish goals in assessment and intervention. There is almost never a single "correct" way to implement goals. This inherent flexibility gives us the freedom to try new procedures or disregard or revamp old ones. Theories clash, opinions differ, and personalities dictate different solutions, making ours a volatile, challenging, constantly changing field. And the 21st century beckons with a promise of more of the same.

Much of the content of this book deals with services provided to school-age children under the provisions of Public Law No. 94-142 and its later revisions and expansions that were discussed in Chapter 2. Under these laws and individual state guidelines, assessment functions as part of the law's charge to "locate, identify and serve all handicapped pupils." So here we have it: one of the key responsibilities of a school speech-language specialist is assessment. And to an inexperienced person, this whole area may be a scary prospect. Most professionals ask themselves, at one time or another, How do I know what to do? What tests should I choose? Should I try dynamic assessment? Curriculum-based evaluation? What about language sampling? I've never even *seen* a child with a traumatic brain injury or Fragile-X Syndrome or swallowing problems or _____ (fill in the blank). After I finish, how do I know if the child should be labeled? How do I interpret the results and write an Individualized Education Program (IEP) that will really improve the child's communication skills? First, be assured that these are normal concerns. Every new speech-language professional feels the same way. Second, it is not only those relatively new to the field who fret about this; in the course of your career, these questions will recur each time you are faced with a student who represents an area with which you are unfamiliar.

To begin, every competent speech-language professional knows that no one set of tests or procedures can fit every student's needs. With the pressure of a large caseload, limited time for assessment, and reduced funding, however, it is frequently tempting to "make do" with the tests that the district already has or to use the same procedure for every child who comes before the Committee on Special Education. Regardless of the temptation, the ethical consideration remains clear: "Individuals shall honor their responsibility to hold paramount the welfare of persons served professionally" (American Speech-Language-Hearing Association [ASHA] Code of Ethics; see Chapter 3). That is, you must always ask yourself, when you plan any

procedure or assessment, if it is in the best interests of the student. (This is the preachy mode.)

Entire textbooks have been written discussing the theory and ramifications of assessment. In 1986, ASHA published an annotated bibliography of more than 100 presentations, texts, and articles on language disorders (Shulman et al., 1986). Currently available from ASHA (1995) is a directory that provides information on over 300 instruments that assess spoken and written language, cognitive communication, fluency, voice, articulation/phonology, swallowing, and oral-motor function along with test batteries and developmental scales for all ages, including the school-age population. The entire issue of *Language, Speech, and Hearing Services in Schools* in April 1996 was devoted to one segment of assessment: observing and interpreting behaviors of the school-age child. In October 1995 in the same journal, authors of five articles presented new language norms for this population. Within the past few years, excellent texts specifically addressing language issues and the school-age population have appeared; for example, those by Paul (1995), Simon (1985a, 1985b), Wood (1982), Wiig and Semel (1984a), and Wallach and Butler (1994). Clearly, assessment issues are alive and well in our profession. Yet even with new or refined information, we continue to struggle to provide appropriate guidelines for when or if a *specific* child should receive speech-language services. Consequently a single chapter like this one can contain only a brief overview of the process involved in choosing and applying procedures to determine if language deficits exist, if they are severe enough to warrant intervention, and if so, how to identify them in enough detail to provide a basis for appropriate intervention. The problem that strikes fear into my author's heart is what to include and what to leave out. (This is the personal mode.)

Therefore I will start with a disclaimer. This chapter can serve only as a very general guide, rather like a house plan in a magazine. It gives you an idea of what the house would look like, but if you want to actually build it, you will need the architectural blueprints. Often the detailed, highly specialized information you need to "zero in" on the subtle problem of a specific student will be absent from this chapter. On a routine basis, you must learn to access the wonderful resources in journal articles; computer webs, comprehensive texts, and sources of condensed versions of information such as the journal *Word of Mouth*, workshops, conventions, teleconferences, in-service opportunities, and, most important, a network of supportive colleagues. Throughout this chapter, I shall refer to a number of written sources that I hope can guide you as you develop your personal professional library. In an attempt to make the amount of information more manageable, I have divided this chapter into three major sections. The first contains a discussion of (for want of a better term) "traditional" approaches to assessment in the schools and a synopsis of measurement terms and concepts. The second features a sampling of some exciting new ways to look at evaluating language, such as an application of Vygotskian developmental theory to the process, curriculum-based assessment, and dynamic assessment. And the third offers four specific cases illustrating the general concepts covered in the preceding two sections. Although many of your students will be female, to simplify the text I have substituted "he" for the awkward "he or she" except in the case studies. Flying in the face of political correctness, I feel that clarity is preferred here.

TRADITIONAL APPROACHES TO ASSESSMENT

Historically, the school speech-language professional has investigated suspected deficits in phonology, morphology, syntax, semantics, voice, fluency, and pragmatics either as a force behind the choice of structure or as an additional and separable part of language in general (Lund & Duchan, 1993). Within these areas of form, content, and use, the specialist has addressed both receptive and expressive skills. In recent years, we have made an additional distinction between language difference and language disorder when we assess the impact of dialect, English as a second language, or contrasting cultural features on a child's communicative competence (Roseberry-McKibbin, 1995). As the principle of inclusion has introduced children with more severe handicapping conditions into the general school population, we have also become responsible for decisions concerning augmentative communication. Therefore, because the range of deficits occurring in the school-age population can be so broad and because all linguistic areas are so intertwined with reading and writing, we must plan assessment with exquisite care. To recommend that a student should or should not receive our services is an awesome responsibility and not to be taken lightly.

The assessment process starts with *case finding*, may proceed to *case selection*, and ultimately may result in a student's being added to your caseload as a speech-language professional. Before embarking on these topics, however, we will take a short detour into the world of measurement. The results of any standardized testing procedure are only as good as the tests themselves. A testing corollary of the computer truism "Garbage in, garbage out" is "Put good food into a contaminated container, and it becomes contaminated too." Therefore, before you trust the interpretation of standardized test results, you must determine to what extent the instrument in question qualifies as a "good" measure *for your purpose*. Part of that process involves understanding what the terms used by the authors of the instrument mean.

I have adapted the most frequently used descriptive terms from a variety of sources; they are listed in Exhibit 6–1. I am assuming that you have had at least some academic training in testing. If you have completed a recent course on the subject, you may find that you can just scan the table. If this is not the case, then you should consult a college textbook on measurement to clarify any terms you do not understand or review other aspects of formal assessment not discussed below. Incidentally, it is a valuable exercise to restate the definitions of the exhibit in your own words. Often you will have to explain these terms to parents, many of whom may have a limited educational background. Casually using these terms in a meeting with a parent who does not understand them can defeat the reason for the conference.

Lund and Duchan (1993) warned that reliability can be adversely affected by factors other than the test items themselves, such as unclear or complicated directions or individual test administrators' interpreting the questions differently. They also cautioned that the model of language on which the test is developed becomes an important question in judging whether or not the questions on the instrument actually measure language—that is, their basic validity. If you frequently deal with dialectical differences or pragmatics—for example, if you wish to discover in which environments different kinds of language are or are not appropriate—you may conclude that the "mismatch" language model is most germane. At other times, you may be more interested in the etiology of a language problem, such as autism, mental retardation, or cerebral palsy (the categorical model). Other commonly used models are those that involve information processing, a neuropsychological basis, auditory processing, or descriptive-developmental aspects. Rather than being identified as models per se, this information is sometimes described as a series of "approaches" and is covered during a historical review of diagnosis in speech-language pathology. The relationship of either to assessment lies in the fact that changing views about what language *is* lead to new tests and procedures. At some point you must evaluate them and decide whether to use them in your practice or disregard them. Sabers (1996) cautioned that "by deciding to use one test over another, the clinician adopts the operational definition of the test's authors" (p. 103). Lest you consider this an esoteric issue, during legal hearings attorneys commonly question specialists like speech-language professionals on the validity of their assessment procedures. A single chapter like this one obviously cannot include any real discussion of these issues, but most texts on language development go into the subject thoroughly, and a review of them can be very helpful as you analyze tests or procedures. I refer you to them. Hutchinson's (1996) article on how to use a technical manual is very helpful for inexperienced clinicians who must choose tests for their districts.

A frequently overlooked avenue of information about a specific test is the publisher of the instrument. If you have specific questions about the normative group or about whether, for example, you can repeat an instruction to

Exhibit 6–1 Common Testing Terminology

Age-equivalent score: the age corresponding to the average raw score on a task obtained by students of a particular age. Most authorities caution against using only this score to determine eligibility.

Anecdotal record: a written report of an incident describing a student's behavior, selected because of its assumed significance. Teachers will often provide ones that are "typical" or "surprising"; anecdotal records are an integral part of interpretation-driven assessment.

Basal: the lowest point in testing from which progress is recorded; all items below this point are assumed to be correct, and credit is given for them, even if the student has not completed those items.

Ceiling: the highest item of a sequence in which a certain number of items have been failed (e.g., six out of eight wrong). It is assumed that all items beyond this point are incorrect, even if they are not administered.

Criterion referenced test: establishes the criteria for acceptable responses; measures skills in terms of absolute levels of mastery (e.g., a multiplication test). Usually criterion-referenced tests cover relatively small units of content. They tell what a student can do, rather than his or her performance in relation to other students. See McCauley (1996) for an application to speech and language.

Derived scores: scores computed from raw scores that allow comparison of a student's performance to the performances of the normative sample (e.g., a percentile rank, a standard score).

Grade equivalent: a score that states the student's achievement in terms of the average expectations for a grade level. A common score in end-of-the-year tests in reading, math, etc.

Mean: the average score of a subject age group on a task. It is computed by dividing the sum of scores by the number of scores: the statistical average.

Mental age: a measure of a child's level of mental development, based on his performance on a test of mental ability and determined by the level of difficulty of the test items passed. If a child, regardless of age, can pass only those items passed by an average 6-year-old, the child will be assigned a mental-age (MA) score of 6 years; see Francis et al. (1996) for a discussion of this topic as it applies to language assessment.

Normative study: the procedure by which the final version of a test is administered to a large sample of subjects. The performances are then statistically analyzed and reported as test norms and derived scores.

Norm-referenced test: a test that compares a student's performance to the performances of a representative sample of peers. It allows an understanding of where the child's performance falls compared to that of others.

Percentile rank: the ranking that indicates the percentage of raw scores within a particular age/grade group that were lower than the raw score in question. If your raw score places you at the 35th percentile, then 34% of your peers scored lower and 65% scored higher than you did. Parents often confuse this term with a percentage.

Practice effect: the change in scores on a test, usually a gain, resulting from previous practice with the test. This is one of the reasons that you should not repeat the same standardized test too soon after it has been given before; usually the waiting period is 6 months to a year. Alternate forms of a test can circumvent this effect.

Raw score: the number earned when correct test items are computed; for example, if there are 16 correct answers, and each is worth 2 points, the raw score is 32. The raw score is usually converted into another type of score.

continues

Exhibit 6–1 continued

Reliability: in general, the consistency with which a test measures a given attribute or behavior, the stability, precision, and accuracy of scores. These can include:

Test-retest: the stability of test scores over time. It is measured by repeat testing of a group of students within a relatively short time.

Content sampling reliability: the internal consistency of a test; a measure of the interrelationship of test items.

Split-half reliability: a measure of a task's reliability obtained by comparing scores obtained on one half of the task with scores on the other half of the test.

Interexaminer reliability: a measure of the variability with which different examiners administer or score a test.

Standardization: the process of administering a test in a systematic and consistent way to a large sample of subjects.

Standardized test: a test composed of selected materials with definite directions for use, predetermined norms, and data on reliability and validity.

Standard score: transforms raw scores into a set of scores having the same mean and standard deviation.

Test norms: the statistical summary of the raw scores received by the normative sample; usually represented in a table.

Validity: the extent to which a test actually assesses the skills that it was designed to assess. Kinds of validity it can include

Content validity: the extent to which a particular domain of content, such as expressive single-word vocabulary, represents a balanced and adequate sampling of what the test purports to measure, such as overall semantic ability.

Face validity: a reference to the apparent content validity of a test that is examined superficially or by an untrained individual.

Criterion-related validity: the extent to which scores on a test are related to some true measure of the behavior being assessed. This is often a question in language tests: Do they really measure language?

Concurrent validity: a measure of criterion-related validity that compares subjects' performances on the test to those on another similar test administered at about the same time.

Predictive validity: a measure of criterion-related validity that estimates the extent to which test performances can be expected to relate to future performances on a criterion measure.

Contrasted groups validity: a measure of criterion-related validity that compares the extent to which a test significantly discriminates between normal subjects and subjects known to possess disabilities for the skills being assessed. This is particularly important in screening.

a student, you should ask, preferably in writing. This serves not only to clear up your confusion but also to alert the publisher that you, as a user and potential buyer of either future tests or "new, improved" versions of the instrument in question, require more detailed or more clearly written information. In other words, if the test directions drive you crazy, complain. If you do not understand, ask. If

the instrument does not include in the normative group members of the body to which your student belongs, do not use the test, and tell the publisher why. (We have reached the cranky mode.)

In addition to the "technical" considerations, all of us, teachers and students alike, should check tests for possible cultural bias. The issue of multicultural sensitivity addressed in Chapter 11 is particularly important in assessment because of the danger of overidentification—that is, of increasing "false positives" and consequent overrepresenting of minority students in special education programs. Federal law states that assessment must be racially or culturally nondiscriminatory. As a beginning, make sure that the normative data reflect the plurality of our population and specifically include the group to which your student belongs. Some commonly administered instruments like the Peabody Picture Vocabulary Test-Revised *PPVT-R*; (Dunn & Dunn, 1981) have been investigated for cultural and/or gender bias (Washington & Craig, 1992; Willabrand & Iwanta-Reuyl, 1994). McFadden's (1996) article on what constitutes "normal" in normative sampling raises some crucial issues regarding overidentification in general. It remains difficult, however, to determine if a test is fair, unbiased, and nondiscriminatory for *every* individual child to whom you administer it. Appendix 6–A contains a list of instruments that either have been developed for a specific population or have alternate responses for members of another group, such as students who use Black English. Be aware that this is only a list and does not represent an endorsement. Because many of the instruments are so new, they have not yet been subjected to the test of time or the scrutiny of researchers. In short, *caveat emptor*: let the buyer beware. As you pursue your professional life, adopt the habit of sharing your experiences of using new tests/procedures with colleagues; this is how the body of information on which we all rely grows.

In judging a test, we should also routinely investigate how easy or complicated it is to *learn*, *administer*, and *score* it. In addition, note the time actually required both to administer it completely and then score it. I remember with a shudder the first time I tried to score the then "new" Clinical Evaluation of Language Fundamentals-Revised (CELF-R; Semel, Wiig, & Secord, 1987). I was familiar with the original CELF (Semel & Wiig, 1980) and assumed I would have no problem scoring the newest version because I had just administered it with no difficulty. Several hours later, I was still flipping pages in the instructor's manual trying to figure out the confidence intervals. I can now score this instrument in minutes, even without computer assistance, but I feel obligated to warn students in my classes that this is not an instrument to score "cold" the night before they have to present results to the Committee on Special Education. The CELF-3 (1995) has simplified the scoring process, leading me to believe that users informed the publisher that changes were in order. Other tests like the Token Test for Children (DeSimoni, 1978) or the Test of Word Finding (German, 1991) require much practice to administer smoothly and correctly. As overwhelming as the "alphabet soup" of test names may seem, be sure also that you can pronounce and spell them: it is the CELF, not the SELF; the TACL, not the TACKLE; and, my favorite student "goof," the Lindamood Test, not Linda's Mood Test.

Apart from these issues, the single most important fact is if the test addresses the suspected, specific deficits of the student for whom the evaluation is planned. In the third major section of this chapter, "Case Studies,"we will plan assessment procedures for four different profiles of student deficits; part of that process will be choosing appropriate standardized instrument(s).

CASE FINDING

Remember that the Education of the Handicapped Amendments of 1986 (EHA) and the Individuals with Disabilities Education Act of 1990 (IDEA), the successors to the Education for all Handicapped Children Act of 1975 (Pub. L. No. 94-142), require schools to locate, identify, and serve students with any handicapping condition. In our field, case finding involves locating school-age and preschool students who are communicatively impaired or who appear educationally at risk because of suspected language deficits. Different ways for the school district to find preschool students will be discussed in the next chapter, but the most typical means for locating school age children are referral or screening. Because your individual state/district will vary in its specific requirements, however, you must make every reasonable effort to keep current with its regulations, often referred to as "the regs." The chair of the Committee on Special Education or your district's director of special education receives this information on a continuing basis. Regardless of the specifics, your initial contact with one of these students forms the foundation of your professional accountability, which continues throughout the intervention process. The spirit of the federal and state guidelines requiring you to consider the needs of the student who may have a handicapping condition should be implicit in all decisions as you plan and complete screening, assessment, and intervention procedures.

Screening

Screening Groups of Students

Frequently the first testing procedure a 4- or 5-year-old encounters is a general preschool or kindergarten screening. *Screening* can be defined as a preliminary method of distinguishing handicapped individuals from the general student population; that is, the means used to identify those in need of further evaluation. Most schools routinely screen all kindergarten or first-grade students; many also screen transfers, regardless of grade, and/or any student who scores below acceptable levels on certain state-mandated achievement tests, such as a second- or third-grade reading or mathematics examination. You, as the speech-language professional, will be responsible for part of this process. In fact, screening often serves as an introduction to the concept of team-based evaluation. Many school districts, for example, divide kindergarten screening into stations overseen by the school nurse (medical history, vision and dental screening), the physical education teacher (gross motor ability), the school psychologist (basic cognitive skills, behavioral concerns), the kindergarten teachers (scholastic readiness, including fine motor skills), and the speech-language professional (fluency, voice, articulation, and language skills). Hearing screening may be done by a speech-language professional, the school nurse, or, in some large districts, an educational audiologist. Chapter 4 contains specific information relating to audiological issues. Because there is often overlap among these professionals, be careful that the procedures and instruments complement rather than duplicate each other. This is particularly important because children at this age (and their parents!) may be very nervous, and testing should not last any longer than necessary.

The portion of a general screening supervised by a speech-language pathologist, remember, is *not* a means to determine if a child has a speech/language deficit. It serves only to identify those students who *appear* to be at risk. Therefore it is not necessary, or even desirable, for any one area of language (e.g., phonology, syntax) to be examined in detail. What is important is that the screening neither over- nor underidentify students with potential speech/language problems. Most school clinicians agree, unfortunately, that they have yet to find the "perfect" screening test/procedure. To compound the difficulty, at one time or another, screenings include students from kindergarten through Grade 12.

Let us begin with the easiest. Almost all versions of *kindergarten* screening include the following, either as part of a standardized screening instrument or through less formal means:

- *Phonology*: usually only the most frequently misarticulated sounds are included (i.e., /s, tʃ, ʃ, z, l, r, ɵ, and f/)
- *Receptive language*: often following two- and three-stage directions (e.g., "Put the ball in the cup, and the spoon in your lap")
- *Expressive language*: usually sentence repetition tasks, story retelling, or talking about an actual incident (e.g., the child's birthday party)
- *Fluency and voice*: evaluated during screening of the previous areas

Some screening instruments, such as the Speech-Ease Screening Inventory (K-1) (Piggott et al., 1985), also include a language sample and tasks addressing vocabulary, basic concepts, similarities/differences, sentence repetition, and linguistic relationships.

For children in the upper elementary grades, articulation screening can be accomplished by having the student count to 20 or say the days of the week or the months of the year. This also provides information about whether recitation of these common series has become automatic. Unfortunately, these procedures do not address underlying receptive or metaphonological deficits that can negatively affect spelling and reading, a connection that will be discussed in Chapter 8.

Some school districts, such as Chappaqua in southern New York State, develop their own instruments. This school district's screening test for Grades 3 through 5 has short sections addressing spontaneous verbal expression (how to play a game/sport, etc.), vocabulary (picture identification, analogies, synonyms, multiple meanings, word retrieval), figurative language (riddles, absurdities), verbal comprehension (story questions, memory for sentences, following directions), and syntax (sentence combining and sentence formulation).

If the district has not developed such a tool, receptive skills are almost always addressed through a standardized instrument, such as a vocabulary test or one involving classroom spatial and temporal terms. If a standardized screening instrument is not used to address expressive language ability, you can play a game, ask questions about the child's interests, or require the student to explain, for example, how to make a peanut butter sandwich. Although screening based on less formal procedures may give you a sense of how the child uses language in naturalistic contexts, judging if the student should or should not be assessed further may be more difficult for the inexperienced speech-language professional. Consequently, in this age group, standardized tests are usually employed for at least part of the screening.

For students in high school, screening is usually based on referral—that is, it is almost never of the "general" variety. It is rare, also, that high school students are being referred for the first time unless they have become seriously ill or injured. Almost always, these students have struggled academically at some point in the past and may even have received services but have not been continued on the caseload of a speech-language professional. As the language demands of the school curriculum increase, however, their ability to compensate reaches the breaking point. Owens (1995) stated, "Language impairment may persist across the lifetime of the individual and may vary in symptoms, manifestations, effects, and severity over time and as a consequence of context, content, and learning task" (p. 22). It has been my experience that high school students, if they receive services from a speech-language pathologist at all, do so as a related service, as part of a learning disabilities label, unless they exhibit a severe communication handicap. Consequently screening is much more likely to focus on classroom pragmatics or an inability to handle curriculum, often with demonstrated weaknesses in both reading and writing. Therefore screening instruments that focus on those areas are most useful. Paul (1995) presented both a student self-assessment form to be used with these students and a checklist adapted from Damico (pp. 481, 483).

As noted above, school districts vary widely in the instruments that they use; a number of them are included in Appendix 6–B. If you are inexperienced and must develop screening procedures, often parts of different instruments can be combined; for example, you might administer the articulation screening procedure from the Arizona Articulation Proficiency Scale (AAPS; Fudala & Reynolds, 1989) or the articulation portion of the original Preschool Language Scale (Zimmerman, Steiner, & Pond, 1979), in addition to a storytelling procedure. For several years, I used both the Computerized Articulation Screening Test, which included articulation, receptive language, and sentence repetition items (Fitch, 1985), and the vocabulary plates from the Joliet 3 Minute Speech and Language Screen (Kinzler & Johnson, 1993). Because the computerized test contained no normative data, we calculated local norms based on six kindergarten classes over 3 years'

time. Be aware that in-depth investigations of likely deficits revealed through screening are planned and take place under quite different circumstances. These will be discussed later under "Case Selection." First, however, let us continue with some additional categories of screening.

Other Types of Screening

Up to this point, articulation/language screening as part of the case-finding process has referred to a brief procedure administered to large groups of students, whether or not deficits were suspected. But screening can also help determine if a student who has been referred for a possible handicapping condition should undergo a complete speech-language evaluation, as in the case of the high school screening discussed above. In this case, you already know that some sort of deficit is interfering with the student's classroom performance. Therefore you want either to eliminate language as a causative factor or to confirm that a likely connection exists. Other types of screening instruments, usually more lengthy, can be used for this purpose. The Bankson Language Screening Test-2 (Bankson, 1977) or the Pre-School Language Scale-3 (Zimmerman, Steiner, & Pond, 1992) are typical of this type. If a language-based disability appears likely, then you continue and assess deficits in greater depth. In many screening instruments, there is a "cutoff" point. Depending on the instrument and the child's age, that point determines whether the child has "passed" or "failed" this part of the screening. In some school districts, if children have not failed the screening but their scores indicate a weakness, they may be placed in groups for "speech improvement." In essence, this designation refers to the children who may benefit from intervention, but who do not qualify for a label. But because of lack of qualified personnel and/or limited funds, many districts have discarded this designation.

Another type of screening addresses a specific deficit area, such as fluency, articulation, or voice. In many cases, you use an instrument specifically devised for this purpose on the basis of a note you have made to yourself, such as "Check for voice problems." Usually a comment like this one does not suggest a full-scale evaluation but only constitutes a reminder to use an additional screening instrument with a narrower focus. Because many screenings take place in the spring and fall, allergies are common; when the pollen disappears, voice quality frequently returns to normal. Voice and fluency screening are often addressed through checklists, self-inventories, or scales found in any text on assessment in speech-language pathology. Case histories, observation, and interviews are particularly important in these areas and will also be discussed later under "Case Selection." Remember, the whole process may cease at this point. First-grade teachers refer many more students for learning disability (LD) evaluations than are actually diagnosed as LD. Consider a child in the first grade who "sounds funny." Screening may reveal only that this 6-year-old does not pronounce medial or final /r/ correctly or that he or she has a dialectical variation (he or she is from Houston, Long Island, or Maine).

Guidelines for Screening Choices

What characteristics of screening procedures and instruments should you consider as you make your choices? Different states/districts may vary in their specific rules for general screening, but most of them specify that this type of testing, regardless of the student's age, must

- be fair/unbiased, nondiscriminatory
- be presented in the child's native language

- be normative or criterion referenced
- be completed by a professional or trained paraprofessional
- be completed within specific time guidelines (e.g., by December 1 of the child's kindergarten year)
- be administered to a group (i.e., not used for an individual student except with the express written consent of the child's parent/guardian)
- test a broad enough span of ages so that it can be given to all children typically in the group or be an alternate test for slightly older or younger students. It is wise to avoid an instrument if the child's age places him or her at the upper/lower limits of the test.
- be valid and reliable
- have clear directions
- be easy to administer. Because kindergarten screening is often the first time a child experiences a "school-type" test, you want your attention on the child's responses, not on difficult-to-manipulate materials.
- be easy and quick to score. Some screening tests can be scored by computer, a real timesaver. If the results do not require interpretation, sometimes scoring can be completed by an aide.

Instruments should also

- screen articulation of age-appropriate phonemes
- screen both receptive and expressive language

If the screening features a standardized instrument, check the instruction manual to verify the acceptability of these factors. If you need additional help in interpreting the information, refer to a standard text on measurement; Hutchinson's 1996 article on what to look for and how to interpret the information in the technical manual is also clear and very helpful. You can also check ASHA's review of the instrument; a number of such reviews appear monthly in *Asha*. Depending on the circumstances, you may choose to emphasize the attributes of one screening procedure/test over another. For example, if you have a huge number of children to screen, you may want to go with one that takes as little time as possible, but if many of your children come from culturally diverse backgrounds, your choice may be quite different. In assessment choices, an enormous "but" seems to lurk perpetually on the horizon; a condition often appears that will dictate a change from an "expert's" preferred method, or from the last time you completed the procedure, or from the way you expected to do it when you walked through the door. Dealing with whatever arises is called "flexibility."

A few last thoughts about screening. First, during the general procedures, you should remain alert to the possibility of a gifted child; this is another reason for choosing an instrument that has a broader age range. Second, the term *screening* can also refer to the procedure of identifying students who fall below a specific reference point on reading or other achievement tests administered to whole grade levels. Although the tests themselves are not screening instruments, you "screen" the results of these tests to identify students who may have undiscovered language deficits (Hill & Haynes, 1992). Last, *screenings* can refer to annual hearing and vision checks of the entire student body.

Although formal screening remains one of the chief ways to locate students who demonstrate communication impairments or who are at risk for them—that is, one of the chief methods of case finding—other types of information are equally important in preliminary assessment or preassessment procedures. They include the careful use of *referrals, observation, interviewing, examination of records,* and *language sampling*.

Referrals

Referrals can come from a concerned parent, from almost anyone within the school community, or from outside agencies or individuals, such as a family physician or preschool program. Because they can include both informal and formal requests, a referral can range from a quick exchange in the teacher's lunchroom ("Please listen to Jonathan") to a written recommendation to the Committee on Special Education that an evaluation take place. Referrals constitute an important part of the assessment process (Kelly & Rice, 1986), and all school personnel who have contact with a student should be encouraged to share their questions and concerns with the speech-language pathologist. Referrals are the most common form of initial identification of the older student (Larson & McKinley, 1995). They usually specify deficits in classroom performance but may not state specifically how these deficits are linked to language. Exhibits 6–2 and 6–3 show two different referral forms, one primarily for elementary and young middle-school students and the other for high school pupils. These forms do address the language link. Presenting an in-service training session in how to use a referral instrument can be a valuable undertaking for you, as the school's expert on speech and language. The meeting may lead to an avalanche of new referrals at first, but it provides an efficient way to sensitize teachers to the ways that speech-language problems can affect classroom performance and behavior.

Exhibit 6–2 Referral Form for Elementary through Middle-School Students

---

Name of student _____ Name of person referring _____
Course/grade _____ Date _____ How long have you had a concern? _____

Please mark any item below if it is of concern (+) or serious concern (++).

Articulation:

_____ student's overall pronunciation is hard to understand
_____ some sounds seem to be missing or in error
_____ student confuses sounds when he/she sounds out words
_____ student confuses sounds when he/she spells

Meaning of Words/Sentences

Student:

_____ has difficulty learning new vocabulary in curriculum
_____ has restricted "everyday" vocabulary
_____ sometimes seems to "search" for words when he/she talks
_____ sometimes uses a "sound-alike" or related word instead of the one he/she wants
_____ overuses particular words, e.g., "thing," "gross,"
_____ has problems understanding more than one meaning of a multiple-meaning word
_____ can't identify the topic sentence in a paragraph
_____ has problems with referents, e.g., pronouns
_____ appears confused by temporal or spatial words
_____ often just doesn't seem to make sense when he/she speaks or writes
_____ often requires many repetitions of directions

Grammatical Form

Student:

_____ leaves off endings of words (walk*ed*), or entire words (he _____ walking)
_____ uses mostly short, simple sentences in speech and/or written work
_____ uses very simple noun and verb phrases
_____ appears confused by sentences containing one or more dependent clauses, e.g., "You may use the computer if you have finished your math, your lab report has been handed in, and you have returned your books to the library."
_____ sometimes confuses the order of words when asking questions or making statements
_____ has problems with irregular forms, e.g., swam, mice, has, etc.
_____ uses incorrect verb tenses in speaking and/or writing
_____ doesn't appear to understand meaning of tense differences, e.g., passive or using multiple auxiliaries, e.g., would have been gone
_____ doesn't recognize grammatical errors even when pointed out
_____ overall, his/her sentences sound like a younger child's

continues

Exhibit 6–2 continued

Social uses of language

Student:

____ is often confused about the routines of the classroom
____ doesn't properly initiate or end conversation with peers
____ doesn't maintain the topic of conversation
____ makes comments that are not organized, difficult to understand the connection
____ stories/explanations often have no point and/or are disorganized
____ persists in one topic of conversation when others want a change
____ doesn't understand implied meaning
____ frequently seems lost during conversation with peers or adults
____ is socially inappropriate
____ appears younger than he/she is
____ doesn't play by the rules

Voice:

____ Student's voice often sounds hoarse or rough
____ Student often speaks too loudly
____ Student often speaks too softly

Fluency

Student:

____ often repeats sounds, syllables, or words when he/she speaks
____ hesitates before he/she begins to talk, sometimes looking distressed
____ blinks, jerks shoulders, moves head before beginning to talk
____ avoids circumstances in which he/she is expected to speak

General comments: Briefly note in what areas of curriculum or instruction you have your greatest concern. If you have used any modifications or other remediation with the student, note them and indicate if they seemed to help or not. Any information you can provide will be of help.

Another type of formal referral is one from the Preschool Committee on Special Education (PCSE). This body deals with children prior to their kindergarten year and oversees their educational needs from birth until the time they enter kindergarten. Here the referral contains much more detailed information, namely results of a full evaluation, the child's present IEP, and a report on the child's progress to date. Usually, although not always, the deficits of these children represent more severe handicapping conditions. Because of space limitations, this chapter will not include typical language profiles of students who represent "special populations." Information in Chapter 5 includes a description of some of the major groups of children eligible for school services. In addition, other sources can be helpful if you need information about specific conditions. Owens (1995), for example, described language implications of traumatic brain injury, mental retardation, language learning disability, specific language impairment, autism, early expressive language delay, and neglect and abuse. Other authors have included severe

Exhibit 6–3 Referral Form, Middle-School through High School Students

---

Name of student _____ Name of person referring _____
Course/grade _____ Date _____ How long have you had a concern? _____

Please mark any item below if it is of concern (+) or serious concern (++).

Reading

The student usually:
____ gains information from independent reading assignments
____ studies for examinations effectively
____ picks out the main idea in paragraphs, chapters, etc.
____ follows written directions without asking for clarification
____ independently accesses information from dictionaries, encyclopedias, and other reference material
____ follows the sequence inherent in written material without difficulty

Writing

In written work, the student usually:

____ does not ramble
____ is unambiguous
____ displays appropriate tone
____ displays adequate handwriting skills
____ displays adequate spelling skills
____ uses correct punctuation and/or capitalization
____ takes adequate notes
       completes take-home assignments that:
       ____ contain descriptions of acceptable quality
       ____ contain explanations of acceptable quality
       ____ contain essay questions of acceptable quality
____ completes a protracted assignment, e.g., a term paper, acceptably
____ uses correct sequencing in written work
____ applies adequate editing skills
       in a test situation:
       ____ produces short-answer questions with adequate written support
       ____ writes essay questions in an acceptable manner
____ displays skills in logic (argumentation)
____ uses age/grade appropriate grammatic complexity

Speaking

The student usually:

____ speaks with no articulation errors
____ speaks fluently
____ uses correct grammar
____ uses age/grade-appropriate complexity
____ discusses everyday topics with adequate skills

continues

Exhibit 6–3 continued

_____ discusses abstract "school" topics with adequate skills
_____ organizes thoughts adequately when speaking
_____ displays adequate vocabulary, including homonyms and multiple-meaning words
_____ makes sense
_____ uses slang appropriately, not dated or overused expressions
_____ keeps to the point, doesn't ramble
_____ does not "search" for word
_____ is not redundant
_____ uses specific vocabulary (doesn't overuse words like "thing," "whatchamacallit," "you know")

Pragmatics

The student usually:

_____ asks clarifying questions
_____ uses humor appropriately ("gets" jokes, tells jokes appropriately, can use sarcasm, can "kid")
_____ understands and uses classroom routines
_____ understands implied meaning
     uses these conversational skills appropriately:
     _____ initiates
     _____ maintains topic
     _____ does not interrupt
     _____ within cultural guidelines, maintains appropriate eye contact
     _____ answers questions
     _____ appears to follow conversation among members of a group of 4 or 5
     _____ can "switch" code between peers and adults in authority
     _____ does not perseverate on a topic when conversational partner wishes to move on
     _____ ends conversation appropriately
_____ uses polite forms
_____ is tactful
_____ reads nonverbal language accurately
_____ can express opinions clearly
_____ can accept another's opinion without anger
_____ can work as part of a small group
_____ can role play
_____ can play a game appropriately following the rules of play

Organization

The student usually:

_____ works independently in the classroom
_____ completes homework
_____ completes in-class assignments
_____ takes notes that are sequenced correctly
_____ takes notes reflecting organizational pattern of lecture
_____ organizes materials in desk, locker, notebooks, and carrier (backpack)

continues

Exhibit 6–3 continued

Listening

The student usually:
____ follows simple oral directions the first time
____ follows complex oral directions the first time
____ follows the organizational pattern of a lecture
____ understands idioms, proverbs, and analogies when presented in context
____ gives some indication that he/she has followed part of the presentation when asking questions
____ can follow orally presented information contained in:
____ films/video tape/ CD-ROM
____ lectures without visual material
____ in-class reports by peers
____ answers questions based on just-presented information
____ distinguishes between inflectional differences that alter meaning
____ recalls and repeats events of an orally presented story/event accurately

Metalinguistics

The student usually:

____ applies rules of pronunciation to unknown words
____ understands and applies prefixes and suffixes to root words
____ recognizes and defines the parts of speech at a grade-appropriate level
____ understands/applies editing rules

General Comments: Briefly note in what areas of your curriculum or instruction you have your greatest concern. If you have used any modifications or other remediation with the student, note them and indicate if they seemed to help or not. Any information you can provide will be of help.

emotional-social dysfunction, motor disorders (cerebral palsy, spina bifida, degenerative diseases), or visual impairment (McCormick & Schiefelbusch, 1984) or have discussed specific syndromes caused by either chromosomal abnormalities (Turner, Fragile-X, 5p-, Prader-Willi, etc.; or metabolic disorders (PKU, thyroid, Hunter syndrome, etc.) (Paul, 1995). Shipley and McAfee (1992) assigned a chapter to assessment of neurologically based communicative disorders. You can also contact organizations that were created to fund research and provide services for families of children who are included in these special groups. Often they provide information about attendant speech-language problems. Remember, school officials frequently rely on your expertise and expect you to assume a leadership role regarding the educational and language implications of these disorders (Hux, Morris-Fríehe, & Sanger, 1993). One more important note: in most school districts, you will provide language support and intervention on a cross-categorical basis— that is, you will group children by what they need to accomplish to make them more competent language learners and users, not by the cause of their deficits.

Observation

The law (IDEA) makes it clear that students must be observed in the classroom if they have been referred for special education services. Unfortunately, observing a student who is suspected of having language deficits is often relegated to a secondary position in the screening/assessment process because of the perceived time involved. Observation, however, is crucial in gaining a clear picture of the student's use and understanding of language within the classroom and other school environments. It is one thing for a student to attend to and reply to a speech-language professional's question in the quiet "speech" room; it is often quite another for the student to perform in the presence of 25 other students in a busy, active classroom. Observing a classroom of "regular" students can also serve as your reality check. It is easy to lose sight of how easily typical students learn, how quick and competent they are. Seeing children with a suspected deficit in the classroom environment where they "live" can be an instructive if painful reminder of how far behind their peers they are. Observation also assumes an additional role in dynamic assessment procedures; these are discussed in the "New Approaches to Assessment" section of this chapter.

Regardless, try to observe the student in as many school locations as possible, particularly if a deficit in pragmatics is suspected. Sites may include "special" classrooms, such as art, music, physical education, or the library, as well as the bus line, the lunchroom, the office, and the hall. Be sensitive to the possibility of culturally based differences if you are observing a child who is not a member of the majority group. Chapter 11 lists a number of cultural factors that can influence a youngster's behavior, such as use of time, individual versus group preference, and organizational style. A typical classroom observation form is included below in Exhibit 6–4; this can be combined with or replaced by one specifically designed for a student who is from a different

culture. Observation is not only part of the screening process but is included in assessing deficits as well. When we discuss the four cases at the end of this chapter, we will look at how observation relates directly to evaluation and developing intervention goals.

A final word about observation in the screening process: try to be alert to information about students wherever it appears. Describe typical *or* unusual behavior, but resist making a subjective interpretation of the behavior without an adequate foundation. When I was a graduate student, another student speech-language pathologist and I were evaluating a 3-year-old. While I took data, my partner administered a standardized instrument to our young client, who was moving around in his chair, was not following directions very well, and appeared anxious. A doctoral candidate and several undergraduate students were viewing the procedure from behind a one-way mirror. The Ph.D. candidate explained to the students that they were observing a most certainly hyperactive, perhaps ADD child. At that point, my partner finished, and I took over. Unaware of what had transpired in the observation booth, this experienced mother of little boys knelt down and asked, "Honey, do you have to go potty?" Clutching his front, our small client frantically yelped, "Yeah!" A short trip to the bathroom later, his ADD with hyperactivity had disappeared. Moral: observe, report, but do not jump to conclusions. At the very least, it can be embarrassing.

In the case of a PCSE referral, it is common that you will be invited to observe the child in his or her preschool setting. At that time, you usually meet with the speech-language professional who is serving the child, as well as the classroom teacher, and you will have an opportunity to ask questions about what you have seen.

Exhibit 6–4 Student Observation

Student _____ Teacher _____ Grade/Subject _____

Date of Observation _____ Time: from _____ to _____ Number of Students in Class _____

If any of the areas below are not applicable, mark a slash through the number:

1. *Position* of student in classroom: front ____ back ____ middle ____ side ____ circle ____

2. Type of *activity*: whole-class lecture ____ small-group lecture ____ cooperative learning ____
   conversational ____ narrative ____ students working independently ____ other: ____

3. *Material read* by student: none ____ text ____ worksheet ____ study sheet ____ test ____
   on chalkboard ____ other : ____ read: aloud ____ silently ____

4. Followed written *directions*: yes _____ no _____ some ____ Comment:

5. *Material written* by student: short answer ____ essay ____ copying ____ note taking ____ Result
   was: acceptable quality ____ not acceptable ____ Comments:

6. Student *attended* (listened): most of time ____ part of time ____ rarely ____ couldn't tell ____

7. Followed orally presented *directions*: yes ____ no ____ some ____ Comments:

8. Student *on task* (completing requirements): most of time ____ part of time ____ rarely ____
   Comments:

9. *Distracted* other *classmates*: yes ____ no ____

10. Student *asked questions*: yes ____: (clarifying ____ asked for new information ____) none ____
    few ____

10. *Responded* appropriately to teacher *questions on material*: yes ____ no ____ part of time ___
    Result: short sentences ____ complex sentences ____ sequenced correctly: yes ____ no ____
    vocabulary : poor ____ rich ____ marginal ____ pragmatics acceptable: yes ____ no ____

11. Number of times student *called on*: ____ volunteered ans/info: ____

12. *Conversation*: initiated ____ took turns ____ polite ____ completed ____ maintained topic ____
    perseverated on topic ____ appeared confused ____ confrontational/antagonistic ____

13. *Student appeared aware of classroom routine*: yes ____ no ____ part of time ____ Comments:

---

continues

Exhibit 6–4 continued

14. Student's reaction to transitions: confused _____ smooth _____ disorganized _____ looked to other students for help _____ Comments:

15. *Modifications present:* list on board/at desk_____ restated information _____ simplified syntax _____ vocabulary/concepts retaught _____modified worksheet/test _____ restatements _____ peer help _____ distractions reduced: visual _____ auditory _____ directions simplified _____

    Teacher: moved around classroom _____ expanded wait time _____ verbal prompts _____ modeling _____ visual prompts _____ mnemonic devices _____ feedback _____

16. Comments, questions, hypotheses, suggestions for follow-up:

School and Other Records

Most schools use a parent information form as part of the kindergarten or first-grade entry process. For the younger student, it usually contains valuable information about language development, medical history, parent educational levels, family members in the household, and so forth. If the student is being seen by a learning disabilities or reading specialist, school psychologist, special education teacher, physical therapist, occupational therapist, social worker, guidance counselor, or other professionals within the school, you should note their perceptions of the student in question. The school nurse usually has current medical information, including developmental information, any prescription drugs the student is taking, and hearing status. The permanent school record can reveal persistent problems in spelling and/or reading, both of which often have a language base (Hill & Haynes, 1992; Temple & Gillet, 1984). Examples of spontaneous (not copied) completed classroom writing assignments should also be analyzed for possible semantic, syntactic, or organizational weaknesses. Written language is decontextualized; that is,

the words alone must convey the message without gestures, intonation, or restatements to help clarify meaning. Consequently a student's language deficits in both syntax and semantics are often more obvious when they are in written form, particularly in the older student.

Language Sampling

Language sampling is not commonly undertaken as part of the screening process in most public school settings. Occasionally, however, formal screening instruments will include a brief sample. This topic will be addressed in more detail in the "Case Selection" section later in the chapter.

Once the screening process has identified a student as a possible candidate for services, there is often a meeting of a school-based team (Child Study Team, Pupil Services Committee, etc.) to determine whether the assessment process should continue under the auspices of the Committee on Special Education. If an evaluation is recommended, there is usually a determination of who will administer what measures. This procedure will be discussed in detail in Chapter 7. During that meeting, however, typically the speech-language pathologist will outline what areas he or she will focus on during his or her evaluation and the procedures that he or she will follow, including the administration of any standardized instruments. This step cannot proceed without written parental permission. How the speech-language professional decides what to do after this meeting will be the subject of the remainder of this chapter.

CASE SELECTION

Selection Criteria

As the result of the screening processes, you may have identified 80 or 90 children who appear at risk and could benefit in some way from your services. Obviously you cannot serve them all, so what factors should you consider when deciding whom to include on your caseload? Most professionals agree that you should reflect on how severe the disorder is in absolute terms, how it specifically affects school performance now and its potential as a causative factor in later problems (its educational significance), the age of the child, the disparity between the child's performance and that of his peers, and the length of time the student has exhibited the problem. Federal guidelines serve as one source of information, as do your particular state and district standards. Recently Medicaid funds have been disbursed to pay school districts for services provided to children in families who receive aid. With the money has come an additional list of rules and regulations. Your professional training, including a number of ASHA position statements, has provided you with yet another set of criteria. Predictably, these criteria can be in conflict with one another.

This problem is discussed in "Issues in Determining Eligibility for Language Intervention," an excellent report published in 1989 by ASHA's Committee on Language Disorders. In brief, it addressed the "economic, administrative and political factors that affect the determination of eligibility for language intervention [and] that are often beyond the speech-language professional's control" (p. 115). The article questioned the definition or model of language on which decisions are based and spoke to such speech-language professional problems as being required

- to use only district-"approved" standardized tests, discrepancy formulas, or other arbitrary criteria to determine eligibility

- to exclude certain groups, such as learning-disabled students, if they are being served by other specialists

- to maintain an excessively large caseload

Other professionals have also expressed concern about these issues—for example, the practice of applying a discrepancy formula (i.e., an arbitrary difference between the student's language abilities and that anticipated based on either chronological or mental age) to determine eligibility. These issues will be discussed later in this chapter under "Standardized Testing." In its entirety, however, ASHA's report provides a detailed discussion that is particularly useful for new school clinicians.

In addition to the above issues, be aware that personal temptation can rear its ugly head. It can be an appealing idea to include on your caseload John, who has a mild, developmental articulation problem but whose school board member parent has been very supportive of programs for children with handicaps, or Jake, a second grader whose teacher is a good friend of yours and has encouraged you to work with him, or Susie, who is a wonderfully likable child who could use just a *little* help. Conversely you may feel a strong desire *not* to include Jimmy who, behaviorally, has been the bane of every teacher he has ever had, or Alicia, whose deficit represents an absolutely new area for you. Often you can rationalize your decision or bury it in your unconscious, but how you deal with these temptations will be a test of your professional character. Remember, you *are* accountable.

Assessing Deficits

Assessing deficits from the traditional perspective is similar to screening in several ways. First, you will gather preassessment information; frequently you can "carry over" facts gathered during screening into this new phase. In addition, you will add data gathered from a case history, interviews, additional observations, an oral peripheral examination if indicated, and, of course, formal and informal testing. Although there is no required order in these steps, usually a case history or interviews are accomplished first.

Case History

As mentioned under "Screening," use the information that is already available in the school records, including the parent form completed when the child entered school. If the school district does not administer regular hearing screenings, be sure you check the date of the most recent one on file. If the parent form is very out of date, however, you may want either to have the parent complete a new form or at least to ask during a parent interview about any recent events, such as names and ages of new siblings; a change in occupations; a divorce; any new medical problems, particularly allergies; or any medi-

cations that may alter behavior. Although a discussion of the case history is often combined with an interview, send the form home to be completed before talking with the parents or other caregivers. This allows family members time to consult records or each other. Be sure to review the completed form yourself before you talk with the parents either on the telephone or in person. Be aware that not all information on a case history form is necessarily accurate, particularly if the student in question has a number of siblings. As a mother of five, I can attest to the fact that the amount of detail regarding my children's development is in inverse proportion to their birth order.

The Oral Peripheral Examination

Exhibit 6–5 presents an abbreviated form that can be used to screen oral peripheral anatomy (form) and physiology (function). In the school population, these examinations are not usually completed unless the deficit could be caused by a physical problem (e.g., neurological soft signs, articulation difficulties, hypo- or hypernasality, drooling, eating problems). Remember that you must *never* conduct an oral peripheral examination without being properly gloved and taking other precautions to prevent the spread of disease.

The Interview

Parent or Caregiver's Interview. As a school speech-language professional, you may not always conduct a full parent interview prior to assessment. The parents have been informed and have given legal permission for an evaluation, but the contact may have been with the school psychologist, the chair of the Committee on Special Education, or the vice principal rather than the speech-language pathologist. Often a phone conference suffices,

Exhibit 6–5 Quick Oral Peripheral Examination

Name _____Date of Birth _____ Age _____ Grade _____ Date _____

Examiner _____ Reason for Exam _____

I. *Oral Cavity and Dental Structures*
  A. Occlusion of anterior teeth
    Normal ____ Overbite ____ Underbite ____ Open bite ____
  B. Alignment with dental arch
    Normal ____ Misaligned ____ Jumbled ____ Spacing abnormal ____
  C. Height and confirmation of hard palate
    Normal ____ Unusually narrow ____ Unusually high ____ Flat palatal vault ____ Other ____
  D. Soft palate
    Normal ____ Large and bulged ____ Other ____
    Abnormal tonsils ____ Narrow faucial isthmus ____
  E. Tongue
    Normal _____ Abnormally large _____ Short _____ Other _____

II. *Function of Oral Structures*

	Easy	Hard	Can't Do
A. Touch hard palate with tongue tip	____	____	____
B. Bulge back of tongue to touch soft palate	____	____	____
C. Thrust tongue	____	____	____
D. Point tongue	____	____	____
E. Groove tongue	____	____	____
F. General control of tongue	____	____	____
G. Smack lips together	____	____	____
H. Pucker lips	____	____	____
I. Lick lips in continuous circle			
K. Pucker and smile alternately	____	____	____
J. Tongue pulls to one side when speaking? Yes ____ No ____			

II. *Frenum*
  A Touch alveolar ridge with tongue tip   ____   ____   ____

IV. *Uvula*   Normal ____ Bifid ____

V. *Velopharyngeal closure*
  A Prolong vowel (ah)   Normal ____ Abnormal ____
  B Short repeated (ah)   Normal ____ Abnormal ____
  C Gag reflex   Normal ____ Hypersensitive ____ Hyposensitive ____
  D Nasality   Normal ____ Hypernasal ____ Hyponasal ____

VI *Diadochokinetic Rate*   Normal ____ Abnormal ____

Comments:

in conjunction with a completed information form. Clinicians who deal primarily with the preschool population are the exception to this. If you are going to meet formally with the parents (or other guardians) before your testing, you must first figure out what you want to ask. Any text on assessment has forms or lists of questions that can be adapted to the particular child's case (Owens, 1995; Paul, 1995; Shipley & McAfee, 1992).

Before discussing questions to ask during an interview, let us look at some general guidelines to help the interaction be as productive as possible. Remember, this is not an inquisition, so do not appear authoritarian or judgmental. Be friendly, open, and noncommittal. Strive for a tone of acceptance and willingness to listen. During an interview, note the way caregivers handle language. Are they glib? Hesitant? Ungrammatical? Critical? Specific? Do they speak in generalities or cliches? Use a dialect? Interacting with parent(s) can be potentially awkward if their educational background is very limited, if you and they represent different cultural groups, or if you do not speak their primary language. Conversely, if one or both parents are M.D.s, Ph.D.s, or educators, *you* may feel intimidated. Regardless of the parents' educational background, always explain the purpose of the interview, why the information is being sought, and the use to which you will put it. Make it clear that you will observe their rights to confidentiality, and expressly state with whom any of the information they provide may be shared. Remember that by law, your parents have a right to all information in their own language. Lund and Duchan (1993) presented an excellent list of questions to ask a cultural informant, as well as other means of working with clients who come from a different background. Garcia (1992) dealt specifically with cultural differences between home and school

language, and Damico and Hamayan's *Multicultural Language Intervention* (1992) has a section on ethnographic interviewing and the use of informants.

Become familiar with the order of questions so you can focus your attention on the caregivers, not on what to ask next. Be prepared for emotional reactions and handle them as tactfully as possible when they occur; parents can be relieved, profane, accusatory, angry, apparently disinterested, or weepy. Caregivers may appear to be primarily interested in not being blamed for the child's problems, or in rationalizing their own or the child's behavior. If this is a first interview, they may be working through their grief at the prospect of losing their "perfect" child. A box of tissues on your desk is as much a part of your professional paraphernalia as your tape recorder. Don't rush! Regardless of your time schedule, try not to appear in a hurry.

Use open-ended questions as much as possible, and avoid leading or "loaded" questions, e.g., "You didn't tell him his speech makes him sound like a sissy, did you?" Provide transitions. For example, if you have completed the section on developmental milestones and are moving into medical concerns, make the change in topic very clear. Be aware that even the most benign question can be intimidating under some circumstances. Suppose you asked about any injuries the child had suffered. The student's mother may be the only one who knows that when he was 8 months old, he tumbled off her bed onto a hard floor. In this instance you could be puzzled by her guarded response. Be prepared also for questions the parents may have for you. Warning! Don't pretend to have information that you do not have. The question you will hear again and again is, "Why is my child like this?" If you don't know, and you frequently won't, say so directly.

During the interview frame direct questions that specifically address any problems in speech-language that the parent has observed in the home. This is equally important whether or not the parent is the referral source. If, for example, a teacher has referred the student, you may be dealing with parents who feel that their child functions just fine at home, thank you. If the parent has referred the child, but the teacher has not expressed concerns, it may be that the child is killing himself at school to keep up, but doesn't fall apart until he reaches his front door. The interview may provide insights into parent expectations that do not match the schools, or a mismatch between home and school language demands. In either case, you have gained information you can use to plan your observations and/or assessment. If reading or spelling is a problem, be sure to ask if there is a history of either late talking or articulation problems, even if they disappeared over time. Another important factor is the existence of relatives who had problems in school. Recent research has indicated that there are some language-based reading problems that appear to have a familial base (Tallal, Ross, & Curtiss (1989); Tomblin (1991).

Don't forget that the family can be a source of strength for both the speech-language professional and student during the young person's school years. Trivette, Dunst, Deal, Hamer, and Propst, (1990) list qualities that characterize the supportive family and suggest that clinicians discover and then encourage the family to use its strengths to assist the child struggling in school. Sometimes we forget to look for and mention what the child, or his family, does well. We will address other aspects of parent counseling in Chapter 9, when we discuss intervention. A final comment: if you forget everything else in these paragraphs of advice, please remember one thing. Listen.

Listen hard. Listen for confusion, for contradictions. Listen for concerns. Listen for cues. Listen for what is between the lines.

Teacher Interviews. Since this interview is often done "off the cuff", much of the information you could gain from a more structured interview is left to be discovered later as you work with the student. Clearly, this is not the most efficient use of your time. Although most college courses in measurement include a form for parent/client interviews, you may not have seen one to use with teachers. One of the most efficient ways to determine a teacher's view of a student's strengths and weaknesses is to use a check list of communicative skills required in the student's grade, for example ones by Damico (1995, p. 187) or Larson & McKinley (1987). Conversely, you can review a list of typical errors associated with language based learning disabilities. I have compiled such a list which appears as Exhibit 6–7 later in this chapter. Another possibility is using the referral forms in Exhibits 6–2 and 6–3 as an outline.

The school nurse represents another source of information about your students which is frequently overlooked. In my experience, if a child is having new problems in the classroom, more frequent trips to the nurse are often the first indication. Stomach aches, headaches, diarrhea, and requests to go home early are common. An increase in absences can also indicate stress. Since school nurses are required to keep a log of student visits, information can be verified. A competent, caring school nurse can be a strong ally, particularly for the inexperienced public school speech-language professional.

The Student Interview. Even young students can be asked specific questions about how they are doing in class. Often children are aware that they are not succeeding, and having someone take their concerns seriously can be wonderfully helpful in establishing rapport. Sometimes students have a very different view from that of their teachers or parents, and this disparity can be clarified in later parent or teacher interviews. As mentioned under "Screening," a student interview is an effective means of gathering information at any age level. It is crucial when dealing with the older student. One of the most direct ways to encourage student communication is to use the pragmatics inventory in Creaghead and Tattershall's work (1985, p. 111). Their questions assess the student's awareness of classroom pragmatic rules, such as "When is it important to be quiet in this class?" and "How important is using correct grammar and spelling when you write for this teacher?" Another list adapted by Paul (1995, p. 503) from Scott and Erwin deals with the student's perception of writing demands; some examples include "Did you write anything in school this month that was more than a paragraph long? What was the assignment?" and "What kinds of writing are easiest for you?"

Observations

As was mentioned under "Screening," observations are absolutely critical in assessing language-based academic problems. In addition to the reasons stated previously, observation provides you with information that will directly relate to intervention. For example, if you observe a seventh grader during a social studies lesson, and it is obvious that he either cannot or will not take notes, you have identified an area that must be investigated further. Are the teacher's sentences too long/complex for him to follow? Does he have problems seeing any organizational pattern in the material that is being presented? Can he write fast enough to keep up, even if he

knows what to write? Does the teacher provide any overheads? Could the student use a partially completed review sheet? Does the vocabulary need to be pretaught? Is the classroom too noisy, too visually distracting, too hot, too cold? Can the student see the chalkboard? Can he read well enough for that to help? Regardless of grade level, students function in a variety of educational environments daily. The more of these in which you can observe the student, the better. Setting up and observing how specific intervention techniques affect the student's deficits is part of observational assessment, discussed in the second major section of this chapter, "New Approaches to Assessment."

Standardized Testing

Hallelujah, we are finally ready to address the topic many of you thought was synonymous with "assessment"! Some of what you will need to absorb in this section of the chapter has been discussed earlier (e.g., testing terminology, multicultural concerns in testing), and you may want to review these areas before continuing.

Generally, assessment of deficits can be divided into two main components: standardized testing and other procedures. Each has its place in the school environment. In recent years, however, the use of standardized instruments has come under increasing fire (Duchan, 1982; Muma, Lubinski, & Pierce, 1982; Siegel & Broen, 1976). Peterson and Marquardt (1990) stated, "No test is ever completely valid, and tests are only valid to the extent that they serve their function" (p. 11). Lund and Duchan (1993) contended that "one cannot judge the adequacy of a child's syntax or semantics without considering what the child is attempting to do" (p. 54); that is, one should not artificially separate form from the overall communicative contexts in which it occurs. They stated, "Part of the unnaturalness of tests comes from the removal of contextual clues in order to assure [that] the child 'knows' the answer only from the language forms given. . . . The language is often characteristically different from language in everyday communicative exchanges" (p. 324). Other concerns have been expressed because, as noted previously, the results of norm-referenced instruments can be misinterpreted or applied incorrectly, particularly to a population not adequately considered in the normative group. Particular concerns have been expressed by members of the African American, Hispanic, Native American, and Asian communities (Westby, 1994).

Another issue in using standardized tests to determine eligibility is the whole issue of assigning a number to a skill as incredibly complex as language comprehension and use. Kamhi (1993), applying Gould's term *reification* to language assessment, defined it as "the process by which something abstract is turned into a material and concrete entity" (p. 111). Once we have done this, he asserted, our human tendency takes over "to rank complex variation into a gradual ascending scale" (p. 111). Muma (1978) warned nearly 20 years ago that because behavior (and by extension, language) is "relative, conditional, complex and dynamic [it follows that] clinical assessment must be relative, contextual, process-oriented and dynamic, . . . not . . . categorical, quantitative or normative. . . . [It] should be about an individual as he functions in natural contexts or deals with systems and processes directly relevant to natural behavior" (p. 211). According to Kamhi, inappropriate quantification and ranking can create and perpetuate potentially damaging misconceptions about competence and skill. We need to develop and use assessment procedures that better re-flect the behaviors we are trying to change in treatment; for example, to reflect the underlying language skills that, when improved, will allow a student to reach his intellectual potential.

Remember also that standardized tests can include both norm-referenced and criterion-referenced tests, used for different purposes. McCauley's (1996) article on the latter clarified the differences. Norm-referenced tests rank individuals, their items are chosen to distinguish among individuals, they address broad content, and they summarize performances into percentile or standard scores. Criterion-referenced instruments distinguish specific levels of performance in a clearly specified domain and are summarized meaningfully using raw scores.

Although you should be keenly aware of the negative aspects of case selection based solely on standardized instruments, this type of testing will undoubtedly remain part of almost any evaluation in the school environment. First, standardized tests are less subjective than informal means and in many cases are less time consuming to administer as well. This is an important consideration because you cannot afford to waste evaluation time on unnecessary or inefficient procedures. In addition, standardized measures have been specifically designed to be administered and scored, and the results interpreted using clearly stated procedures. Finally, issues of validity, reliability, correlation to other tests, and the presence of a normative group for comparison purposes (for norm-referenced measures) have been considered in their construction. Federal, state, and district guidelines often require that a child's scores on two or more standardized measures must fall 1.5 (or in some cases 2.0) standard deviations below the mean before a label indicating a handicapping condition can be assigned.

Plante and Vance (1994) raised questions about these guidelines that maximize diagnostic accuracy when the standard deviations for two tests are markedly different. But this criterion, though not perfect, is still accepted more readily by professionals in our field than either age-equivalent scores or a measure of discrepancy. *Caution, caution:* just because a test says it is standardized, it does not automatically follow that all the issues above have been addressed properly. When the above researchers investigated 21 tests of language skills that included norms for children aged 4 and 5, only 38% of them met half or more of the following 10 psychometric criteria, (see definitions in Exhibit 6–1).

- description of normative sample
- sample size
- item analysis
- means and standard deviations
- concurrent validity
- predictive validity
- interexaminer reliability
- description of test procedures
- description of tester qualifications

All standardized tests have specific ways to be administered that must be followed if the accuracy of the scores is not to be compromised. It is part of your professional responsibility to review the directions carefully and practice as necessary before administering any instrument "for real." These instructions may address some or all of the following: the permissible age range for the student; where the examiner and the student should sit in relation to each other and the test materials; how much training the examiner must have; whether test questions can be repeated; what prompts, if any, can be given; where to begin and end the testing procedure; the form the

answers must be in (standards for the response); how the scoring is to be computed; time limits of the test; how long an examiner can wait for a question to be answered; training questions; and permissible reinforcers. A word of encouragement: you will be astonished at how quickly you become proficient once you gain some experience.

Types of Standardized Tests. As discussed previously, there are two main categories of standardized tests, (a) norm referenced and (b) criterion referenced.

Norm-referenced tests are designed to determine relative ranking based on a comparison with members of the student's peer group. Typical examples of this type in our field include the CELF-3, the PPVT-R, and the Language Processing Test (Richard & Hanner, 1985). One use of this type of test is to verify that the student's performance is inferior to that of his or her peers. If the instrument has a number of subtests—as in the case of the CELF-3, which has 11—it can also help identify specific areas within language that are deficient, such as receptive semantics or expressive syntax. Norm-referenced tests are usually administered to answer the general question "Does this child have a problem?"

Criterion-referenced tests measure a child's performance in terms of mastery. Evaluating Communicative Competence and the Test of Problem Solving (Zachman, Barrett, Huisingh, Orman, & Blagden, 1991) are typical of this type; others include language sample analyses, pure-tone threshold screening, and percentage of intelligible words (Weiss, 1980). Almost all classroom examinations, ranging from weekly spelling tests to end-of-the-year examinations in chemistry or earth science, are also criterion referenced. Tests of this type answer the questions "Does this student have these specific skills?" and "What is the child's *specific* problem?"

Reporting Scores Using Standard Deviations. After choosing and administering standardized tests, scores are reported orally and as part of a written report. An example of a speech-language diagnostic report is presented in the "Case Studies" section of this chapter (Exhibit 6–16). Standardized results often include terms such as *percentile rank, stanine, NCE score, deviation quotient, z or T score,* or *standard score* based on a mean of 100, 50, or 10, this last one sometimes called a *scaled score.* When you share these results with other professionals, these terms usually pose no problem. To expect a parent to interpret what they mean, however, is expecting too much, particularly if the information is presented in the emotionally stressful atmosphere of an initial meeting of the Committee on Special Education.

One way to make results more understandable is to translate each score into one based on the approximate standard deviation as follows. Scores that fall between –1 and +1 S.D. are considered within normal limits. Most school districts do not consider a child to have a handicapping condition unless the score falls at least 1.5 or, in some districts, 2.0 standard deviations below the mean. The example below shows test scores and their translations into approximate standard deviations:

Test	*Test Score*	*Standard Deviation*
PPVT	Percentile rank 12	–1.0 to –1.5
CELF-R Formulated Sentences subtest	Standard score 6	–1.0 to –1.5
CELF-R Expressive Language	Standard score 71	–1.5 to –2.0
Language Processing Test	Standard score 42	–0.5 to –1.0
Year-end reading score	Stanine 3	–1.0

There are precise numerical tables available to translate values exactly, but you can use the bell-shaped curve chart that follows in Figure 6–1 to make the quick approximations given above. Caution: some standard scores, called *linear standard scores,* are computed from the mean and standard deviation of the sample; others, called *normalized standard scores,* are based on percentile ranks and their relationship to the z score in a normal distribution. To make the comparisons above, the tests must be using the same unit of measurement.

Interpreting Scores Using Other Means. As mentioned before, other common ways to determine eligibility are based on *discrepancy,* *age delay,* or *descriptive* approaches. *Discrepancy* is usually defined in terms of a "significant language delay." Either the child's chronological age (CA) or "mental" age (MA) can serve as the comparison. If you choose the former, be aware that all cognitively challenged children will automatically be labeled as speech impaired even if their language is on a par with their intellectual level. Choosing MA as the comparison, however, also presents problems because using MA could eliminate students with mental retardation, even if they clearly need help in applying language skills to school situations.

There are additional problems with using MA as the basis of comparison. First, the means used to calculate mental age can be af-

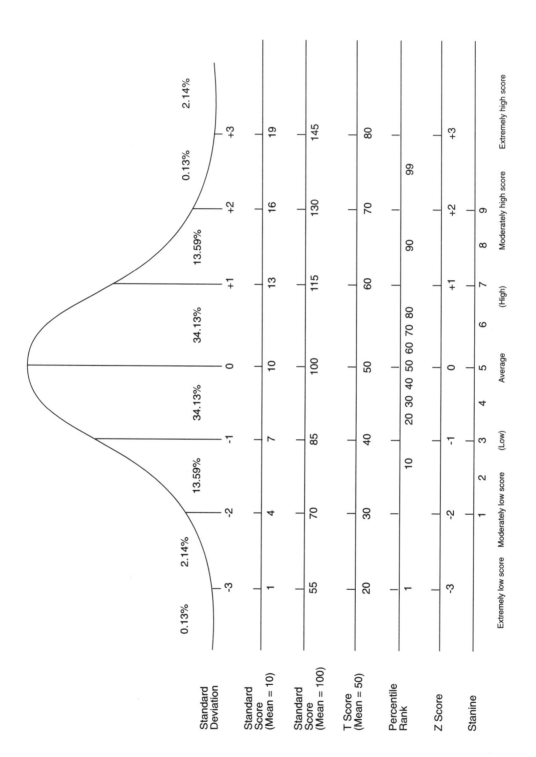

Figure 6–1 Bell-Shaped Curve Used To Convert Test Scores to Standard Deviations

fected by environmental factors, achievement history, motivation, ethnicity, and the problems inherent in any kind of standardized testing, such as validity or reliability issues. Often an IQ score is used as a measure of MA, and critics have stated for years that this measure may be contaminated because language skills themselves are used to determine the number. Not sure what this means? Think of it this way. Suppose you need to know if "Medicine X" lowers blood pressure. Before you can say that it does, you have to determine what "normal" blood pressure is. So you take readings, but only from people who are already on the medication. Clearly, you have contaminated your results. Francis et al. (1996) discuss this issue in detail. It is necessary to understand how IQ is measured before you can discuss comparisons with the school psychologist or in a meeting in which you have to justify services based on discrepancy.

Others criticize discrepancy scores (and, by extension, standardized testing in general) because they are often based on a single area of language, such as phonology or syntax, but ignore others, such as pragmatics or the relationship of language to reading or writing. Indeed, no commonly accepted normative data for the latter three areas exist. Consequently, although a child may be judged as having weaknesses in syntax, the discrepancy in this specific area may not be considered large enough to warrant labeling the student. This can occur even though the youngster's overall communicative skills are too weak to allow success in the school environment. Closely linked to this criticism is the fact that deficits in some areas of language are potentially more serious than others in terms of their effect on school performance at different grade levels.

An *age delay*, the second means of comparison, varies across grades and/or stages of development. Clearly, a child who is "one year behind," whether the comparison is to CA or MA, has a potentially higher degree of deficit if she is a 6-year-old first grader than if she is a 15-year-old in the 10th grade. Charts have been developed that present a sliding scale, but they are more often used with preschool than with school-age students.

Descriptive approaches are almost always used as an addition to normative data. You can employ them to indicate how the child applies (or does not) apply language in a specific school situation; for example, when describing how a lack of organizational skills can be devastating to a high school student, regardless of subject area. A severity rating can also be considered as an example of a descriptive approach if it is based on a subjective decision of the speech-language professional. This may be the case if you evaluate a student's voice as having "severe" hypernasality, or his articulation as "moderately" deficient if "it is intelligible with careful listening." A fluency disorder can also be described as mild, moderate, or severe. Other severity ratings, however, are linked to percentiles or standard scores. Customarily, a mild to moderate level is equated with a score between 1.0 and 1.5 standard deviations below the mean, a moderate level with a score between 1.5 and 2.0 standard deviations below the mean, and a severe level with a score 2.0 or more standard deviations below the mean. The value of descriptive approaches is that they often make more sense to parents and teachers.

Language Samples

Like almost every aspect of assessment, language sampling has its advantages and disadvantages. Some of the advantages are obvious. A language sample not only allows you to say with absolute surety that a child can produce a structure or word spontaneously, but it can also provide more specific information concerning intervention goals because, as Blau, Lahey, and Olesiuk-Velez (1984) stated, it includes both the content and context of language. Owens (1995) added, "If the goal of language intervention is generalization to the language used by the child in everyday situations, it is essential that the speech-language professional collect a language sample that is a good reflection of that language in actual use" (p. 120). In addition, spontaneous language sampling allows you to make an informal judgment concerning any possible voice, fluency, or articulation problems in connected speech. So if language sampling is such a good idea, why isn't it used routinely by all speech-language specialists?

Typical of relatively inexperienced clinicians, many of my speech pathology students are scared to death of language samples or language sampling procedures in general, let alone the prospect of eliciting one from a school-age child. First, they worry that the child will not talk. Second, they fear that even if they do manage to collect a decent sample, their background in grammar will be insufficient to analyze the child's language correctly. Next, unlike standardized instruments, no script exists to tell them exactly what to say. Finally, clinicians often do not know the child well, and may not know him at all. Perhaps this common early experience is the reason that I have always compared language sampling in the schools to regular exercise. Every school-based speech-language professional understands how important taking a language sample is to the diagnostic procedure, knows how to do it, but tends to avoid it as much as possible.

Another obstacle to language sampling among school-based speech-language professionals, in addition to general reluctance, is the obvious time constraints when one is dealing with caseloads of 40 to 60 students; this is particularly crucial when intervention time must be sacrificed because one is evaluating another student. Some school clinicians also cite the lack of accepted norms/procedures for the older school-age population. Few can dispute that historically this age group, compared with preschoolers, has been treated with benign neglect by those involved in basic language research. Fortunately, there is new interest in this area. The October 1995 issue of *Language, Speech, and Hearing Services in Schools* features five articles that provide new normative data for school-age children; let us hope that this trend continues.

Even if the data existed, however, the problem of obtaining a truly representative sample would remain. Hux et al. (1993) warned that school speech-language pathologists who create their own abbreviated procedures may have "forfeit[ed] the benefits offered by standardized procedures with respect to reliability and validity" (p. 90). This quote appears at the end of an interesting survey conducted by the three authors that reported on both the analysis and the collection procedures of 239 school-based speech-language pathologists in California, as well as their attitudes toward formal language sampling. Although the survey respondents recognized the importance of language sampling and reported using a variety of published standardized and nonstandardized guidelines to analyze the samples, most of them employed self-designed procedures. Usually these procedures measured mean length of utterance (MLU) and the overall pragmatic, syntactic, morphological, and semantic aspects of language. The most popular elicitation technique was conversation, distantly followed by descriptions, story retelling, explanations, question-answer formats, and story-generation activities. The majority of respondents, however, employed language sampling only with younger or more severely involved students, not with older or mildly impaired ones.

If you have decided to take a language sample as part of an assessment, here is one procedure you might follow: first, collect information to determine the best time and location for the sample; next, decide what linguistic area you wish to tap. Third, determine the means to elicit it. Following elicitation, interpret the sample. Finally, report the results.

Determining Time and Location The question of where and when will depend on the underlying purpose of your sample. Wallach and Butler (1994), Paul (1995), Owens (1995), and Simon (1985a) have all spoken to this issue. Other authors have indicated that the most representative samples occur when children's language is evaluated in seminaturalistic and naturalistic situations (Lund & Duchan, 1993; Nelson, 1990). However, within these situations, what is your purpose? Are you interested primarily in the student's pragmatic behavior in a typical school setting? Or, because the student's written grammar is so poor, is your main focus the complexity (or lack of it) in his or her oral language? Do you feel, as Nelson (1994) suggested, that you should identify "the curricular contexts where language-related problems are evident" (p. 174)? Van Kleeck (1994) suggested taking a sample while the student pushes the limits of his competence as he uses language to work through problems. Indeed, many experts suggest that clinicians take several samples in different environments because a child's production will obviously undergo changes as he switches from the school setting to a casual setting outside the classroom in conversation with friends. Taking samples in different environments can also serve to indicate if the child can "switch code" as he moves from one setting to another. Even if you are primarily interested in expressive language, remember that, as Nelson (1985) stated, "it is often observed that children who have difficulty comprehending connected discourse or text also have difficulty expressing their own thoughts in a connected fashion" (p. 84). In other words, do not treat comprehension as a separate issue.

If you are not sure which (if any) of the above areas to target, first review pertinent records, or complete your teacher or student interviews and your student observation(s). If this is the student's initial evaluation, other school personnel will be investigating the student's academic achievement, learning characteristics, social and physical development, and management needs as required by federal and state statute. Often these assessments contain valuable information concerning language, such as the pragmatic implications of social development, the possible language basis of a reading profile, or the extent of cultural literacy. On the other hand, if the child has already been labeled as having a learning disability in oral expression, listening comprehension, written expression, basic reading skills, reading comprehension, mathematical calculation, or mathematical reasoning, set up a language sample that will add to your knowledge of how the language problem specifically affects performance in each area.

You must also become aware of the changing demands and alterations in basic teaching methods that take place in the curriculum across the years, often an area of weakness for the inexperienced speech-language pathologist. Even if there is growth in a student's language skills, it often does not keep pace with the new skills needed to learn curricular material. Bashir (1989) stated that as the nature of a language disorder changes, it can ultimately affect a young child's academic, social, and vocational growth. As professionals in the field of speech and language, we must be able to adapt the student's goals to match the school's language requirements. Exhibit 6–6 contains information from Bashir & Scavuzzo (1992); you can use it to help language sampling (and assessment in general) remain sensitive to the demands of the changing school environment. Although Bashir's article does not encompass the language demands of the high school student, you should be able to extrapolate them from your own experience, including the requirements of the workplace, whether it is a full-time job after graduation or the local hamburger palace during the school year.

Choosing the Area of the Limited Sample. Do not forget the reason for this digression into Bashir's work; you are deciding where and under what conditions to elicit a language sample. Bashir's article suggests the role of the curriculum in your choice; that is, the language skills required to succeed academically. However, there is another way to select the means and area of your language sample: areas of weakness. A brief review of the "symptoms" of school problems and their relation to basic causes can also be helpful in deciding what area of language to target in testing. Globally, "The single most significant deterrent to educational growth remains the inability to use oral and written language, to speak and to read" (Stark & Wallach, 1980, p. 6). Within this inability lie the classic divisions you have learned by heart: phonology, morphology and syntax, semantics,

and pragmatics. Nelson (1989) added that a student's processing capabilities (receptive skills) should include metalinguistic skills: that is, the ability to talk about and manipulate language. As a *school* speech-language professional, however, do not forget that the reason for addressing underlying language weaknesses is to enable the student to improve performance within the educational environment. You must also consider the relationship among and within the language areas. It is possible for a child to use a syntactically complex construction (embedding) at the same time that he exhibits very limited use of morphemes or basic verb construction, as in " I don't know he be on yet" (Wood, 1982, p. 14). Although the information in Exhibit 6–7 is hardly exhaustive, it represents a compilation of typical problems experienced by children with language-based learning problems. Incidentally, it would be rare for a student to display all the behaviors under any single heading.

Eliciting the Sample. Now to elicitation. Between preschool and high school come all the other grades, each with its own set of language expectations. Prior to student teaching, you, like many clinicians, may have had experience taking language samples from mostly preschool children. After a few times, you probably became relatively comfortable engaging in conversation while playing with a Fisher-Price Airport set. You also developed a sense of what to listen for, such as Brown's morphemes or simple syntactical structures. Facing a slouching, uncommunicative 14-year-old across the table represents a distinctly different experience. Over the past decade, however, the literature has featured excellent examples of different ways to elicit samples that do relate to children in kindergarten through high school, as well as reports

Exhibit 6–6 Language Demands and the Curriculum

Kindergarten through Second Grade

- Child is expected to use language to
  1. follow directions
  2. self-regulate
  3. speak in small groups
  4. generate early oral narratives
  5. learn the relationships between phonology and reading and apply those skills to access knowledge. (If these skills are not securely in place by this time, the student will have difficulty using texts to acquire content information.)

Third to Fourth Grade

- Learning begins to focus on content and problem solving, rather than being child centered.
- Reading shifts from learning to read to reading to learn.
- Sentence structure increases in length and complexity.
- Comprehension of reading material shifts from literal/factual understanding to making inferences and drawing conclusions.
- Understanding of written material includes how information is organized in a text (e.g., titles, chapters, headings, subheadings, appendices, table of contents).
- There are greater demands on comprehension, with growth in word meaning, especially multiple meanings.

- The student is expected to
  1. become an active partner in learning
  2. apply previously acquired skills and information to classroom discussions and dialogues

Fifth through Eighth Grade

- Child must adapt to
  1. different teaching styles and different styles of instructional language
  2. lecture formats for learning content materials, with student sharing responsibility for acquiring information through dialogue and independent reading
  3. different comprehension demands as content becomes more technical, as in science, literature, and math
- Child must accommodate to the increased language demands of expanding subject areas, such as social studies, history, science, and math.
- Curriculum requires further development of written language and creation of different types of compositions, such as summaries, essays, research papers, poetry, and spontaneous writing.
- Child must be able to self-organize work and develop effective study and note-taking skills.
- There are demands for different communication styles necessary for effective interaction in the classroom and with peers.

Source: Adapted from Bashir (1989), Language intervention and the curriculum. *Seminars in Speech and Language*, 10, 181–191.

---

of the effects of such variables as contextual support, listener's knowledge of information, age, and mental capacity on obtaining a representative sample.

It is beyond the scope of this chapter to detail specific stories, techniques, and rationales, but the literature abounds with valuable suggestions like this treasure from Masterson and Kamhi (1991): Hold two balloons of different colors and sizes in front of the student. The larger balloon is filled with helium and the smaller with air. You hold one in each hand and then release them. The student tells you what happened and then describes it to another child who was not in the room at the time. Among other results, the authors

Exhibit 6–7 Some Common Classroom Behaviors Resulting from Possible Language Deficits

Phonology
- Students may
  1. take longer than their "typical" classmates to recognize that language is a code, that the code is print, and that individual sounds correspond to the smallest segments
  2. have poor spelling skills, even of phonetically regular spelling words
  3. confuse vowel sounds, particularly short vowels (e.g., "tin" vs. "ten")
  4. have weak decoding skills in reading
  5. have difficulty creating or hearing rhyme
  6. not be able to identify how many syllables are in a word (e.g., to clap three times for *butterfly*, twice for *butter*)
  7. have poor skills in sound manipulation (metaphonology), as in sound blending or phoneme segmentation ("t" plus "ap" is *tap*; *sink* without the "s" is *ink*)
  8. have difficulty organizing, storing, and retrieving words from memory on the basis of their phonological properties
  9. have a history of a phonological disorder as a preschooler
- In connected speech, students may
  1. omit sounds or syllables in words
  2. substitute one sound for another
  3. insert an extra sound
  4. have difficulty imitating speech sounds, particularly in multisyllabic words or in difficult phrases (e.g., "Fly free in the air force")

Morphology
- Students may
  1. experience difficulties with irregular verb forms (e.g., *swung*)
  2. use incorrect verb tenses in speaking and writing
  3. leave out words (e.g., "He going")
  4. use plurality incorrectly, particularly irregular forms
  5. have problems in perceiving and discriminating among various pronunciations of the plural morpheme (e.g., *cats, dogs, glasses*)
  6. make errors in article use

  7. have difficulty with changes in spelling of irregular forms that persists into adulthood
  8. have difficulty understanding/using affixes
  9. have persistent problems with comparative/superlative forms
  10. have persistent difficulty in spelling/pronunciation changes dictated by derivational affixes (e.g., *medicine, medical, medicinal*)

Syntax
- Students may
  1. have receptive and/or expressive syntactic deficits
  2. use few sentence complexities (clauses or multiple verbs), instead using short, syntactically simple sentences, usually subject-verb-object
  3. not elaborate noun or verb phrases beyond a simple level
  4. have particular difficulty interpreting relative and adverbial clauses (e.g., those containing *if, before*) after age 7 or 8
  5. not use correct subject/verb agreement (e.g., "They is going")
  6. use incorrect pronoun forms (e.g., substituting an object pronoun for a subject pronoun, as in "Him and me are friends")
  7. confuse word order, particularly in questions
  8. habitually use incomplete sentences when writing
  9. have problems in perceiving, acquiring, and recalling the rules for modals and auxiliaries (e.g., *must, will, should, could, have, had*)
  10. confuse "Wh" words
  11. have persistent problems in understanding and using the passive
  12. sequence adjective strings incorrectly (e.g., a "green, big ball")
  13. have problems using negatives correctly
  14. have difficulty understanding the relationship between direct and indirect objects

continues

Exhibit 6–7 continued

15. not understand subtle differences in tense meaning (e.g., the differences between "I study all the   time," "I studied all the time," and "I will study all the time")
16. repeat a grammatically correct sentence incorrectly
17. not identify as incorrect an utterance with a syntactic error

- Written grammar may be poorer than spoken grammar.
- Metalinguistic skills may be particularly weak in this area of language, even if the student's spontaneous production appears the same as that of normally achieving children. For example, students may have difficulty in structured tasks requiring syntactic manipulation:

1. changing a statement to a question
2. given a word, using it in a sentence
3. completing a sentence like " I will go tomorrow because . . . "
4. syntactic compression tasks such as putting two statements together (e.g., taking, "The baby fell" and "The baby cried" and combining them to make "The baby that fell cried"

Semantics

- Deficits occur either receptively or expressively or both. Student may

1. have a limited vocabulary
2. overuse certain words, (e.g., *cool, dumb, stuff, thing*)
3. have difficulty understanding and using synonyms, antonyms, and homonyms (e.g.: giving a word that has a similar meaning when asked for an opposite)
4. not use context to differentiate meaning, (e.g., *die* versus *dye*)
5. overuse one meaning of multiple-meaning words
6. not understand analogies
7. have problems interpreting figurative language, including common idiomatic expressions
8. confuse "Wh" words (e.g., when asked when they eat lunch responding, "In the lunchroom")

9. experience difficulty understanding complex sentences because they do not understand the meaning of clausal connectors (e.g., *since, nor, if*)
10. have problems with reference, particularly pronouns
11. experience difficulty with abstractions (e.g., words like *democracy*)
12. struggle with time relationships, particularly those with shifting references (e.g., "the day before yesterday," "a week from Friday"
13. have difficulty with spatial concepts, e.g., *on* vs. *in* (younger students) "at school" vs. "in school" (older students)
14. substitute inaccurate words (e.g., *lemon* for *orange)*
15. offer limited information in verbal reports
16. exhibit symptoms of word-finding problems: rambling, using inexact, ambiguous, or nonspecific words; appearing disorganized or hesitant
17. using circumlocutions, repetitions, disjointed phrases, and fillers that may be rooted in a faulty semantic reference system
18. have inadequate understanding of relational meanings beyond word meanings

Pragmatics

- Students may

1. have difficulty understanding implied messages (e.g., not recognizing what the teacher wants when he says, "This room is noisy")
2. not get jokes
3. have problems asking for or understanding need for assistance or clarification
4. have difficulty with ritualistic greetings/farewells (e.g., starting a conversation without saying hello or walking away without closing conversation)
5. have problems with topic initiation and maintenance, often changing subject or perseverating on a topic that the listener wishes terminated
6. have difficulty concentrating on

continues

Exhibit 6–7 continued

conversations among peers/adults
7. not alter the message depending on their knowledge and relationship to the listener (e.g., age, familiarity, social status, sex)
8. display disorganized content within or among utterances
9. express socially inappropriate emotional reactions
10. have limited interpersonal relationships
11. be inappropriately loud or passive in classroom situations
12. maintain poor eye contact that is not culturally based
13. have difficulty with implied cause-and-effect relationships
14. appear immature and/or silly

15. have difficulty in adhering to classroom etiquette (e.g., interrupting another student to answer, shouting out an answer, answering in a disrespectful manner to teachers and administrators without any awareness)
16. cheat or lie to cover up incomplete or undone class work
17. misread a speaker's verbal or nonverbal signals that are part of the message
18. use conflicting verbal and nonverbal messages
19. not repair communicative breakdowns
20. not honor correct turn-taking behavior, either conversationally or otherwise
21. not provide the listener with necessary information

reported that more complex language occurred when the child explained what had happened to someone who was not a participant (absent referents) than when the child explained it to someone who was. They also gave examples of specific stories that clinicians can employ and ways that explanations can be used to elicit a good sample. If you are inexperienced in eliciting samples, be sure to consult the literature for techniques that match the age/interests of your student. The references at the end of this chapter and the references that appear at the end of any article on language sampling will include some that may be exactly what you need. Note: if you have not already done so, make the transition from seeing a journal article as something you take a test on (the student mode) to seeing it as a source of information you can use tomorrow (the professional mode).

One aspect of this complex procedure is worth noting. Practice helps enormously; trust me, the more you do it, the easier it becomes. If you have not worked around children the ages you will be working with in

your student teaching, run, do not walk, to the nearest school, day care center, or Girl Scout troop and volunteer. It is not necessary to work with children who have handicaps; just learning how to talk with children of different ages alone or in groups will remove some of your anxiety. Watch children's shows on television. What cartoons or TV programs are "in"? If you are still talking about Ninja turtles when second graders are crazy about Power Rangers, you enter a conversation with two strikes against you. In case this appears utterly overwhelming, remember, you do not have to do it all at once. Assessment continues to take place long after the formal evaluation is over. Indeed, a competent speech-language professional creates ongoing hypotheses during every intervention session. This fact, incidentally, is one of the underlying assumptions of dynamic assessment, which will be discussed later in this chapter.

Obviously, the reason you take a sample is to investigate some particular aspect of spontaneous language. But I cannot stress strongly enough that dividing language into rather arbitrary "components" for assessment purposes is potentially dangerous, whether for a language sample or otherwise. It is easy to lose sight of the effect of communicative intent, nonverbal cues, or use of scripts on overall language competence. That said, most clinicians find it helpful to provide a profile of the student's strengths and weaknesses and to include categories like "syntactic complexity," "spatial concepts" (semantics), or "age-inappropriate phonological processes." In a way, they are acting like a doctor who, while evaluating a patient's overall health, orders a blood test because she suspects anemia. The symptom that caused the patient to make an appointment may have been fatigue, but the physician suspects problems in the blood as the underlying cause and "isolates" this body system to test. Incidentally, if the "she" referring to the physician made you pause, please recognize your reaction for what it is: an unconscious culturally determined preconception that doctors are male (see Chapter 11!).

Where do I stand on the issue of language samples? Although they are not routinely used in the school population except in the preschool group, and although most districts do not require them, I think that a speech-language professional, at the very least, must make notations about semantic strengths/weaknesses, presence or lack of syntactical complexity, and morphological implications of the student's spontaneous language. Problems in pragmatics should also be described. Lists of structures for checking morphology and syntax are given in the sections that follow. In lieu of lists like these, you may prefer to feature "typical" utterances. In any case, samples based on oral language should also be compared with the student's written work, particularly in the upper grades. These suggestions are made with full knowledge that they do not represent the ideal or even the preferred mode. They do, however, reflect the reality of school practice, warts and all.

The kind of language interpretation that follows is not meant to be used as "proof" that the student should be labeled. It is more narrow. It only helps to discover the child's strengths and weaknesses as he verbally approaches a *specific* task. It points us toward intervention that addresses any academic problems that are syntactically based. It is quite possible that you could use a language sample primarily to investigate the child's pragmatic abilities as he interacts with peers. A month or two later, you might want to look at the child's semantics as he reports cause and effect while describing a third-grade science experiment. In actuality, you are continuing to assess the student long after the formal evaluation is over, creating and testing ongoing hypotheses as you work with the child.

To illustrate language sampling, we will present *one* way to sample *one* area; we will assume that the student has problems using form; that is, morphology and/or syntax. I will present an adaptation and expansion of a procedure based on Fugiki and Willbrand's (1982) suggestion that "a combination of spontaneous language sampling and sentence completion or elicited imitation" is likely to be most effective in clinical language evaluation (p. 48). You will first decide the most pertinent setting—whether the student should be alone in the intervention room or part of a group in his class—and then arrange your chosen materials to engage the student as you take the sample. From your sample you will note the form, content, and use your student makes of language. On the basis of this information, you can probe for elements that appear to be omitted or in error. If later you think you are still missing a key part of the puzzle, you may have to set up a means to check, preferably through a naturalistic approach.

Illustration: Sampling for Morphologic Analysis. Our first task will be to review some basic morphological terms in Exhibit 6–8. (Although syntax and morphology analyses are usually combined, for clarity we will separate them.)

Exhibit 6–9 is an illustrative language sample representing a younger child that is subjected to a morphological analysis.

We will enter the results of the analysis on a simple chart as in Exhibit 6–10 under these headings: morphological structures used, those omitted or those in error. At this point we can decide other structures we need to elicit. Appendix 6–B contains a list of standardized tests that can be used in part or in their entirety, if you need the standardized "numbers" for a report. Those included in Exhibit 6–11 measure some aspect of morphology. Using only a portion of a test can save much time in testing and focuses only on those test items that are likely to appear as intervention goals. After completing this process we can describe the child's strengths and weaknesses in the general area of morphology, but only under the conditions and limitations that existed at the time the sample was taken. In Chapter 8 we will also discuss the implications of morphological limitations as they apply to the older school-age child, particularly their connection to spelling and advanced vocabulary growth.

In some morphological analyses, one calculates the exact percentage of times that the child used each structure. If, as in Exhibit 6–10, you do not do this, at least note whether inconsistencies exist. These are often the clue for the child's rule as in the case of his use of regular/irregular past tense markers.

After you complete an initial analysis, attempt to elicit all omitted or substituted structures using portions of the tests listed in Exhibit 6–11 or your own elicitation techniques.

Illustration: Sampling for Syntactic Analysis. Our next step is to perform the same type of analysis, but featuring syntax rather than morphology. Please note that in a real sample, these two linguistic areas are usually combined; they are separated here only for teaching purposes.

Again, it will first be helpful to review some syntactical terms (Exhibit 6–12). Be aware that this exhibit represents only the "bare bones" of information you can use to describe syntactical form. For older students, and/or for written examples, you may need more sophisticated information. Remember, you are a speech-*language* professional, and operating without a solid metalinguistic foundation is like sailing across the ocean without charts or a sextant. On very old maps, unexplored oceans were marked "There be dragons." Our particular dragon is labeled "misdiagnosis," and it is a frightening prospect indeed.

As a school speech-language professional, you will probably find it most helpful to check five general areas in determining syntactical skills: (a) the elaboration of noun phrases, (b) the elaboration of verb phrases, (c), the use of negatives, (d) question forms, and (e) complexity as determined by conjunctions. For younger children, or those delayed to that level, all language development texts contain the developmental order of each of these areas through Brown's Stage V++. For students in the upper grades, indicate also which of the four different sentence types the student has employed: exclamatory, interrogative, imperative, and declarative. You may also calculate T-units and C-units, which are described later in this section.

Exhibit 6–8 Morphology Terminology

Inflectional morpheme: adds grammatical information to free morphemes, such as number, tense, or possession (*goes, walked, Mama's*, etc.).

Derivational morpheme: signals a change in part of speech (*run* [verb] + *er* = *runner* [noun] or meaning (*tie* + *un* = *untie*, the opposite). For the older language-learning-disabled (LLD) student, derivational morphemes are the more difficult.

Prefix/suffix: morphemes added at the beginning or to the end of a root word (*un-, sub-, mis-,* or *-ful, -ence, -ment*). These are very difficult for the LLD older student, who does not usually see the connection between *microscope, microbiology,* and *microwave.*

The list below contains the most common morphological structures that are assessed. Those marked with an asterisk (*) are listed in Brown's 14 morphemes (Brown, 1978) and form the basis for morphological analysis for the preschool population. Brown's stages are used as normative data.

The following refer to **Verbs:**

*Copula: linking verb that usually joins a subject to a complement; often is a form of *to be*. The other copular forms are the verbs of the senses (*look, hear, taste, smell, sound*) and ones like *appear, seem, become, grow, prove, and remain,* which can be substituted in a sentence by some form of *be* and still make sense ("It looks good = "It *is* good"; "The rumor proved true" = "The rumor *is* true").
*Auxiliary: the helping verb used with a main verb to indicate action or tense (*is* going, has *been* running).
*Contractible auxiliary: helping verb that can to be contracted ("He *is* going" = "He's going").
*Uncontractible auxiliary: helping verb that cannot be contracted ("He *was* going," or the answer to the question "Who's going?" ["He is"; you can't just say, "He's"]).
*Contractible copula: linking verb that can be contracted ("He *is* ill" = "He's ill").
*Uncontractible copula: linking verb that

cannot be contracted ("He *was* ill," or the answer to the question "Who's ill?" ["He *is*"; you can't just say, "He's"]).
*Regular past tense: completed action formed with the suffix ed (*walk* + *ed* = *walked*).
*Irregular past tense: completed action formed without the suffix *ed.* Can be formed by changes in the vowel (*run/ran*), consonant (*leave/left*) or total change of word (*go/went*). LLD students have difficulty with these, particularly the spelling rules associated with them.
*Present progressive: "She *is* walking" (*walk* + *ing*). Can be omitted by the younger child or used in place of more complex forms by the older. LLD students may omit the auxiliary that goes with it.
*Third-person singular, present tense: "She *walks.*"
Lexical: a kind of verb that adds content or meaning to the utterance, the type you usually mean when you say that verbs show action or a state of being. The complication comes for LLD students when they confuse the perfective auxiliary (all the forms of *have*) or the *do* auxiliary (including *does, did*) with the lexical form: "I have six cats" (lexical) versus "I have *fed* 6 cats (auxiliary), or "I did the dishes" (lexical) versus "I did want that new dress" (auxiliary).
Catenative: early infinitive/modal form [*gonna, wanna, gotta, hafta*]; its use persists even in formal language in the LLD student.
Participle: verb form that functions as an adjective (*broken* branch, *running* shoe). Metalinguistically, this is very difficult for LLD students.
Gerund: verb form that functions as a noun ("*Swimming* is fun"; "*Running* can be exhausting"). This form is also a metalinguistic puzzle for LLD students.

The remaining terms deal with other parts of speech:

*Article: a noun modifier that denotes specificity. It is often omitted by young

continues

Exhibit 6–8 continued

children. Older LLD kids may not use *an* before a word beginning with a vowel or may confuse *a* and *the* (e.g., they may not understand the difference between "a book" and "the book").
*Plural: denotes more than one. This can be omitted, particularly in certain dialects. Errors persist in the irregular forms in LLD students.
*Possessive: denotes ownership
Adverb: supplies information about time, place, manner, degree or cause of action. The "ly" suffix is rarely used by the LLD student.
Preposition: connects nouns or pronouns with other parts of the sentence. The idiomatic use of these causes problems (on time, in a hurry, etc.)
*in, on are part of Brown's 14 morphemes.

Adjective: description words. The order of these may be confused in the LLD child.
Conjunction: a class of connectors that indicate the relationship between the joined parts of an utterance. Typical of the LLD child is the overuse of "and" as well as the lack of more sophisticated ones, e.g., although, however.
Comparatives/superlatives: a means of comparison. Irregular forms cause problems with the LLD child.
MLU: mean length of utterance, used to compute the average length of the child's utterances by either the number of morphemes or words divided by the total number of utterances.

Exhibit 6–9 Language Sample: Morphology

SLP	Billy
Hi, Mike, what did you do this weekend?	Billy and me goed to zoo.
What fun! Who's Billy?	Billy mine brother, mine little brother. He two.
What did you see?	We seed 3 lion. And 2 tiger. But no monkeys.
What did you do?	We climb way, way, way up.
Where?	On a ur, um, uh, hill.
Where was the hill?	In zoo.
Was something there?	Yeah, elephants up there. They feeding the baby. The baby mama mean! She runned at fence. She goed, "ROWRRRRR!"
Wow, that's exciting!	Bill and me afraid.
Do you want to go back again?	We can't.
Really?	Daddy say we can go when Grandma come.

Exhibit 6–10 Language Sample: Morphological Analysis

Mean length of utterance (MLU) by morphemes: 76 morphemes, divided by 17 utterances = 4.47 (age appropriate).

Structures Present in Obligatory Context and Correctly Used
- present progressive
- *in, on*
- plural (inconsistently)
- article *a* (inconsistently)

Structures Omitted
- contractible copula
- uncontractible copula
- possessive

- articles *the, a* (inconsistently)
- uncontractible auxiliary (*were*)
- regular past
- third-person singular present tense

Structure Substituted for
- irregular past

Structures Not Present, But No Obligatory Context
- contractible auxiliary

Additional Information
- pronoun substitution: *mine* for *my, me* for *I*

Now look at the sample in Exhibit 6–13 and identify those syntactic structures that are omitted, contain errors, or do not appear (are not obligatory) in the context of the sample. Exhibit 6–14 contains the analysis and interpretation of the sample, and Exhibit 6–15 contains a representative list of standardized instruments that can be used in whole or part to gain more information about error structures identified in the sample.

An interesting aspect of this sample is that Luis's use of English may be influenced by his Hispanic background and his first language, Spanish. In the background information it was revealed that his mother does not speak English. Consequently you will want to make a differential diagnosis between those structures that may be typical of dialectical influence as opposed to those that may indicate a language problem. After you have elicited these structures, check the results against a standard list of morphological differences common to Hispanic speakers. These include but are not limited to lack of possessive marker ("the shirt of my brother" vs. "my brother's shirt"), substitution of the regular past *ed* ending for the irregular form, omission of the third person singular, lack of obligatory *do*, and omission of articles. Charts you can use to address dialectical differences common in speakers of Asian, Black English, or Hispanic background can be found in Lund and Duchan (1993), Owens (1995), Shipley and McAfee (1992), and Roseberry-McKibbin (1995) among others.

The increasing complexity and length of both spoken and written language (linked to semantic meaning) is the hallmark of a competent language user in the schools. Often, a deficit in this area is not obvious because students may not make errors during conversational speech. If their language is simpler and less elaborate than that of their peers, however, it may provide "an insufficient base both for the understanding of literate language and for age-appropriate writing skills" (Paul, 1995, p. 410). Once a student is beyond Brown's Stage V, you must develop new means to describe length and complexity. Based on the work of Loban (1976), Scott (1988), and Paul (1981, 1995), I suggest the following steps, with the terms defined below.

Exhibit 6–11 Evaluation Instruments Addressing Morphology

Asterisk (*) marks tests with a chart for Black English use.

1. *Multilevel Informal Language Inventory* (Goldsworthy & Secord, 1982) Spontaneous or elicited; contains most of Brown's 14 morphemes
2. *Clinical Evaluation of Language Fundamentals-Revised* and *Clinical Evaluation of Language Fundamentals-3* (Semel, Wiig, & Secord, 1987a, 1987b, 1989) *Word Structure subtest:* irregular and regular plurals and past tense, possessives, third-person singular, comparative/superlative, auxiliary + *ing*, reflexive, possessive pronouns
3. *Bankson Language Test-2* (Bankson, 1990) Pronouns, present progressive, regular and irregular past, third-person singular, auxiliary, copula
4. *Carrow Expressive Language Inventory* (Carrow, 1974) Auxiliaries, third-person singular, copula, articles, plurals, pronouns, present progressive, *in*, *on*, irregular and regular past
5. *Patterned Expressive Syntax Screening Test* (Young & Perachio, 1993) All of Brown's 14 morphemes arranged developmentally
*6. *Structured Photographic Expressive Language Test-Preschool* and *Structured*

Photographic Expressive Language Test-2 (Werner & Kresheck, 1983a, 1983b) Auxiliaries, copula, plural, present progressive, irregular and regular past, third-person singular
7. *Clinical Evaluation of Language Fundamentals-Preschool* (Wiig, Secord, & Semel, 1992) Plural, possessive, third-person singular, regular and irregular past, present progressive, copula, auxiliary, pronouns
8. *Test of Language Development-Primary: 2* (Newcomer & Hammill 1991a, 1991b) *Grammatic Completion subtest:* possessive, third-person singular, regular and irregular past and plurals, present progressive, comparative/superlative
9. *Preschool Language Scale-3* (Zimmerman, Steiner, & Pond, 1992) Irregular and regular plurals, possessives, *in*, *on*, irregular and regular past, present progressive, auxiliary, copula
10. *Test for Examining Expressive Morphology* (Shipley, Stone, & Sue, 1983) Uses cloze; present progressive, irregular and regular past and plurals, third-person singular; age ranges given for each structure
11. *Berry-Talbott* (Berry, 1966) Uses nonsense words; most of Brown's 14 morphemes
12. *Northwest Syntax Screening Test* (Lee, 1971) Most of Brown's 14 morphemes

- calculate MLU in words (not morphemes) using T-units or C-units of *both* spoken and written samples;
- divide the T-units or C-units into complex, coordinating, and simple segments;
- using these segments you may
  —calculate the subordination index
  —divide clauses into early or late types
  —calculate the number of disruptions;

- determine whether the results indicate general age-appropriate development.

Because Paul indicates "using MLU per T-unit rather than per sentence will provide a more valid assessment of utterance length" (Paul, 1995, p. 411), the first step will be to divide the sample into T-units. In brief, a T-unit is one main clause with all the subordinate (dependent) clauses and non-clausal phrases attached to or embedded in it. All coordinated clauses (those connected by *and,*

Exhibit 6–12 Syntax Terminology

Noun Phrase

Most speech-language professionals include five components in the noun phrase. All but the noun itself (sometimes called the *head*) are optional. In the utterance "Daddy come!" "Daddy" is a noun phrase. These components appear in a predetermined order:

Initiator + Determiner + Adjectives + Noun + Postmodifier

Three of the components come before (in front of) the noun, but they all modify the noun:

Initiators (e.g., *only, just, almost, nearly*)

Determiners: these can include quantifiers (e.g., *both, some, any*), articles, a possessive pronoun (e.g., *our, my*), a demonstrative pronoun (e.g., *this, those*), or numbers

Adjectives of any type: nouns marked for possession (*Mommy's*); ordinal numbers (*first, third*); nouns used as adjectives (*truck stop, turkey farm*).

Next comes the **noun** itself [students].

After the noun comes **postnoun modifiers**, which can include

Prepositional phrases ("in the snow"; "up a tree")

Relative clauses ("that I used to know," "that Mom always gave me")

Adverbs (*here, there*)

Appositives ("Judy, *our leader,* . . .")

Therefore a noun phrase may be as simple as a single word or as complicated as "half that scrumptious, calorie-loaded pie that they served me" or "only his incredible convertible in the driveway."

Noun phrases become more elaborate as the child's syntax becomes more sophisticated. All the elements listed above can occur in a child by Brown's Stage V.

Verb Phrases

Like noun phrases, a verb phrase can be composed of a single word; the *go* in "Daddy go" is a verb phrase. The verb phrase also has a head, in this case the verb, and six optional functions. The head can also be called the *main verb*. It is important to note that the copula serves as the head; that is, the main verb. The optional categories that can be added to the main verb are modal auxiliaries, perfective auxiliary, auxiliary (*be* form), negative, passive, and the postverb modifiers.

Therefore in front of the main verb can come

Modals: a kind of auxiliary verb that expresses attitudes or intentions (*can, may, shall, should, would, could, might, must*)

Perfect: the forms of *have* verbs that denote action that has been or will be completed by a certain time (*have* gone)

***Be* auxiliary:** (*am, is, are, was, were, be, been*)

Negative: *not* or its contracted form *n't.* If there is a modal, the negative comes between the modal and perfective forms ("could not have gone").

Passive: in its simplest explanation, the passive represents a two step process: First the passive is marked by *been* or *being* (he *has been*") plus an addition to the head, usually *ed* or *en* (He has been eaten by cannibals," or "He is being nibbled to death by ducks").

After the verb come **postverb modifiers,** which can include

Prepositional phrases ("in the bucket")

Noun phrases (a "new coat")

Adverbial phrases ("to the store," "too late," "with a vengeance")

So a verb phrase can be as simple as "*go*," but as complicated as "might have been studying in the bedroom all night" or "would not have been eaten by the children."

Negatives

Negation can include any form of negation (*no, don't, not*). It does not appear in a set sequence like noun and verb phrases. If a sentence contains auxiliaries of any type, the negative comes after the first element in a verb phrase ("He is not happy"; "The cat should not have been let loose"). When there is no auxiliary, this rule does not work ("I type not"). In this case, we have to add a form of the auxiliary *do* in front of the main verb ("I don't type"; "I do not type").

Question Forms

There are three forms of questions: *yes/no (Y/N), what/who/when/where/why/how (WH),* and *tag*

continues

Exhibit 6–12 continued

questions (questions added to the end of a declarative sentence, intended to seek agreement rather than information). Stages of acquiring question forms, based on Brown's stages, with examples of each, are listed in order below:

Stage I: Intonation only ("Go?", "Mama?"); use of *what* and *that*.

Stage II: Y/N with intonation but no auxiliary verb ("Doggie nice?" "Mama go?"); use of *why* and *where*

Stage II: Y/N with auxiliary and inversion ("Is Doggie nice?"). WH with no inversion of auxiliary ("Where she is going?").

Stage IV: WH with inversion of auxiliary ("Where is she going?"); inversion of subject and either the main or auxiliary verb in positive questions only; use of *when, how*, and *why* completely correct.

Stage V: Inversion of subject/auxiliary with negative questions also ("Can't I go?" "Isn't she going?"); use of tag questions [She's going, isn't she?]; use of obligatory *do* in questions ("Do you want to go?"); LLD children confuse the order of questions much beyond the ages expected.

Conjunctions:

Conjunctions are important primarily because they are used in more advanced clause structures. They, and the clauses they connect, are an indication of complexity. Conjunctions as clausal connectors can be one of two types: *coordinating* (and, but, or), used to conjoin clauses, or *subordinating* (as, if, since, because, that, etc.), used to introduce subordinate clauses.

Clauses: Each clause must contain both a subject and a verb. There are a number of different types.

Simple:

She's going.

Simple with compound subject, verb, or object:

The girl and boy are going.
She *jumped and ran.*
She likes *burritos or tacos.*

Compound clauses

The girl is running, and the boy is hopping.
The man laughed, but the boys frowned.

Object clauses (uses verbs like *hope, know, think, feel, hate, like, remember*; answers the question "What"); also called **Propositional complement**

She knew *that they did it.*
I hope *that you are ready to go.*
I like *how you did that.*
I think *(that) I want this one.* (*That* can be present or absent; it is still an object clause)

Relative clauses, right embedded

The boy hit the door *that had been left open.*
I want the puppy *that we saw last night.*

Relative clauses, center embedded

The puppy *that you wanted* was sold.
The girl *who has long red fingernails* won't wash any dishes.

Embedded questions: contain "Wh" words, but not in interrogative sentences. Also called **WH clauses**.

I like *how you did that.*
She told him *why she wanted to go.*
I hope you know *when your homework is due.*

[Compound]/{complex} clauses

{She went shopping and then she took in the movie} [that was playing at Shopping town].
{They ran but they missed the bus} [that had already left].
{I know [that you wanted a scholar], but I hate school}.

Multiple clauses of other types

I think I know what you mean. (Embedded question within objective clause)
Since I went to college, I have watched little

continues

Exhibit 6–12 continued

television except when the Olympics are on. (Adverbial clause, main clause [independent], embedded question)

Subordinate (dependent) clauses include:
- Relative clauses
- Object clauses

Infinitive clauses (generally do not include the early infinitive forms *gonna, wanna, gotta*). In early ones, the subject is the same as the main sentence and is often deleted ("He has to move"; "She wants to get out"). Later ones are embedded clauses that have a different subject from the main clause, so that the embedded clause subject is expressed ("I want it to go chug"; Dad made this for me to ride").

Adverbial clauses ("since I was going," "after he comes back," "because I am over 21")

Exhibit 6–13 Language Sample: Syntax

Head Start Teacher	Client
Hi, Luis, what did you do over the weekend?	Saturday I walk to store to get some pants that aren't dumb.
What do you mean?	My Aunt Angela give me pants on my birthday but they are ugly.
Ugly?	Yeah. With stripes. And they is more ugly than ur, uh, warts. Nobody like them.
Did you find some you like?	Yeah, jeans. (Points to ones he has on) See?
(Looks at them) They are nice. Did you look at anything else?	Yeah, at boots.
Did you get some?	We couldn't. My mama say that they are too much money so we go home.
I'm sorry; maybe next time.	Where you shop?
I like catalogues. I was shopping just before you came in to see me.	How you are shopping in them?
I look at pictures to find something I like and then I look at how much it costs. (Points to page) Here, you look. Do you like this shirt?	No. I no like that one. My sister maybe would like it.
(Teacher starts to turn page)	No turn yet. (Luis points to another shirt) My sister like big shirts. Bought some with her own money (Indicates a blue one). This is the shirt of my sister.

Exhibit 6–14 Language Sample: Syntactic Analysis

MLU by morphemes = 5.35 (age appropriate)

Present in Sample		*Omitted/In Error in Sample*
	Noun Phrase Elaboration	
a few adjectives		
increasing length of noun phrase		
object clauses		
postnoun modifiers		
relative clauses		
	Verb Forms	
present progressive		irregular past
copula (error in number)		regular past
modal (*would*)		third-person singular verb marker
uncontractible auxiliary (*are*)		
	Negative Forms	
no and *no* plus verb		*no* substituted for *don't*
aren't, couldn't, nobody		
	Question Forms	
intonation for *yes/no*		no inversion of subject and
where, how		auxiliary verb
		no inversion for WH sounds
		no obligatory *do* in questions
	Conjunctions	
and		
but, so joining clauses		
	Other Errors	
		possessive, articles
		omission of pronoun

but, when, etc.) are separated into T-units, unless they contain a coreferential subject deletion in the second clause. For example, compare these two ways of constructing an utterance. "He runs and he drops it." (2 T-units) vs. "He runs and drops it." (1 T-unit because *he,* the subject of *drops,* has been deleted). Breaking down an utterance into T-units help avoid overestimating the length of an utterance separated primarily by "and . . . and . . . and . . ." The subordination index is the average number of dependent and main clauses *per T-unit,* usually ranging from 1 to 4. Let us identify the subordination index and how many T-units are in each clause (the T-units appear within the parentheses).

"Today we're gunny go to Disney Land and my mom and dad are gunna go too

Exhibit 6–15 Evaluation Instruments Addressing Syntax

1. *Test of Language Competence-Expanded Edition* (Wiig & Secord, 1989)
   Recreating Sentences subtest
   Coordination, complex sentences

2. *Multilevel Informal Language Inventory* (Goldsworthy & Secord, 1982)
   Spontaneous or elicited; coordination of both words and clauses, complex clauses, participles, gerunds, passives plus earlier verb forms

3. *Clinical Evaluation of Language Fundamentals-3* (Semel, Wiig, & Secord, 1995)
   - *Formulated Sentences subtest:* phrases, simple sentences, coordinated sentences, complex sentences, and sentences requiring three clauses
   - *Recalling Sentences subtest:* simple sentences, coordinating and complex sentences, including relative clauses, passive sentences (three types), and interrogative; noun and verb phrase elaboration
   - *Sentence Assembly subtest:* simple sentences, coordinating and complex sentences, declarative, interrogative, imperative, and passive sentences
   - *Sentence Structure:* negatives, phrase elaboration, compound and complex clauses, interrogatives. Note: this subtest addresses receptive language; it can be used to check comprehension of structures missing in the child's repertoire.

4. *Bankson Language Test-2* (Bankson, 1990)
   Negatives, questions, simple verb forms

5. *Carrow Expressive Language Inventory* (Carrow, 1974)
   Negatives, auxiliaries and other verb forms, passive, interrogatives, complex dependent clauses

6. *Patterned Expressive Syntax Screening Test*
   Delayed imitation. All sentence types, arranged developmentally

7. *Structured Photographic Language Test-Preschool Structured Photographic Language Test-II*
   Verb tense, auxiliaries, copula, infinitive, dependent clauses (complex), interrogatives

8. Clinical Evaluation of Language Fundamentals-Preschool (Semel, Wiig, & Secord, 1987a)
   Infinitive, coordination, relative and subordinate clauses, verb tenses, auxiliaries, interrogative

9. *Test of Language Development II-Intermediate*
   - *Sentence Combining:* Complex and coordinated clauses, elaborated noun and verb phrases, passive
   - *Word Ordering:* relative clauses, elaborated noun and verb phrases, passive, infinitive clauses, interrogatives

10. *Test of Language Development II-Primary*
    - *Sentence Imitation:* noun and verb phrase elaboration, complex clauses

11. *Clark-Madison Test of Oral Language*
    Noun phrase, verb phrase elaboration; 97 structures targeted in 66 sentences

12. *Developmental Sentence Scoring*
    Verb forms, a few compound and complex sentences, WH and Y/N questions

13. Test of Adolescent Language
    - *Speaking Grammar subtest:* Complex and coordinated sentences with multiple embeddings, noun and verb phrase elaboration, infinitive clauses, embedded questions, negatives, interrogatives. Much higher level than the other tests.
    - *Writing Grammar subtest:* sentence combining: coordination, complex clauses, elaborated noun and verb phrases

and my cousin George is gunna come later after his dad gets off work but he's a real pain and he always wants his own say and he has to go to the bathroom all the time and one time we were at the movies and it was the best part and my mom made me take him to the men's room and boy was I mad because when we got back the movie was all over except for the mushy stuff."

T-1 Today we're gunna go to Disney Land (1)

T-2 (and my mom and dad are gunna to too (1)

T-3 (and) my cousin George is gunna come later after his dad gets off work (2)

T-4 (but) he's a real pain (1)

T-5 (and) he always wants his own way (1)

T-6 (and) he has to go to the bathroom all the time (1)

T-7 (and one time we were at the movies (1)

T-8 (and) it was the best part (1)

T-9 (and) my mom made me take him to the men's room (1)

T-10 (and) boy was I mad because when we got back the movie was all over except for the mushy stuff (3)

Subordination Index = 13/10 = 1.3

Owens uses C-units as well as T-units to describe length or complexity, and they can be helpful in evaluating the younger elementary child (Owens, 1995). They are similar to T-units, but they also include incomplete (partial) sentences in answer to questions and aphorisms. Using the example above, each of the 10 T-units is also a C-unit. If more utterances which count as C-units are added to the sample, you can see the difference.

Clinician: How old is George, Larry?

Larry: Eight. (0 T-units, 1 C-unit)

Clinician: What movie did you go to see?

Larry: It had Bruce Willis but I don't remember the name. (2 T-units, 2 C-units)

Clinician: How was it?

Larry: Totally, completely awesome, man! (0 T-units, 1 C-unit)

Both units become longer as verb and noun phrase elaboration take place (e.g., "run" vs. "would have been running like mad" or "cat" vs. "the short-haired gray cat with the folded down ears and stumpy tail").

The next step is to analyze the complexity of the T-units themselves by separating simple utterances from those that are complex or coordinated. Paul divides complexity into early and late types. The early ones (MLU 3.0–4.0) include simple infinitive clauses with the same subject (He wants to go), object clauses (prepositional complements), embedded questions without infinitives (WH clauses), simple conjoinings, multiple embeddings, and embedded plus conjoined sentences. Later occurring types (MLU 4.0–5.0) include infinitive clauses with different subjects (He wants me to go), relative clauses, gerunds, embedded questions with infinitives (He knows where to go), and unmarked infinites (the "to" is deleted: Look at him go).

Since space limitations in this chapter prohibit a detailed discussion of disruptions, I refer you to the original reference for calculating disruptions, "A procedure for Classifying Disruptions in Spontaneous Language Samples," by Dollaghan and Campbell (1992), in *Topics in language Disorders*, volume 12, pps. 56–68. This is well worth your time to investigate if your student appears to have word-finding problems or just "gets tangled up" when he speaks. As a general rule of thumb, the authors report that in a 100 word sample, the number of pauses and mazes, etc., produced by a typical student was 5.9 with a standard deviation of 1.8. Therefore, they suggest that the possibility of word-finding deficits be investigated if a student's sample exceeds 7 or 8 disruptions.

After your calculations, how can you tell if your student is exhibiting adequate length or complexity for his age or grade? Although researchers have published data on T-units, C-units, and the subordination index, often their methodology number of subjects, and definition of basic terminology differed enough to make comparisons and/or compilation into charts difficult. One researcher, for example, divided T-unit data by narrative or expository categories. Table 6–1, therefore, should be viewed as representing only a general developmental progression, not as a source of specific numerical values (Scott, 1988; Loban, 1976; Paul, 1995; and Owens, 1995).

As I stated at the beginning of this chapter, I think lists can be often be more helpful than detailed reports of research. Therefore I will close this section with some general guidelines to help you assess, understand, and describe the effects of increasing length and complexity.

Scott (1988) showed that MLU per T-unit increases slowly throughout the school years. Loban's research indicates that important differences exist between oral and written length. In the sixth and seventh grades, the length of oral T-units is longer than those in the student's written samples; in the eighth and ninth grades, they are about equal, but by the tenth through twelfth grades, T-units of written work are longer than oral ones (Loban, 1976). In sum then, if this gradual change is not taking place, you may need to work on expanding complex forms during intervention.

By the time a child is age 4 or 5, 20% of the spontaneously produced sentences contain complex structures. Therefore, you can compute or estimate the percentage as a quick check of syntactic elaboration. If your student is producing complex structures, Paul points out that you only have to transcribe only those portions which contain complexity of some sort, compute the approximate percentage, and classify the forms into late or early types listed above. By the time students enter school, they should be using an average of 6 to 8 different conjunctions (usually *and*, *if*, *because*, *when*, and *so*) within a 15-minute sample (Paul, 1981, 1995). If these structures, which result in clauses, are not present in a spontaneous sample, try to elicit those that are absent using part of a standardized test or other elicitation procedures.

Table 6–1 T-Units, C-Units, and Subordination Index by Grade

Grade	Length of T-Units in Words		Length of C-Units in Words		Subordination Index	
	Spoken	Written	Spoken	Written	Spoken	Written
3–4	7.6–9.0	5.2–8.6			1.2–1.3	1.0–1.3
5–6	8.1–9.6	7.3–9.0	9.8	9.0	1.3–1.4	1.2–1.4
7–8	9.7–10.7	8.9–10.4			1.3–1.4	1.3–1.5
9–10	10.7–10.9	10.1–11.8	10.9	10.1	1.3–1.5	1.4–1.5
11–12	11.1–11.7	10.7–14.4	11.7	13.3	1.5–1.6	1.5–1.7

Pragmatics, Semantics, Fluency, Voice and Metalinguistics: A Note on Assessment

Because of space limitations, I cannot provide detailed procedures for assessing pragmatics, semantics, voice, and fluency. Voice and fluency are best addressed through specific measures and techniques found in detail in texts covering those topics. Because episodes of dysfluency are often intermittent, you should always check for its presence in multiple locations and at different times. Semantics and pragmatics can be approached much as we approached the syntactic analysis we have just completed; that is, first determine the hallmarks of normal development, typical error patterns, and implications of the student's performance in the area within the classroom using Exhibit 6–2 or 6–3, 6–4, 6–6, and/or 6–7.

Because students must also develop a conscious understanding of the linguistic code, it is crucial to evaluate the whole area of metalinguistics when dealing with the school-age population. *Metalinguistics* can be defined in its simplest terms as the understanding of and ability to use language to discuss and manipulate the forms of language. This includes understanding and altering phonological segments as children learn early decoding skills, and later explaining and applying the rules of spelling, subject-verb agreement, topic sentence, dependent clause construction, and so forth. Not only are these abilities essential in learning to read, but as the student reaches upper grade levels, the skills must become increasingly sophisticated. Often included under the same heading, but sometimes considered separately are the allied skills of metacognition and metapragmatics. Metacognition deals with students' defining how they think ("Let's see, first I have to multiply, then subtract, and then bring down the next number"); metapragmatics involves a conscious knowledge of the often subtle rules of social communication ("Teacher, he's pushing into line and says it's his turn when he knows it's mine"). Teaching written expression as a developmental process can be considered an entirely multilinguistic task. Often the most direct way to assess a student's abilities in this area is by observation or by asking the student to explain what he or she is doing and why. Recently some instruments have been published that address these areas; they are listed separately in Appendix 6–C. Metalinguistics is an integral part of dynamic assessment, which is discussed later in this chapter under "New Approaches to Assessment."

After you review screening and/or school records, complete your interviews and observation(s), and plan an effective means to sample the student's language. On the basis of those data, choose standardized measures to fill in the blanks and provide the "numbers" that may be required by your state/district. Of course you may find that you can combine this with your analysis of syntax or phonology, although not necessarily.

NEW APPROACHES TO ASSESSMENT

Given the amount of information presented so far, it may be hard to believe that there are more ways to approach assessment. From a student perspective, you may well be wondering if we really need more. In my experience, yes, but the reason is neither simple nor straightforward. According to Westby, Stevens Dominguez, and Oetter (1996), much of the information gained through the traditional procedures outlined earlier in this chapter is quantitative, and of little use in guiding intervention. Therefore, drawing on research from the psychology of learning, professionals in our field are creating new methods of assessment in which the line between intervention and evaluation is blurred. Although I have created this section of the chapter to underscore the differences between traditional assessment approaches and "new" approaches, the separation is largely artificial because new theories always owe something to their predecessors. In fact, I hope you will discern that many of the concepts and procedures discussed in this section are ones you have met before dressed in new clothes.

Authors have adopted various names to describe new concepts of assessment: dynamic, interactive, observational, judgmental, ecological, portfolio, or, when applied to the school population, curriculum based. Space does not permit a detailed description of every type, or its place in the developmental history of these approaches, but the citations noted throughout this section contain definitions, discussion, and examples of each if you need more specific information. For clarity, my description of them will refer to them as if they were all developed to be used in the school environment, but in actuality, many of them were not originally designed with the school-age population in mind. The feature they all appear to share, however, is a multistage, ongoing analytical procedure. In one form or another, the proponents of each type look at a student's language as it relates to the communication expectations of the classroom but do not stop at this point. They continue to identify points of match and mismatch between the ability of the student and the demands he or she faces and then to design strategies that support the student's attempts to learn. These steps of testing, teaching, and retesting are repeated with a conscious, concerted effort to decrease dependence on the clinician's help (Nelson, 1994; Palincsar, Brown, & Campione, 1994; Schneider & Watkins, 1996; and Westby et al., 1996). Obviously, two of the substantial differences from traditional assessment involve the ongoing nature of the process; that is, assessment has no real end point and the assumption that "the focus of assessment should shift from identifying the conditions that cause failure to identifying those that are likely to lead to academic success." (Paratore, 1995, pp. 67–68).

Before we delve into the historical roots of interactive assessment, let us look at why it has been so appealing for the school-based speech-language professional. First, the general concept of curriculum-based assessment has itself grown out of an increased use of the collaborative intervention model that you will find discussed in detail in Chapter 8. In simplest terms, the previous practice of removing students from the regular classroom (pull-out) was based on the assumption that professionals could "fix" the child's deficits outside class by using intervention approaches specific to the handicapping condition(s). By definition, these techniques were quite different from those used to teach typical children. As a result of this appropriate therapy, proponents predicted, failure would be prevented, and students could reenter the class when they had caught up with their peers. Problem: for many students, it simply never happened.

As a result, many speech-language professionals have endeavored to provide speech-language services within the regular classroom to the greatest extent possible (push-in), using the regular curriculum as "therapy" material. Advantages and disadvantages of this intervention approach are discussed in Chapter 8. To return to our subject of assessment, however, it appears logical that if you expect a student to succeed using a specific curriculum, then the curriculum itself must be part of the evaluation process. For the student with language based learning disabilities, "Curriculum-based language intervention . . . involves starting with an inventory of areas where change is needed most" (Nelson, 1994, p. 106). Nelson listed and defined the different curricula that language can affect, namely "official," "cultural," "de facto," "school culture," "hidden," and "underground." She recommended identifying "zones of significance," contextually based areas that at least two informants have selected as priorities. The following methods are all used to identify zones of significance:

1. interviewing the participants (teachers, parents, the students themselves) to elicit intervention priorities

2. carefully studying artifacts (written language samples)

3. observing the student in the classroom to determine strengths and weaknesses as they relate to the linguistic, commu-

nicative, and cognitive demands of the curriculum

4. closely observing the student as "scaffolding" and "miscue analysis" (Goodman, 1983) take place

As mentioned previously, "new" concepts build on those that have come before. The basic premise of miscue analysis is that the errors a student makes while reading aloud are not accidental; that is, the inaccuracies reflect the decoding process gone awry in a specific way. Therefore, by analyzing errors as a student reads curriculum-level material aloud, you can gain insights into areas that should be addressed during intervention. Another of the underlying assumptions of curriculum-based assessment is that scaffolding is effective. Scaffolding can be thought of as focusing on a level of understanding just slightly more advanced than the low-achieving student is presently capable of using. In a nascent model developed in 1969, Feuerstein proposed the concept of mediated learning, the means by which an experienced adult selects, focuses, and feeds back a learning experience to children, leading to children's gradual internalization of the structure as their own. Feuerstein developed the concept of the Learning Potential Assessment Device (LPAD) to measure a low-achieving student's ability to profit from such instruction. It is, in effect, a way to "depict the modifiability of cognitive structures and the source of difficulties in learning" (Palincsar et al., 1994, p. 133). Although later researchers acknowledged their debt to Feuerstein, they were not fully satisfied with the model because it did not involve the curriculum in any meaningful way: LPAD was "divorced from the content and context of classrooms" (p. 134).

Some 35 years before that, in 1934, Vygotsky postulated a seminal theory based on the importance of social interaction in learning. He developed the concept of a *zone of proximal development* (ZPD), defined as "the difference between a child's actual developmental level as determined by independent problem solving and the level of potential development as determined through problem solving under adult guidance or in collaboration with more capable peers" (Schneider & Watkins, 1996, p. 157). Assuming this, then, if we are to understand the child's present level of development, we cannot use a "static" test; we must look at those processes that are in a state of flux, of maturation. Predictably, other researchers refined the theories of Vygotsky and Feuerstein; Carlson and Weidl modified specific test procedures to include an interactive component, and Campione and Brown focused on determining how easy it was for students to learn from others and the amount of flexibility they displayed in transferring their new skills to similar situations (Palincsar et al., 1994).

Westby et al. (1996) suggested that we use ecological assessment, which considers the combined effects of physical, social, and psychological context on a student's classroom performance and therefore includes "insights, knowledge and impressions of professionals and parents who work with the children" (p. 145). Such assessment should be conducted in multiple natural, familiar settings (home, school) and should include multiple domains (speech-language, sensory, motor, cognitive, social/emotional, temperament, etc.). Because professionals representing different backgrounds have distinct insights, the overall picture that emerges will lead to an intervention plan that should address all the child's needs. Westby et al. described in detail the NEW TeamS model; although it was originally developed for preschoolers and below, she suggested that the principles apply to

an individual of any age. The goals of this program all reflect an awareness of a child's ZPD. According to Westby et al., using intervention within ZPD maximizes the development of the child's competence and confidence. Implicit in the application of this transdisciplinary approach to the school environment is the presence of language-based tasks that are directly related to the curriculum.

One of the concerns of speech-language professionals unfamiliar with curriculum-based intervention, however, is that they will become tutors. Admittedly, with a deadline for an assignment approaching rapidly, the temptation to help one of your students get a passing grade is a real one. But a restatement of the saying "Give the man a fish, and he eats for a day; teach a man to fish and he eats for a lifetime" is clearly applicable here. The intent of these assessment/intervention procedures is in its sequence of procedures. First we must discover what the student's abilities are at present as he struggles to complete a particular task. Then we want to determine how much and, most important, what kind of help (support, scaffold, model) this particular student needs to be able to succeed at a more advanced stage of the activity. After this step comes the one that differentiates this view of assessment from previous ones; as we guide the student, we work to discover his *potential to change his approach* to the task. Our assessment/intervention continues until the student can use the strategies he has learned independently in an untrained but related situation. In essence, we have taught him or her how to fish. If this sounds like the definition of *generalization*, it is, but our focus is on discovering and working within the ZPD, not in using assessment information (weaknesses) to apply a diagnostic label, compare the student's results to a norm, or determine if he qualifies for services within our area of professional expertise.

Another reason speech-language professionals have become increasingly interested in trying these new assessment approaches is that the reading and writing processes are so clearly an appropriate application. As Wallach and Butler (1994) note, "Learning to read and write is part of, not separate from, learning to speak and comprehend language" (p. 11). Reading can be, and has been, divided into a series of subskills, often taught in a bottom-up fashion, with children learning letter-sound correspondence and then decoding words containing different syllable types. Several grades later, the reading process, now largely applied below the level of consciousness, is used to comprehend the meaning of passages, paragraphs, and chapters. Researchers have become particularly interested in two aspects of language-based strategies: first, teaching students how to recognize the opportunity for using one or more of them, and second, helping them discover specific ways to apply the strategies to new, different material or subjects. These strategies can include understanding how to activate prior knowledge, use text structure and schemas, or connect ideas to infer meaning. In reciprocal teaching, students and instructors take turns in discussing a shared text. A similar sequence exists for evaluating and teaching the writing process. One of the ways to evaluate and teach writing skills is through portfolio assessment, defined as "a purposeful collection of student work and records of progress and achievement assembled over time . . . permit(ing) the documentation of children's performances across a range of literacy tasks, texts, and settings, . . . (and) allow(ing) students to display their literacy knowledge under the real conditions of daily classroom demands." (Paratore, 1995, p. 68). This clear connection between intervention and evaluation is the differentiating characteristic and the strength of dynamic assessment. In your role as speech-language professional, you determine the student's level, teach, retest, move the level up a notch, teach, retest, and repeat the sequence over and over again.

Some critics have complained that these approaches rely too heavily on the skill of the clinician and the "intuitive nature" of the assessment (Palincsar et al., 1994, p. 134). Although the criticism may be justified, any approach that demands careful observation should have a place in evaluation. In the first part of this chapter, I stated repeatedly that assessment is not a one-time event, that each time you meet with a student you should gain new insights and make new hypotheses. The skill to do this will grow as you gain experience. "Book knowledge" will gain new meaning as you apply new ideas and techniques to the assessment and intervention processes; it is one of the reasons you will never be bored.

CASE STUDIES

By necessity, much of the information covered so far in this chapter has been contained in general statements; it has been my experience, however, that students absorb information better if they can apply general information to a specific case.

Therefore Eileen Gravani, the author of Chapters 2 and 7, and I have developed four profiles to illustrate steps to follow as you: (a) plan and implement assessment procedures, (b) develop IEP goals, and (c) detail how to address them in intervention. In other words, the students you are introduced to in this chapter will appear again in Chapters 7 and 8. I am sure you know that in the real world every student and case is unique, but as you gain clinical experience you begin to recognize that patterns of deficits appear to exist. Therefore approach these cases as illustrative models only; they should not be taken as a checklist to use for every similar student. As new instruments become available or as new research provides insights and methods to improve the quality of assessment, they should be adopted.

For each case, we will provide a description of the child and the reasons he or she has been brought to your attention as a school speech-language professional (e.g., referral, screening). Using what you have learned in this chapter, your job is to take a few minutes and think about what *you* would do to assess this student. Try to cover all the bases: think how the apparent problem(s) could affect classroom performance, and decide what information you need and could access from records, interviews, observation, and less formal procedures. I have given you one set of possible outcomes of the process as it relates to assessment. Be aware that there are dozens of other solutions that could address the issues just as effectively. You have probably been warned about using "cookbook" techniques in assessment, and I agree. However, as someone who has cooked, literally as well as figuratively, for a long time, a cookbook is not altogether a bad analogy. If you want to bake a cake, there are whole books full of good recipes to consult, but it is up to you to consider your budget, what the occasion is, how much time you have, what

is in the cupboard, who is allergic to nuts, if the cake is a good "keeper," who is on a diet, or even if a pie is a better choice. As you read my solution for each of the first three cases, you may come up with recipes that are better than mine.

CASE 1: STEVEN

Steven, called "Mr. Smiles" by his first-grade teacher, Ms. Rose, was referred to you by her in late February because he had been struggling academically all year, particularly in reading and spelling. Ms. Rose is an experienced teacher with a master's degree in reading. She regularly takes courses and attends workshops addressing the needs of the underachieving child because she enjoys the challenge of working with students in her lowest reading group, which this year includes Steven. Even compared with these classmates, however, he is making limited progress. In her written referral for a possible evaluation, she states that she is not sure if he will (or should) pass into second grade. She also noted in the referral that he is a delightful, hard-working, popular child. It has been my experience that January and February are very heavy months for referrals. With the excitement of the holidays over, teachers begin to think about possible retentions.

We will assume that no full-scale meeting of a Child Study Team was deemed necessary until I had done some initial investigation. My first task (and yours) is to figure out what we know and what we need to find out.

Without letting your eyes cruise down the page, think: What questions would you ask Steven's teacher? His parents? Steven himself? What other sources of information could you tap? Is there anything specific you might look for during your classroom observation? On the basis of these accumulated data, what procedures/instruments would you then plan to test his language?

Here are my answers: Although I had planned to begin by conferring with Ms. Rose, she was not available, so I checked Steven's records instead. According to his kindergarten screening results, Steven's vision, hearing, and gross motor skills were within normal limits, but he had been placed on a "watch" list because of borderline scores on the articulation and sentence repetition tasks of the language section of the screening. It is frequently instructive to check individual items that were in error, but only the scores of the speech-language screening had been retained; the actual protocol (test sheet) for this part of the screening had been discarded. The speech-language professional who had administered the screening had resigned midyear and moved to another state, so no details were available. The "school readiness" portion of the screening administered by the kindergarten teachers, however, was intact and indicated that Steven counted to 20, knew eight colors, and recounted personal information (name, age, etc.) but that he was not able to identify any letters.

Routine hearing screening of everyone in Steven's first-grade class 2 months before Ms. Rose's referral indicated that Steven's results were, as before, unremarkable. Steven's attendance in both grades had been excellent. In this particular school district, end-of-the-year tests are not used in kindergarten, and those administered to first graders are not scheduled until May, some 3 months in the future.

My interview with Ms. Rose began with a discussion of those "borderline" kindergarten screening scores. Steven's kindergarten teacher told her that even with lots of practice, Steven didn't seem to "get" sound-sym-

bol relationships. Please note this exchange because, in schools, much information is shared informally. It is very common for one teacher to check for insights into a student's problems with a colleague from the preceding year. Often this information does not appear in written form, so you have to ask.

Discussing current problems, Ms. Rose commented that while most first graders use at least two related sounds (phones) as they attempt to spell an unfamiliar word, Steven used only one, always in the initial position. The other letters he printed bore little relation to the sounds in the word (e.g., "kappe" for "Cortland"). The actual printing of letters did not appear to be difficult for him. Although Steven always paid attention, from September to December he often copied his friend's work in language arts as if he were not sure what to do. When Ms. Rose moved his seat away from his friend after Christmas vacation, Steven seemed lost, and his performance worsened. His spelling tests earned low average marks. Ms. Rose remarked that the grades represented Steven's hard work memorizing the simple words at home; three weeks later, however, he could not pass the identical test.

Because the borderline scores occurred in articulation and receptive language, I asked specifically about Steven's ability to pronounce sounds in words during spontaneous conversation. Ms. Rose responded that some sounds, mostly r's, were "a little funny" and that Steven also "gets his tongue tangled up when he tries to pronounce a long word with lots of syllables." Occasionally she could not understand him. Because I also wondered about the reason for Steven's poor performance on the sentence repetition task, I asked Ms. Rose if she had noticed any memory problems. She reported she wasn't sure; he seemed to follow directions for art projects and "science" experiments fairly well, but at other times he seemed very confused. Ms. Rose added that Steven remembered classroom rules and followed them better than many of his classmates.

Before making an appointment to observe Steven, I determined the subjects and time during the day when his deficits were most likely to be evident. Later that week, I observed him first during his reading instruction and then as he took part in a language arts writing activity. Steven attended well during the reading lesson. He experienced real difficulty, however, in sounding out words, even though Ms. Rose reviewed most of the sounds before each child read a short passage aloud. There appeared to be no pattern to his errors when he guessed a word. I noted that Steven looked very carefully at the pictures on the page and also listened intently to the questions Ms. Rose asked that gave clues about what was coming next.

The language arts lesson featured pictures representing the main points of the story they had just finished. The pictures had been cut apart, and the children were told to put them into the correct sequence. After this had been accomplished, Ms. Rose called on Steven to retell the story from the pictures. His rendition was adequate, if brief. Although his attempts at clarifying questions were not always successful, his pragmatics were appropriate. Overall, Steven had far less difficulty with this activity than the previous one, and his obvious fatigue at the end of the reading lesson disappeared.

Before the observation, I had interviewed Steven's kindergarten teacher, Ms. Warren, who agreed that Steven was a child who tried hard every minute. She reiterated that he just didn't seem to grasp the sound-symbol con-

nection and added that his parents were concerned. At their request, another hearing test had been completed. Ms. Warren said that Steven really liked finger plays but didn't remember the words, although he knew all the actions. The "watch" status had not been pursued because of the speech-language professional's departure in January. Steven's art and physical education teachers were interviewed briefly also; both felt that his memory was fine and described him as a delightful, popular child.

Both parents were very tense during their interview, alternating between expressing fear that something was wrong with Steven and commenting that they were sure he would catch up soon because he tried so hard. They confirmed that all developmental milestones had been met at typical times, except speech, which was "a little slow in coming." There was no family history of language problems. Mom volunteered that although Steven would "sit for hours" playing legos, he was easily frustrated when they tried to teach him a few letters. He loved looking at books by Dr. Seuss but didn't seem to get the idea of rhyme. Both his behavior and his health were good, but he was usually exhausted when he came home from school. At the close of the meeting, the parents asked that Steven be tested. After appropriate meetings and procedures outlined in Chapter 7, I audiotaped a brief language sample during recess and another language arts lesson. It revealed somewhat restricted vocabulary, some articulation errors, a few morphological omissions in longer sentences, and not many examples of syntactic complexity. Now, what do you recommend? Make a list before reading on.

On the basis of information gained through observations, interviews, and screen-

Tests	*To Tap Information Concerning*
Clinical Evaluation of Language Fundamentals-Preschool (CELF-Preschool; Wiig, Secord, & Semel, 1992)	word structure and receptive syntax (be sure he can understand complex forms)
Peabody Picture Vocabulary Test-Revised (PPVT-R; Dunn & Dunn, 1981)	single-word receptive vocabulary
Expressive One-Word Picture Vocabulary Tests-Revised (EOWPVT-R: Gardner, 1990)	single-word expressive vocabulary
Structured Photographic Expressive Language Test-2 (SPELT-2; Werner & Kresheck, 1983b)	morphology/syntax based on errors in screening, omissions/errors in language sample, and confirmation of errors in the CELF-Preschool
Goldman-Fristoe Test of Articulation (Goldman & Fristoe, 1986)	articulation errors

ings, I administered the following standardized tests for the reasons noted:
No fluency, voice, or formal pragmatics assessment appeared necessary. A Weschler Preschool and Primary Scale of Intelligence (WPPSI) revealed overall intelligence within normal limits, with performance subtests slightly better than verbal ones.

Articulation

Errors of *individual* phonemes were confined to gliding, distortion, and vocalization of /r/ and /l/, with fewer errors in single words than in words in sentences. The misarticulations in the Goldman-Fristoe Test of Articulation were also confirmed in Steven's connected speech; as a time-saving measure, the language sample also served as a speech sample. Because the quality of /l/ production was superior to /r/, deficits in single words may represent a developmental lag in liquids.

As his teacher had noted, Steven also struggled with multisyllabic words not related to gliding or vocalization, possibly indicating difficulty in sequencing speech sounds during processing (receptive phonology) or when he tried to produce a complex series of phonemes (Swank, 1994). According to Hodson, six-year-olds should be significantly more successful in producing common multi syllabic words than five-year-olds. She also states that kindergarten skills such as the ability to recognize and produce rhyme are related to reading and spelling, weaknesses noted by both kindergarten and first grade teachers. Extension testing as part of intervention should include both areas; in the schools, such in-depth investigation is usually not done as part of the initial diagnostic process because of time limitations.

As intervention progresses you will want to check if Steven can segment words into syllables or blend segments into words. This is especially important because Steven must be able to store phonological representations long enough for the meaning of the word to be recognized. Limitations can impede comprehension (and consequent production) of complex morphological and syntactical forms as the child grows older.

Spelling concerns should be addressed partly by determining what phonological skills he is bringing to the task, i.e., what stage of spelling he is in (probably early phonemic) and then moving him into the next stage, even though it may not be grade appropriate (Temple & Gillet, 1984).

Language

Steven's performance on the SPELT-II indicated areas of weakness of both derivational and inflectional morphemes, particularly those forms which are not as salient. In a typical example Steven omitted the "ed" ending from a verb when it is pronounced as "t", as in walked; this morpheme is harder to perceive than the regular past tense marker in climbed ("d") or planted ("ed"). In sentence repetition tasks, he left out small words, omitted endings, and reversed the order of words, indicating again that memory for sounds is weak.

Being able to sequence events correctly appeared to be related to the availability OF visual cues; when Steven could observe the steps in a science experiment, see block patterns, or follow the movements of the art or P.E. teacher, he was much more successful

than when he had to rely solely on his auditory memory.

Steven's vocabulary scores are within acceptable limits with little discrepancy between receptive and expressive skills.

An example of a speech-language diagnostic report based on Steven's case, including test results and their interpretation, appears as Exhibit 6–16. Compared with university or hospital clinic evaluation reports, it may appear abbreviated. When I was first employed in the schools, my reports were detailed, comprehensive, and lengthy—very lengthy. In a Committee on Special Education meeting one day, the chair asked a question, the answer to which had been covered in my report. When I referred to this fact, the chair responded with "I don't have the time to read your reports; I only read your recommendations." Although my initial reaction was anger, I came to realize that if a report was so long that nobody (teachers, administrators, other specialists) reads it, then I was defeating my own purpose. Teachers *wanted* to know what I had discovered; it was my job to make my explanation free of jargon and as brief as the case would allow. Therefore only if another speech-language professional really needed exhaustive detail did I provide it. You will see that the report in Exhibit 6–16 includes some of the information you have just read. Other details, however, have been omitted or condensed. As you work through the succeeding cases, write a report for each of them, or discuss with another student what should be included.

CASE 2: JAMES

James is a youngster in third grade, the child of an African American military family who just moved into the district from another

Exhibit 6–16 Report of Speech-Language Evaluation

Sunnyside School

Cortland, New York

Identifying Information:

Name: Steven Smith

Address: 123 Main Avenue

Cortland, NY

Date of Birth: 9/11/8–

Grade/Teacher: First: Ms. Rose

Date of Evaluation: March 10, 199–

Background Information:

Steven, age 6–6, was referred for a speech-language evaluation by the Child Study Team on March 3, on the basis of academic problems reported by Ms. Rose involving the language arts curriculum, particularly reading and spelling. Both she and Ms. Warren, his kindergarten teacher, cite deficits in articulation and formation of some grammatical endings, and the lack of age/grade-appropriate sound-symbol relationship.

Steven's developmental and medical history are unremarkable; he has passed two recent hearing screenings. His mother reports that Steven can attend for long periods building with legos but is "antsy" and frustrated when she attempts reading activities with him. This examiner's observation of Steven during reading instruction and a language arts activity confirmed Ms. Rose's concern. Steven attended well but could not sound out words that had just been taught. His story sequencing ability was adequate, but his syntax during the story retelling was faulty. On the basis of these factors, the following standardized and nonstandardized evaluation procedures were chosen to assess possible deficits in word structure, vocabulary, and articulation. Results are listed below.

Test	Subtests	Standard Score	Percentile Rank
CELF-Preschool			
	Linguistic Concepts	9	37
	Basic Concepts	12	75
	Sentence Structure	8	25
	Recalling Sentences in Context	4	2
	Formulating Labels	9	37
	Word Structure	7	16
Receptive Language Score		98	45
Expressive Language Score		83	13
Total Language Score		90	25
Age Equivalent: 5-0			
PPVT-R		90	26
Age Equivalent: 6-0; Stanine: 4			
EOWPVT-R		92	30
Age Equivalent: 5-9; Stanine: 4			
SPELT-2	—	6	
% Correct: 76			
Goldman-Fristoe Test of Articulation		—	11
Stimulability		—	35

continues

Exhibit 6–16 continued

17 errors; /l/ and /r/ in all positions

Review of Steven's written language indicated adequate letter formation but correct use of only the initial sound in spelling of words; other letters were added but bore no resemblance to the sounds in the word (e.g., "kappe" for "Cortland").

Relationship of Standardized Scores to Standard Deviation:

Between – 1.0 and +1.0 (normal range): *CELF-Preschool:* Overall Receptive Language score, Total Language score, Linguistic Concepts, Basic Concepts, Sentence Structure, Formulated Labels, and Word Structure; *Peabody Picture Vocabulary Test-Revised; Expressive One-Word Picture Vocabulary Test-Revised;* Stimulability subtest of the *Goldman-Fristoe Test of Articulation.*

Between -1.0 and -1.5 (mild to moderate deficit): Expressive Language score of the *CELF-Preschool;* overall score of the *Goldman Fristoe Test of Articulation*

Between – 1.5 and -2.0 (moderate to severe deficit): Recalling Sentences in Context subtest of the *CELF-Preschool; SPELT-2*

Above +1.0: none

Articulation: Errors of *individual* phonemes were confined to gliding, distortion, and vocalization of /r/ and /l/ (*rug* becomes *wug; little* becomes *wittle,* and the "r" sound in *car* is distorted); these errors were confirmed in Steven's connected speech. These sounds are late developing, and Steven could improve his production of them by imitating the speech-language professional, so these individual sounds are not of concern at this time. Steven also struggled with multisyllabic words, possibly indicating difficulty in sequencing speech sounds during processing (putting them into his memory) or when he tried to produce a complex series of sounds (*aminal* for *animal*). Six-year-olds should be significantly more successful in producing common multisyllabic words than 5-year-olds, so this does constitute a deficit. Nonstandardized tasks revealed that Steven has little concept of rhyme or breaking words down into syllables; both of these skills are required for reading and spelling.

Language: Steven's performance on the SPELT-2 indicated areas of weakness of both derivational and inflectional morphemes, particularly those forms that are not as salient. In a typical example, Steven omitted the "ed" ending from a verb when it is pronounced as "t", as in *walked;* this morpheme is harder to perceive than the regular past tense marker in *climbed* ("d") or *planted* ("ed"), which he did produce. In sentence repetition tasks, he left out small words, omitted endings, and reversed the order of words, indicating again that memory for sounds is weak.

Being able to sequence events correctly appeared to be related to the availability of visual cues; when Steven could observe the steps in a science experiment, see block patterns, or follow the movements of the art or P.E. teacher, he was much more successful than when he had to rely solely on his auditory memory.

Steven's vocabulary scores are within acceptable limits, with little discrepancy between receptive and expressive skills.

Summary Statement:

Steven exhibits deficits in speech and language characterized by omission of word endings (morphology) and age-inappropriate skills in manipulating and comprehending sounds and sound sequences, including syllables and rhyme (receptive and expressive phonology). These deficits can negatively affect his learning to read and spell.

Recommendation:

Steven should be labeled as handicapped in speech and language by the appropriate district committee. (Note that this evaluation was done prior to the meeting of the labeling body; if the evaluation had been completed as a result of their deliberations, then the recommendation would specify the kind and frequency of intervention and whether it was to take place during individual or group sessions.)

state. Because he is a transfer student, he was administered the CELF Screening Test (Semel, Wiig, & Secord, 1989); his score fell below the cutoff score established by the district. As a quick check of articulation, he was instructed to count to 20 and recite the days of the week and the months of the year. During these tasks, James started the recitation of the days of the week with Wednesday, named the months of the year in random order, omitting October and February entirely, and employed some articulation characteristics of Black English dialect. In spontaneous conversation James appeared shy and hesitant, frequently used interjections (*err, ah, um*), and appeared to apply some morphological and syntactic rules of Black English, such as eliminating the plural marker if a number was given ("two shoe") and eliminating the third-person singular present tense verb ending ("he walk"). Second-grade records from his previous school revealed that he was a slightly below-average student; older files were not available because they had been lost during transfers between earlier schools. His older brother Douglas's screening results were unremarkable, although I noted he also used some Black English forms; Douglas is in fourth grade.

In this quite different case: what questions would you ask James's teacher, Ms. Dwyer? His parents? James himself? What other sources of information could you tap? Is there anything specific you might look for during your classroom observation?

In James's case, Ms. Dwyer will have limited information, but she (or the reading specialist) will have reviewed what past records are available and completed enough testing to place him in an appropriate reading group. In our conference, his classroom teacher noted that his oral reading skills seemed

"about average"; she also related this additional information based on his "permanent record": standardized tests given at the end of second grade resulted in scores one standard deviation below the mean in reading comprehension. Because this score falls within normal range, albeit low normal, James would not qualify for special reading services. Mathematical computation, spelling, and basic decoding skills in reading were all also within normal limits. Note that you can often save yourself time by checking with the classroom teacher concerning previous years' accomplishments, particularly if you do not understand what the scores or subtests of these educational instruments imply (i.e., what they measure).

Ms. Dwyer reported that "so far" James appears to be a quiet, almost shy child who rarely asks for help, even though he seems to have problems following directions some of the time. Her class is divided into heterogeneous groups, and although he hasn't made any close friends yet, James gets along well with the other children, and his "different way of talking" doesn't seem to matter. Right now you should be asking yourself what she means by this statement; it is typical of information that sometimes falls into your lap during an interview. In clarifying the comment, Ms. Dwyer appears to be referring to elements of Black English in both articulation and language. She adds, however, that James often seems to have a really hard time finding the word that he wants, and almost acts as if he were stuttering.

I observed James during a science lesson and later as part of a small group working on map skills (social studies). James was attentive during the lesson but did not volunteer any answers. He experienced difficulty with a worksheet of definitions based on the science lesson but did not seek help. During the other small-group activity, the students were required to follow directions and find a "hidden treasure" on a map of the United States. James consistently struggled with left/right concepts and compass directions. He spoke little and did not ask clarifying questions; there were few hesitations or interjections. The school nurse's records indicate that James passed the hearing screening; he has never appeared at her office because of illness.

Neither parent was available during the day for a meeting (a not uncommon occurrence), but a telephone conference with James's mother revealed that she was concerned about James's educational progress, particularly because Douglas had never had any problems in the same school. She said that James had always been a healthy child, had met all developmental milestones at age-appropriate levels, but often looked to his brother for help with his homework or to interpret events in general. When asked about possible stuttering behavior, she said that it seemed to her that James had trouble figuring out what word he wanted, not in trying to "get a word out." She described her son as a likable child who rarely got into trouble.

Now, based on the above, what procedures/instruments would you plan to test his speech/language?

One of the key issues here is James's apparent use of Black English; all standardized instruments must be carefully checked to be sure that they were normed on a substantial number of male African American students his age. The possibility of stuttering will require multiple observations/samples because dysfluency can occur intermittently. A language sample taken early in the assessment process should give a general idea what areas of language to test formally.

One language sample was recorded during a planning session for a school party; James and two other students had to think of several ideas for a theme and a list of items to be purchased. I elicited a second sample on a Friday afternoon when I played a game with James and three other boys, one of whom was on my caseload. James's use of interjections, circumlocutions, hesitations, and proforms (nonspecific words like "whatzit", "whatchamacallit", "thing," etc.) was particularly noticeable during the planning session as he attempted to name items like party favors, cupcakes, and Hi-C. To the nonprofessional, some of these behaviors could indeed be mistaken for stuttering, but no hallmarks of that disorder were present, such as repetition of sounds, syllables or phrases, long hesitations, or "blocking." Occasionally he seemed confused with the planning time line—for example, not understanding when "a week from Friday" was.

His use of some Black English morphological/syntactical/phonological forms was consistent but not pervasive; that is, he did not use many dialectical forms, but the ones present were used in all applicable cases. His vocabulary appeared limited and his syntax somewhat simplified; his MLU by words appeared inflated by circumlocutions. Both Ms. Dwyer and his mother confirmed that these samples "sounded like the way James talked," a useful quick check for the validity of a specific language sample.

I will ask again, given this additional information, what procedures/instruments would you plan to test his speech/language?

On the basis of the information gained through observations, interviews, and screenings, I administered the following standardized tests for the reasons noted:

Tests	*To Tap Information Concerning*
Test of Language Development (TOLD)-Primary: 2 (Newcomer & Hammill, 1991b)	compare overall receptive and expressive language; check sentence repetition for syntax and morphology errors (Black English?)
Comprehensive Receptive and Expressive Vocabulary Test (CREVT; Wallace & Hammill, 1994)	test has Black English norms; check additional single-word receptive and expressive vocabulary to confirm TOLD; check ability to define single words: word-finding problems?
Test of Word Finding (German, 1991)	identify specific word-finding problems
Goldman-Fristoe Test of Articulation (Goldman & Fristoe, 1986)	articulation errors check against Black English dialectical forms
Test of Relational Concepts-Revised (Edmonston & Thane, 1993)	spatial, temporal, and other "school" concepts
Clinical Evaluation of Language Fundamentals-3 (CELF-3; Semel et al., 1987b)	check automaticity through Rapid Naming subtest

---

No voice or formal pragmatics assessment appeared necessary. WPPSI revealed overall intelligence within normal limits, with performance subtests superior to verbal ones. James's scores and their interpretation are reported in Table 6–2.

I should explain that some of the instruments in Table 6–2 were *not* chosen before testing began. The first tests to be administered were the CREVT and the TOLD 2–Primary. James's performance on the receptive portion of the CREVT was within normal limits. However, during the expressive subtest of that instrument, it was clear that James struggled to find words to define items he clearly knew. With the exception of Oral Vocabulary, the TOLD 2–P results appeared to indicate that James's overall language skills were roughly within normal limits, pro-

viding his use of Black English morphological, phonological, and syntactic substitutions were taken into consideration. His performance on the Oral Vocabulary subtest indicated the same behaviors as on the CREVT. Combined with the other reported indications of probable anomia, the Test of Word Finding was administered. Its results confirmed word-finding deficits. This test, however, does not address automatic recall of common sequences like the days of the week, a problem during initial screening. Therefore the Rapid Naming subtest of the CELF-3 was administered; the results clearly identified automaticity as weak also. Because of James's reported problem with some concept words, the Test of Relational Concepts was administered, even though the upper age limit for this instrument is 8 years, some 2 months

Table 6–2 Scores and Interpretation of Testing

Test	Subtests	Standard Score	Percentile Rank
TOLD-Primary: 2	Picture Vocabulary	9	37
	Oral Vocabulary	5	5
	Grammatic Understanding	9	37
	Sentence Imitation	7	16
	Grammatic Completion	7	16
	Word Discrimination	12	7 5
	Word Articulation	7	16
CREVT	Receptive	92	30
	Expressive	75	5
	General	80	9
Test of Word Finding			
	Total Score	76	15
	Word Finding Profile	Slow and inaccurate namer	

Goldman-Fristoe Test of Articulation
    All errors attributable to Black English dialect

Test of Relational Concepts   Above age ceiling; some spatial, temporal concepts are in error

CELF-3

Rapid Naming:	no standardized scores
Time:	typical of just below 6-year-old
Errors:	typical of child between ages 6 and 7

Interpretation:
Relationship of Standardized Scores to Standard Deviation:
Between −1.0 and +1.0 (normal range): TOLD-Primary: 2: Picture Vocabulary, Grammatic Understanding, Sentence Imitation, Grammatic Completion, Word Discrimination, Word Articulation; Receptive Score of CREVT
Between −1.0 and −1.5 (mild to moderate deficit): General Score of CREVT
Between −1.5 and −2.0 (moderate to severe deficit): Oral Vocabulary subtest of the TOLD-2 Primary; Expressive Score of CREVT
Above +1.0: none

---

younger than he. James's errors appeared only in spatial and temporal concepts, specifically left/right, ordinal numbers, and before/after. Finally, to confirm that Black English usage did account for the marginal scores in articulation, the Goldman-Fristoe Test of Articulation was administered; as suspected, all articulation errors were so identified. I also checked James's spelling capabilities and found that they were entirely grade appropriate; that is, his articulation difference did not appear to affect a related classroom subject. Please note that the results of one test lead to using another; if you have a battery of tests you "always" administer, you can miss important information. Diagnostics is a form of puzzle solving in which you ask yourself at every stage of the process, Where do I go next?

Using this information, write a summary statement: How would you characterize James's use of language in the classroom?

I classified James's errors in morphology, syntax, and articulation as a language difference, not a language deficit. Equally on the basis of the scores of the standardized instruments and the interpretation of nonstandardized procedures, James's most serious deficit appeared to stem from word-finding problems, which directly affected his scores in expressive vocabulary. Semantically, he demonstrated weaknesses with some age-inappropriate temporal and spatial concepts. This case is an example of one in which some errors can be explained by dialect but in which others represent real deficits. Therefore see this case as a cautionary tale: just because you recognize the use of dialect, do not jump to the conclusion that it necessarily represents the sole explanation for every deficit you identify.

CASE 3: CHRISTINE

Christine is 14 and is in the second semester of her freshman year in high school. In late March, she was referred to the Committee on Special Education because of consistently poor grades in nearly all subjects since September. Christine has been a student in the same district since kindergarten so her records are complete. In grade school (K–5) she held a B average. In middle school (Grades 6–8), her average was C to C+. During the fall semester of her freshman year, her average had slipped to D to D+. She had been placed on the "Watch List" by her ninth-grade team during that semester. The team did not want to overreact because it is not uncommon for students to experience problems during the transition from middle school to high school, with its seven academically challenging classes and seven different teachers a day. By March of the spring semester, however, she was clearly failing several courses. Her team members report that she

works hard, often completing extra credit assignments, but has great difficulty understanding material either from lectures or textbooks. Her outlining skills are poor, and she does not seem able to grasp more complex material. She does not analyze or synthesize curriculum material adequately, even compared with those classmates who exhibit generally low average ability.

What would you ask these teachers? Her parents?

Entering the high school as a speech-language professional means going into an entirely new world. Teachers usually consider themselves specialists within their area (math, English, biology, etc.) and often find it difficult to adapt curriculum material to meet the needs of students with language based learning problems. They are frequently sensitive to possible criticism that they passed a student who clearly did not have a grasp of the material. In the most extreme case, they can be blunt: "Look, I teach ____; if they can't do the work, they don't belong in my class." The focus for the speech-language professional shifts to student survival—and keeping the youngster from dropping out. To compound matters, for every student you serve, you must also interact with five to seven instructors. Because scheduling can be daunting, it is extremely helpful if teachers meet in teams. Typically, they meet early in the morning, and your time for questions will be very brief.

In this atmosphere, I learned that they considered Christine "a really nice girl" who works hard and wants to do better than she does. She appears to get along fine with classmates, although she does not appear to have any particularly close friends in her classes. Christine's parents had already met with the team three times and, although willing to help, said that Chris had already dropped all extracurricular activities, spent 3 to 4 hours a night on homework, and was getting very discouraged. She had consistently received after school help from a number of her teachers and had also worked with a peer tutor. That assistance was discontinued when the other student reported that Christine's notes from class were so disorganized, it took most of their assigned time just trying to make head or tail of what Chris had managed to get down on paper. When none of the typical remedies appeared to be helping, Christine was referred for an evaluation.

School records indicated a steady downhill slide in grades and an increase in teachers' comments that Christine often did not appear to understand cognitively difficult or "dense" material. She had been switched from a precollege program to one in general education to lessen classwork complexity. Her comprehension of both texts and lectures was extremely limited, and although spelling and grammar were correct, her writing employed only simple vocabulary and structure, mostly declarative subject-verb sentences and few dependent clauses. End-of-year test results in reading comprehension were in the very low normal range. During middle school, her seventh-grade English teacher suggested that Christine be tested for a learning disability, but there was no indication that any testing had been undertaken.

A conference with her parents indicated that developmentally and medically, Christine was average. Her mother said that "it broke her heart" to see that no matter how hard Christine worked, she was still failing. Because Chris had dropped her extracurricular activities, her social life had changed, and she was now alone much of the time and often "depressed." Chris's mother was a high school graduate, but her dad had left school at the end of 10th grade because it "got too hard." He was concerned that his daughter would end up the same way and would not be able to get a good job. When I asked about the recommendation for testing, the parents said that Chris did not want to, so she went to summer school instead and passed seventh-grade English that way.

I observed Chris in her social studies class while I was working with another student on a project. She was attentive but frequently checked with her neighbor during the short lecture; twice I heard her ask, "What did he say?" Her difficult-to-read notes filled the page, margin to margin. There was no sign of "chunking" of information, such as headings or outline configuration. A free study period followed the lecture, and Chris was clearly having a problem finding the answers to chapter review questions in her book. Mr. Dunn, the social studies teacher, showed me the essay question from Christine's last test. It was short, and paragraph development was inadequate, with no transitions among paragraphs; overall, her answer did not support any discernible argument. Mr. Dunn commented that this example was actually a little better than most of her work. He confirmed that Chris was a hard worker but that she just did not seem to "be with the program."

Later, in my room, when I asked about her problems in school, Christine said that she "read and read and read" the material but that it was too hard. She added that those "long sentences, they start and stop" bothered her the most. She used to like to write, but in high school they wanted "pages and pages and pages," and she did not know what to say. When she borrowed a friend's notes from class, it helped her to study; using her own did not help at all.

The school psychologist determined that Christine's overall IQ was 92; she suggested that language testing be done before any decisions be made about a possible label.

So, now it is up to you. How will you evaluate Christine? I hope you feel a sense of urgency about this third case; when a student is 14, depression about school can have very serious repercussions.

No voice, formal pragmatics, fluency, or articulation assessment appeared necessary. Christine's scores and their interpretation are reported in Table 6–3.

Given the scores in this third case, formulate a summary statement, and make some notes on how you would report this information verbally to the committee who asked you to evaluate her.

Evaluation data point to Christine's having significantly poorer skills in understanding complex language compared with her verbal expression. This, combined with fair memory skills and a "good girl student" personality, may be reasons why she has not been identified before, i.e., in everyday conversation, she sounds pretty typical. Clearly, Christine possesses language skills that have allowed her to cope with academics through eighth grade; why is she having problems now? It has been my observation that many students can compensate for their language deficits throughout a number of grades. Often the odd-numbered grades resulted in a higher "fallout." In other words, some students manage pretty well in kindergarten, but cannot keep up with the demands of first grade; others make it until they have to start reading for

meaning in the third grade or are required to gain information independently in the fifth. And on it goes, with a new group who seem all right until seventh grade or, like Christine, until their first year in high school. Incidentally, this phenomenon appears to continue even beyond this point, as subtle language deficits surface during 11th grade, the freshman or junior years in college, and the first year of graduate school. Indeed, it is not uncommon for students to be identified as having a language-based learning disability during their college years.

Certainly, one of Christine's most significant areas of weakness is dealing with complexity. On the basis of observation, analysis of written work, and the results of standardized and criterion-based testing, Christine appears to have adequate understanding of single-word vocabulary, can repeat syntactically correct sentences, and can even manipulate them if the words are present. Although not a strength, her grasp of semantic concepts appears sufficient. When she is confronted with clausal connectors in syntactically complex sentences, however, she struggles, missing 8 out of 10 on the ECC. This deficit directly affects her ability to understand logical connections (*because*), dysjunctions (*but, although, except*), temporal issues (*before, after, when, while*), and the

Tests	To Tap Information Concerning
Clinical Evaluation of Language Fundamentals-3 (CELF-3; Semel et al., 1995)	overall receptive and expressive language
Peabody Picture Vocabulary Test-Revised (PPVT-R; Dunn & Dunn, 1981)	receptive vocabulary
Evaluating Communicative Competence (ECC; Simon, 1986)	"school" language skills

Table 6–3 Scores and Interpretation of Testing

Test	Subtests	Standard Score	Percentile Rank
CELF-3	Concepts and Directions	4	2
	Word Classes	8	25
	Semantic Relations	7	16
	Formulated Sentences	6	9
	Recalling Sentences	10	50
	Sentence Assembly	9	37
	RECEPTIVE LANGUAGE	78	7
	EXPRESSIVE LANGUAGE	90	25
	TOTAL LANGUAGE	83	13
PPVT-R		87	20
	Age Equivalent: 12-10; Stanine: 3		
ECC	Note: ECC is a criterion-based instrument.		

ECC Inadequate performance in: *Receptive Tasks*
Inference in Paragraphs
Expressive Tasks
Clausal Connectors
Opinion
20 Questions
Barrier Games

Interpretation:
Relationship of Standardized Scores to Standard Deviation:
Between –1.0 and +1.0 (normal range): CELF-3: Overall Expressive Language and the subtests Word Classes, Semantic Relations, Recalling Sentences, and Sentence Assembly
Between –1.0 and –1.5 (mild to moderate deficit): CELF-3: Total Language Score and Formulated Sentences subtest
Between –1.5 and –2.0 (moderate to severe deficit): CELF-3: Concepts and Directions subtest
Above +1.0: none

conditional (*if, then*). Unfortunately, there is scarcely a high school subject that does not routinely use these connectors. In the ECC, she displayed acceptable skill in comprehending and remembering single facts and directions, but her ability to use inference was strikingly lower; that is, when she had to use the information and apply it, she faltered. She stated an opinion but provided no elaboration; similarly there was no logical progression to her questions when she was trying to identify an object that had been removed,

and she failed to use enough detail to differentiate between two similar pictures in the barrier task. On the basis of this profile, it would seem prudent to evaluate a longer writing sample from English class and calculate the number of clauses per T-unit and the subordination index and compare them to spoken samples as discussed earlier in this chapter in Table 6–1. Discovering what level of visual support leads to improvement would be helpful also (e.g., using partial outlines, semantic webs).

You will meet Steven, James, and Christine again in Chapter 7 when we develop an IEP for each of them, and finally in Chapter 8, when we discuss intervention plans.

CASE 4: MEGAN

For this case, you are on your own. I will describe Megan, but you will develop assessment procedures, choose evaluation instruments, and fabricate probable test results. On the basis of these, you will write an IEP and describe some appropriate intervention goals. At each stage, you may want to check with classmates in a cooperative learning group and/or to discuss your results, conclusions, and plans with your instructor.

Megan, a redhead with big brown eyes, is 13 and in the sixth grade. She was labeled as mentally retarded when she entered school, based initially on WPPSI results and confirmed later by WISC-R scores. Her parents, aware of her mental status since birth, were actively involved in all aspects of an early intervention program. Megan was a student in a typical preschool for 3 years, with speech-language services integrated into her daily routine. She has been mainstreamed since first grade. Considering her combined IQ of 70, with verbal/performance scores of 70 and 71 respectively, she has held her own very well. Her most recent report card (modified program) features grades mostly in the B range in science, social studies, language arts, and math. Achievement scores in these subjects place her at the early fourth-grade level. She is pragmatically appropriate in social situations, although in recent years she has interacted more successfully with adults than her peers. Her mouth breathing and sometimes careless hygiene may be part of the reason that sixth-grade students do not seek her out. In addition, her classmates' behavior reflects the language and interests of early adolescence, and Meg is still very much a child. She often seeks out younger students to talk with during lunch and recess.

Her teacher, Mr. Walters, reports that Megan appears to enjoy school and works hard. As noted above, most of her subject areas reflect at least a 2-year lag, but he comments that there are a number of other students whose skills place them in "the low group" too. All "solid" subjects are taught in the classroom by Mr. Walters; with the rest of the class, Megan leaves the room for art, music, and physical education. She is an average student in music and does fairly well in art if the lesson deals with crafts but struggles if the activity features something like perspective. She is having increasing difficulty in gym class as her classmates develop more skill, but her teacher at this time does not recommend adaptive P.E. Megan has a very difficult time taking notes and relies on teacher-designed study questions to prepare for examinations. Her parents report that they spend an hour or two every night helping Megan with her homework or studying for tests.

Math was Megan's favorite subject until fifth grade. Her good rote memory made simple addition, subtraction, and multiplication tasks easy for her. Long division and double-digit multiplication, however, present difficulty, exacerbated by Megan's failure to keep columns of figures straight on her paper. Word problems have always been hard and are getting harder. Following directions has become more difficult too. If they are single-step, logical, and clearly laid out, Megan can cope, but when they are long or contain words like *if* or *except*, she flounders. Semantically, she exhibits problems comprehending figurative language, multiple-meaning words, comparisons, and inference in written material; understanding oral language containing those same elements appears easier. Her basic decoding and spelling skills are adequate, representing third- to fourth-grade skills. Automatic series, such as days of the week or months of the year, are fine. Her spontaneous writing consists of simple one-clause declarative sentences containing few complexities and having straightforward sequence as the only form. In her narratives, mostly stories about her family, there is little sense of motivation, detail, concept of a plot, or use of intraparagraph connectors. Her speech is intelligible, but a persistent gliding of liquids, now more of a distortion, as well as problems with multisyllabic words, sometimes makes her hard to understand, particularly to someone who does not know her.

Megan's organization skills leave much to be desired; her desk is a disaster, with papers stuffed everywhere. Her glasses, which she needs to read, are often "lost." Mr. Walters is not sure if she really does forget where she has taken them off, or if she just does not like to wear them because they constantly slide down her nose. Students around her have learned to keep extra pencils and paper handy because Megan can never find hers.

Megan is due for a triennial evaluation in a month or so. Her parents and Mr. Walters all are worried about her ability to function in the seventh grade. They are particularly concerned with her changing classes each period, the increased amount and complexity of the material in upper middle school, and her ability to switch from one teaching style to another, particularly when the teachers at this level see themselves as being responsible for covering a specific amount of material in "their" subject. Mr. Walters and Megan's parents have also expressed concern about the availability of assistance for Megan, as well as a possible lack of coordination among her teachers.

The following is an excerpt from Megan's oral language sample:

My family is going camping. It is fun! We will drive to Pennsylvania and then go the campground. First we will unload the car and set up our tent. Then we can go for a hike. We will probably go to the big pond. I like to go there because I catch salamanders and see some little fish. The baby salamanders are small and very fast. They're orange. At dinnertime, we cook hamburgers and hot dogs. We also cook potatoes and corn. Later we sing around the campfire and eat s'mores. We stay at the campfire until it's time for bed. Camping is a lot of fun. I like it.

The following is an excerpt from Megan's spontaneous written sample:

My sister Jess has a dog. His name is Sam. Sam is a little black puppy.
One day he made a hole under the fens. He squesed through. He ran down the street. He fell into a hole. The hole was very deep. He tried to get out but he couldn't.
Jess came out to get him. My mom and Jess looked for him. Jess herd barkking and she falloed the sound. She saw Sam. They reskued him. We were happy. The end.

On the basis of an analysis of the two samples and the information contained in the case history, what are your standardized testing recommendations for Megan? Remember, with a student who is mentally retarded, the published age range on instruments should match her approximate MA, not necessarily her CA. Listed below are some common instruments to consider; be careful, not all of them may be either appropriate or advisable. You may also want to consider others not on the list. Typically, the *total* time you have available for administering standardized measures in the schools is about 2 hours. Therefore choose instruments that meet your purposes but whose administration time fits into this time frame. Be prepared to provide well-thought-out, specific reasons for your choices. Check with your instructor before proceeding to the next step.

Possible Evaluation Instruments for Megan are listed below:

- Goldman-Fristoe Test of Articulation (Goldman & Fristoe, 1986)
- Goldman-Fristoe Test of Articulation combined with the Khan-Lewis Phonological Analysis (Khan & Lewis, 1986)
- Arizona Articulation Proficiency Scale-Revised (Fudala & Reynolds, 1989)
- Test of Language Development-2 (TOLD-2), either Primary or Intermediate (Newcomer & Hammill, 1991a, 1991b)
- Clinical Evaluation of Language Fundamentals-3 (CELF-3; Semel et al., 1995)
- Structured Photographic Expressive Language Test-2 (SPELT-2; Werner & Kresheck, 1983b)
- Expressive One-Word Picture Vocabulary Test-Revised (EOWPVT-R; Gardner, 1990)

- Peabody Picture Vocabulary Test-Revised (PPVT-R; Dunn & Dunn, 1981)
- The Word Test (Huisingh, Barrett, Zachman, Blagden, & Orman, 1990)
- Test of Problem Solving-Adolescent (Zachman et al., 1991)

After choosing the instruments, project probable scores. At the close of Chapter 7, you will be asked to develop an IEP for Megan.

Before leaving this chapter, I have a final word of both caution and consolation. First the consolation: regardless of whether the assessment model you adopt falls into the traditional or new variety, it is an ongoing process; each time you work with a student, you will discover something about what he knows how or he learns that will affect your future plans. Therefore, if you have missed something in the initial assessment, you will have ample opportunity to evaluate new information and state a new hypothesis. Now the caution: be aware that each time you interact with a student, the yellow light should always be blinking: attention, attention, important new assessment information lies ahead.

NOTE

1. *Word of Mouth* can be obtained by writing to P.O. Box 13716, San Antonio, TX 78213.

REFERENCES

Adler, S. (1991). Assessment of language proficiency in LEP speakers. *Language, Speech, and Hearing Services in the Schools, 22*(2), 12–18.

American Speech-Language-Hearing Association. (1986).

American Speech-Language-Hearing Association, Committee on Language Disorders. (1989). Issues in determining eligibility for language intervention, *Asha, 14,* 113–118.

American Speech-Language-Hearing Association. (1995). *Communication development and disorders in multicultural populations.* Rockville, MD: Author.

Bankson, N. (1977). *Bankson Language Screening Test-2.* (BLST-2) Baltimore: University Park Press.

Bankson, N. (1990). *Bankson Language Test-2.* (BLST-2) Baltimore: University Park Press.

Bankson, N., & Bernthal, J. (1990). *Bankson-Bernthal Test of Phonology.* Chicago: Riverside.

Barrett, M., Huisingh, R., Zachman, L., LoGiudice, C., & Orman, J. (1994). *The Listening Test.* East Moline, IL: LinguiSystems.

Barrett, M., Zachman, L., & Huisingh, R. (1988). *Assessing Semantic Skills Through Everyday Themes.* (ASSET) East Moline, IL: LinguiSystems.

Bashir, A. (1989). Language intervention and the curriculum. *Seminars in Speech and Language, 10*, 181–191.

Bashir, A.S., & Scavuzzo, A. (1992). Children with language disorders: Natural history and academic success. *Journal of Learning Disabilities, 25*, 53–65.

Berry, M. (1966). *Berry-Talbott Language Tests 1: Comprehension of Grammar*. Rockford, IL: publisher.

Blank, M., Rose, S., & Berlin, L. (1978). *Preschool Language Assessment Instrument*. (PLAI) Orlando, FL: Grune & Stratton.

Blau, A., Lahey, M., & Oleksiuk-Velez, A. (1984). Planning goals for intervention: Language testing or language sampling? *Exceptional Children, 51*, 78–79.

Bliss, L., & Allen, D. (1983). *Screening Kit of Language Development*. (SKOLD) East Aurora, NY: Slosson.

Blodgett, E., & Cooper, R. (1987). *Analysis of the language of learning: The practical test of metalinguistics*. East Moline, IL: LinguiSystems.

Boehm, A. (1986). *Boehm Test of Basic Concepts-Preschool*. Available from The Psychological Corporation, Order Service Center, P.O. Box 9954, San Antonio, TX 78204.

Bracken, B. (1984). *Bracken Basic Concept Scale*. San Antonio, TX: The Psychological Corporation.

Brinton, B., & Fujiki, M. (1992). Setting the context for conversational speech sampling. *Best Practices in School Speech-Language Pathology, 2*, 9–19.

Brown, R. (1978). *A first language: The early stages*. Cambridge, MA: Harvard University Press.

Burt, M., & Dulog, H. (1978). *Bilingual Syntax Measure I and II*. Available from The Psychological Corporation, Order Service Center, P.O. Box 9954, San Antonio, TX 78204.

Carrow, E. (1974). *Carrow Elicited Language Inventory*. Austin, TX: Learning Concepts.

Carrow-Woolfolk, E. (1981a). *Carrow Elicited Language Inventory*. (CELI) Chicago: Riverside.

Carrow-Woolfolk, E. (1981b). *Test for Auditory Comprehension of Language-Revised*. (TACL-R) Chicago: Riverside.

Compton, A., & Kline, M. (1981). *Compton Speech and Language Screening Evaluation: Spanish Adaptation*. Available from Carousel House, P.O. Box 4480, San Francisco, CA 94101.

Creaghead, N., & Tattershall, S. (1985). Observation and assessment of classroom pragmatic skills. In C. S. Simon (Ed.), *Communication skills and classroom success* (pp. 105–134). San Diego: College Hill.

Damico, J. (1985). Clinical discourse analysis: a functional language assessment technique, In c.s. Simon (Ed.),*Communication skills in the classroom success: Assessment of language-learning disabled students* (pp. 165–206). San Diego: College Hill.

Damico, J., & Hamayan, E. (1992). *Multicultural language intervention : Addressing cultural and linguistic diversity*. Buffalo, NY: EDUCOM Associates.

Damico, J., & Oller, J. (1985). *Spotting language problems: Pragmatic criteria for language screening*. Available from Los Amigos Research Associates, 7035 Galewood, Suite D, San Diego, CA 97120.

DeSimoni, F. (1978). *Token Test for Children*. Chicago: Riverside.

Dollaghan, C.A., & Campbell, T.F. (1992). A procedure for classifying disruptions in spontaneous language samples. *Topics in Language Disorders, 12*, 56–68.

Duchan, J.F. (1982). The elephant is soft and mushy: Problems in assessing children's language. *Speech, language and hearing*. In N. Lass, L. McReynolds, J. Northern, & D. Yoder (Eds.), Philadelphia: W. B. Saunders.

Dunn, L., & Dunn, L.M. (1981). *Peabody Picture Vocabulary Test-Revised*. (PPVT-R) Available from American Guidance Service, P.O. Box 99, Circle Pines, MN 55014-17962.

Edmonston, N., & Thane, N. (1993). *Test of Relational Concepts-Revised*. (TRC-R) Tucson, AZ: Communication Skill Builders.

Fisher, H., & Logemann, J. (1971). *Fisher-Logemann Test of Articulation Competence*. Boston: Houghton Mifflin.

Fitch, J. (1985). *Computer Managed Screening Test*. Tucson, AZ: Communication Skill Builders.

Fluharty, N. (1978). *Fluharty Preschool Speech and Language Screening Test*. Chicago: Riverside.

Francis, D., Fletcher, J., Shaywitz, B., Shaywitz, S., Rourke, B., & Sabers, D. (1996). Defining learning and language disabilities: Conceptual and psychometric issues with the use of IQ tests. *Language, Speech, and Hearing Services in Schools, 27*(2), 132–143.

Fressola, D., & Hoerchler, S. (1989). *Speech and Language Evaluation Scale*. Columbia, MO: Hawthorne Educational Services.

Fudala, J., & Reynolds, W. (1989). *Arizona Articulation Proficiency Scale*. (AAPS) Los Angeles: Western Psychological Services.

Fujiki, M., & Willbrand, M. (1982). A comparison of four informal methods of language evaluation. *Language, Speech, and Hearing Services in Schools, 13*(1), 42–52.

Garard, J.E., & Weinstock, G. (1981). *Language Proficiency Test*. Available from Academic Intervention Publications, 20 Commercial Blvd., Novato, CA 94949-61913.

Garcia, G. (1992). Ethnography and classroom communication: Taking an "emic" perspective. *Topics in Language Disorders, 12*, 54–66.

Gardner, M. (1983). *Expressive One-Word Picture Vocabulary Test-Upper Extension*. Available from Academic Intervention Publications, 20 Commercial Blvd., Novato, CA 94949-61913.

Gardner, M. (1990). *Expressive One-Word Picture Vocabulary Test-Revised*. (EOWPVT-R) Available from Academic Intervention Publications, 20 Commercial Blvd., Novato, CA 94949-61913.

Gardner, M., & Brownell, B. (1985). *Receptive One-Word Picture Vocabulary Test*. (ROWPVT) Available from Academic Intervention Publications, 20 Commercial Blvd., Novato, CA 94949-61913.

Gardner, M., & Brownell, B. (1987). *Receptive One-Word Picture Vocabulary Test-Upper Extension*. Available from Academic Intervention Publications, 20 Commercial Blvd., Novato, CA 94949-61913.

German, D. (1991). *Test of Word Finding*. Chicago: Riverside.

Goldman, R., & Fristoe, M. (1986). *Goldman-Fristoe Test of Articulation*. (GFTA) Available from American Guidance Service, P.O. Box 99, Circle Pines, MN 55014-17962.

Goldsworthy, C., & Secord, W. (1982). *Multilevel Informal Language Inventory*. (MILI) Available from The Psychological Corporation, Order Service Center, P.O. Box 9954, San Antonio, TX 78204.

Goodman, K.S. (1983). Analysis of oral reading miscues: Applied psycholinguistics. In F. Smith (Ed.), *Psycholinguistics and reading* (pp. 158–176). New York: Holt, Rinehart, & Winston.

Hammill, D., Brown, V., Larsen, S., & Wiederholt, J. (1994). *Test of Adolescent Language-3*. (TOAL-3) Austin, TX: Pro-Ed.

Hammill, D., Larsen, S., & Wiederholt, J. (1988). *Test of Written Language-2*. (TOWL-2) Austin, TX: Pro-Ed.

Hill, S., & Haynes, W. (1992). Language performance in low-achieving elementary school students. *Language, Speech, and Hearing Services in Schools, 23,* 169–175.

Hodson, B. (1980). *Assessment of Phonological Processes-Spanish*. Available from Los Amigos Research Associates, 7035 Galewood, Suite D, San Diego, CA 97120.

Hresko, W., Reid, K., & Hammill, D. (1991). *Test of Early Language Development*. (TELD) Austin, TX: Pro-Ed.

Huisingh, R., Barrett, M., Zachman, L., Blagden, C., & Orman, J. (1990). *The Word Test-R Elementary*. East Moline, IL: LinguiSystems.

Hutchinson, T. (1996). What to look for in the technical manual: Twenty questions for users. *Language, Speech, and Hearing Services in Schools, 27*(2), 109–121.

Hux, K., Morris-Friehe, M., & Sanger, D. (1993). Language sampling practices: A survey of nine states. *Language, Speech, and Hearing Services in Schools, 24,* 84–91.

Johnston, E., & Johnston, A. (1990). *Communication Abilities Diagnostic Test*. Chicago: Riverside.

Kamhi, A. (1993). Assessing complex behaviors: Problems with reification, quantification, and ranking. *Language, Speech, and Hearing Services in Schools, 24,* 110–113.

Kelly, D., & Rice, M. (1986). A strategy for language assessment of young children: A combination of two approaches. *Language, Speech, and Hearing Services in Schools, 17,* 83–94.

Khan, L., & Lewis, N. (1986). *Khan-Lewis Phonological Analysis*. Available from American Guidance Service, P.O. Box 99, Circle Pines, MN 55014-17962.

Kinzler, M., & Johnson, C. (1993). *Joliet 3 Minute Speech and Language Screen*. Tucson, AZ: Communication Skill Builders.

Larson, V., & McKinley, N. (1995). *Language disorders in older students*. Eau Claire, WI: Thinking Publications.

Lee, L. (1971). *Northwest Syntax Screening Test*. (NSST) Evanston, IL: Northwestern University Press.

Lindamood, C., & Lindamood, P. (1979). *Lindamood Auditory Conceptualization Test-Revised*. Chicago: Riverside.

Loban, W. (1976). *Language development: Kindergarten through grade twelve*. Urbana, IL: National Council of Teachers of English.

Lund, N., & Duchan, J. (1993). *Assessing children's language in naturalistic contexts* (3rd ed). Englewood Cliffs, NJ: Prentice Hall.

Masterson, J., & Kamhi, A. (1991). The effects of sampling conditions on sentence production in normal, reading-disabled, and language-learning-disabled children. *Journal of Speech and Hearing Research, 34,* 549–558.

Mattes, L., & Santiago, G. (1991). *Bilingual Language Proficiency Questionnaire*. Available from Academic Communication Associates, 7035 Galewood, Suite D, San Diego, CA 97120.

McCauley, R. (1996). Familiar strangers: Criterion-referenced measures in communication disorders. *Language, Speech, and Hearing Services in Schools, 27*(2), 122–131.

McCormick, L., & Schiefelbusch, R. (1984). *Early language intervention: An intervention*. Columbus, OH: Merrill.

McDonald, E. (1968). *Deep Test for Articulation*. Pittsburgh: Stanwix House.

McFadden, T. (1996). Creating language impairments in typically achieving children: The pitfalls of "normal" normative sampling. *Language, Speech, and Hearing Services in Schools, 27*(1), 3–9.

Morgan, D., & Guilford, A. (1984). *Adolescent Language Screening Test*. Austin, TX: Pro-Ed.

Muma, J. (1978). *The language handbook: Concepts, assessment, intervention*. Englewood Cliffs, NJ: Prentice-Hall.

Muma, J., Lubinski, R., & Pierce, S. (1982). A new era in language assessment: Data or evidence. In N. Lass (Ed.), *Speech and language: Advances in basic research and practice* (Vol. 7, pp. 135–147). New York: Academic Press.

National Hispanic University. *Chinese Oral Proficiency Test*. Oakland, CA: National Hispanic University.

Nelson, K. (1985). *Making sense: The acquisition of shared meaning*. New York: Academic Press.

Nelson, N. (1989). Curriculum-based language assessment and intervention. *Language, Speech, and Hearing Services in Schools, 20*(2), 170–184.

Nelson, N. (1990). Only relevant practices can be best. *Best Practices in School Speech-Language Pathology, 1,* 15–27.

Nelson, N. (1993). *Child language disorders in context*. Columbus, OH: Merrill.

Nelson, N. (1994). Curriculum-based language assessment and intervention across the grades. In G. Wallach & K. Butler (Eds.), *Language learning disabilities in school-age children and adolescents* (pp. 104–131). New York: Macmillan.

Newcomer, P., & Hammill, D. (1991a). *Test of Language Development 2-Intermediate* (TOLD-2 Int.) Austin, TX: Pro-Ed.

Newcomer, P., & Hammill, D. (1991b). *Test of Language Development 2-Primary* (TOLD-2 Primary) Austin, TX: Pro-Ed.

Owens, R. (1995). *Language disorders: A functional approach to assessment and intervention* (2nd ed). Needham Heights, MA: Allyn & Bacon.

Palincsar, A., Brown, A., & Campione, J. (1994). Models and practices of dynamic assessment. In G. Wallach & K. Butler (Eds.), *Language learning disabilities in school-age children and adolescents* (pp. 132–144). New York: Macmillan.

Paratore, J.R. (1995). Assessing literacy: Establishing common standards in portfolio assessment. *Topics in Language Disorders, 16*(1), 67–82.

Paul, R. (1981). Analyzing complex sentence development. In J.F. Miller (Ed.), *Assessing language production in children: Experimental procedures* (pp. 36–40). Needham Heights, MA: Allyn & Bacon.

Paul, R. (1995). *Language disorders from infancy through adolescence: Assessment and intervention.* St. Louis: C.V. Mosby.

Peterson, H., & Marquardt, T. (1990). *Appraisal and diagnosis of speech and language disorders* (2nd ed). Englewood Cliffs, NJ: Prentice Hall.

Piggott, T., Barry, J., Hughes, B., Eastin, D., Titus, P., Stensel, H., Metcalf, M., & Porter, B. (1985). *Speech-Ease Screening Inventory.* Austin, TX: Pro-Ed.

Plante, E., & Vance, R. (1994). Selection of preschool language tests: A data-based approach. *Language, Speech, and Hearing Services in Schools, 25,* 15–24.

Richard, G., & Hanner, M. (1985). *Language Processing Test.* (LPT) East Moline, IL: LinguiSystems.

Riley, A. M. (1991). *Evaluating Acquired Skills in Communication.* (EASIC) Tucson, AZ: Communication Skills Builders.

Roseberry-McKibbin, C. (1995). *Multicultural students with special language needs: Practical strategies for assessment and intervention.* Oceanside, CA: Academic Communication Associates.

Sabers, D. (1996). By their tests we will know them. *Language, Speech, and Hearing Services in Schools, 27,*(2), 102–108.

Sawyer, D. (1987). *Test of Awareness of Language Segments.* Austin, TX: Pro-Ed.

Schneider, P., & Watkins, R. (1996). Applying Vygotskian developmental theory to language intervention. *Language, Speech, and Hearing Services in Schools, 27*(2) 157–170.

Scott, C. (1988). Spoken and written syntax. In M. Nippold (Ed.), *Later language development* (pp. 49–96). Boston: College Hill.

Semel, E.M., & Wiig, E. (1980). *Clinical evaluation of language functions.* San Antonio, TX: Psychological Corporation.

Semel, E., Wiig, E., & Secord, W. (1987) *Clinical Evaluation of Language Fundamentals-Revised.* (CELF-R) Available from The Psychological Corporation, Order Service Center, P.O. Box 9954, San Antonio, TX 78204.

Semel, E., Wiig, E., & Secord, W. (1995). *Clinical Evaluation of Language Fundamentals-3.* (3rd ed.). Available from The Psychological Corporation, Order Service Center, P.O. Box 9954, San Antonio, TX 78204.

Semel, E., Wiig, E., & Secord, W. (1989). *Clinical Evaluation of Language Fundamentals Screening Test.* Available from The Psychological Corporation, Order Service Center, P.O. Box 9954, San Antonio, TX 78204.

Shahzade, A., Becze, D., Christian, S., Eirich, M., Falkenthal, S., Fennell, J., Goncalves M., Levine, H., Prolman, B., & Tuch, T. (1984). *Cambridge Kindergarten Screening Test.* Allen, TX: DLM.

Shipley, K., & McAfee, J. (1992). *Assessment in speech language pathology: A resource manual.* San Diego: Singular.

Shipley, K., Stone, T., & Sue, M. (1983). *Test for Examining Expressive Morphology.* (TEEM) Tucson, AZ: Communication Skill Builders.

Shulman, B., Chapman, P., Cheney, M., Driver, A.G., Dye, C.L., Millikan, C.D., Reed, K.R., & Starcher, L. (1986). Child language disorders: An annotated bibliography. *Asha, 28*(1), 33–41.

Siegel, G., & Broen, P. (1976). Language assessment, in L. Lloyd (Ed.), *Communication assessment and intervention strategies* (pp. 73–122). Baltimore: University Park Press.

Simon, C. (Ed.). (1985a). *Communication skills and classroom success: Assessment of language-learning disabled students.* San Diego: College Hill.

Simon, C. (Ed.). (1985b). *Communication skills and classroom success: Intervention methodologies for language-learning disabled students.* San Diego: College Hill.

Simon, C. (1986). *Evaluating Communicative Competence.* (ECC) Tucson, AZ: Communication Skill Builders.

Simon, C.S. (1987). *Classroom communication screening procedures for early adolescents: A handbook for assessment and intervention.* Tucson, AZ: Communi-Cognitive Publications.

Southwest Communication Resources. (1988). *Look, listen, and learn.* Available from Southwestern Communication Resources, P.O. Box 788, Bernalillo, NM 87004.

Stark, J., & Wallach, G. (1980). The path to a concept of language-learning disabilities. *Topics in Language Disorders, 1,* 1–14.

Tallal., Ross, R., & Curtiss, S. (1989). Familial aggregation in specific language impairment. *Journal of Speech and Hearing Disorders, 54*(2), 167–173.

Temple, C., & Gillet, J. (1984). *Language arts learning process and teaching practices.* Boston: Little, Brown.

Tomblin, B. (1991). Familial concentration of developmental language impairment. *Journal of Speech and Hearing Disorders, 54,* 587–595.

Toronto, A. (1976a). Developmental assessment of Spanish grammar. *Journal of Speech and Hearing Disorders, 41*(2), 150–171.

Toronto, A. (1976b). *Screening Test of Spanish Grammar.* Evanston, IL: Northwestern University Press.

Trivette, C., Dunst, C., Deal, A., Hamer, A., & Propst, S. (1990). Assessing family strengths and family functioning style. *Topics in Early Childhood Special Edition, 10,* 16–35.

Trudeau, G. (1985). *Multicultural Vocabulary Test.* Available from Los Amigos Research Associates, 7035 Galewood, Suite D, San Diego, CA 97120.

van Kleeck, A. (1994). Metalinguistic development. In G. Wallach, & K. Butler (Eds.), *Language learning disabilities in school-age children and adolescents: Some principles and applications* (pp. 53–98). New York: Macmillan.

Wallace, G., & Hammill, D. (1994). *Comprehensive Receptive and Expressive Vocabulary Test.* (CREVT) East Aurora, NY: Slosson.

Wallach, G.P., & Butler, K.G. (1994). Creating communication, literary, and academic success. In G. P. Wallach & K.G. Butler (Eds.). *Language learning disabilities in school-age children and adolescents: Some principles and applications* (pp. 2–26). Needham Heights, MA: Allyn & Bacon.

Wallach, G., & Butler, K. (Eds.). (1994). *Language learning disabilities in school-age children and adolescents: Some principles and applications.* Needham Heights, MA: Allyn & Bacon.

Warden, M., & Hutchinson, T. (1992). *The Writing Process Test.* Chicago: Riverside.

Washington, J., & Craig, H. (1992). Performances of low-income, African-American preschool and kindergarten children on the Peabody Picture Vocabulary Test-Revised. *Language, Speech, and Hearing Services in Schools, 23,* 329–333.

Watson, D.L., Omark, D.R. & Gomez-Huebner, M. (1984). *Basic Elementary Skills Test.* Available from Los Amigos Research Associates, 7035 Galewood, Suite D, San Diego, CA 97120.

Weiss, C. (1980). *Weiss Comprehensive Articulation Test.* (WCAT) Chicago: Riverside.

Werner, E., & Kresheck, J. (1983a). *Structured Photographic Expressive Language Test-Preschool.* (SPELT-Preschool) Available from Janelle Publications, P.O. Box 12, Sandwich, IL 60548.

Werner, E., & Kresheck, J. (1983b). Structured Photographic Expressive Language Test-2. (SPELT-2) Available from Janelle Publications, P.O. Box 12, Sandwich, IL 60548.

Westby, C. (1994). Multicultural issues. In J. Tomblin, H. Morris, & D. Spriestersbach (Eds.), *Diagnosis in speech-language pathology.* San Diego: Singular.

Westby, C., StevensDominguez, M., & Oetter, P. (1996). A performance/competence model of observational assessment. *Language, Speech, and Hearing Services in Schools, 27,* (2). 144-156.

Wiig, E., & Secord, W. (1989). *Test of Language Competence-Expanded Edition.* Available from the Psychological Corporation, Order Service Center, P.O. Box 9954, San Antonio, TX 78204.

Wiig, E., Secord, W., & Semel, E. (1992). *Clinical Evaluation of Language Fundamentals-Preschool.* (CELF-Preschool) Available from The Psychological Corporation, Order Service Center, P.O. Box 9954, San Antonio, TX 18204.

Wiig, E., & Semel, W. (1984a). *Language assessment and intervention for the learning disabled.* Columbus, OH: Merrill.

Wiig, E., & Semel, E. (1984b). *Test of Word Knowledge.* New York: Macmillan.

Wiig, E., & Semel, W. (1992). *Language assessment and intervention for the learning disabled* (2nd ed.). New York: Macmillan.

Willabrand, M., & Iwata-Reuyl, G. (1994). Gender bias in language testing. *Asha, 36,* 50–52.

Wood, M. (1982). *Language disorders in school-age children.* Englewood Cliffs, NJ: Prentice Hall.

Woodcock, R. (1980). *Woodcock Language Proficiency Battery (Spanish Form).* Chicago: Riverside.

Young, E., & Perachio, J. (1993). *Patterned Elicitation of Syntax Test (Revised) with Morphophonemic Analysis.* (PEST) Tucson, AZ: Communication Skill Builders.

Zachman, L., Barrett, M., Huisingh, M., Orman, J., & Blagden, C. (1991). *Test of Problem Solving-Adolescent.* (TOPS-Adolescent) East Moline, IL: LinguiSystems.

Zachman, L., Huisingh, M., Barrett, M., Orman, J., & Blagden, C. (1989). *The Word Test-Adolescent.* East Moline, IL: LinguiSystems.

Zachman, L., Barrett, M., Huisingh, M., & Jorgensen, C. (1984). *Test of Problem Solving-Elementary.* (TOPS-Elementary) East Moline, IL: LinguiSystems.

Zimmerman, I., Steiner, V., & Pond, R. (1979). *Preschool Language Scale-Revised.* (PLS-R) San Antonio, TX: Psychological Corporation and Harcourt, Brace, Jovanovich.

Zimmerman, I., Steiner, V., & Pond, R. (1992) *Preschool Language Scale-3.* (PLS-3) Available from The Psychological Corporation, Order Service Center, P.O. Box 9954, San Antonio, TX 78204.

Appendix 6–A

A Sampling of Instruments That Address Multicultural Differences

Name of Instrument	Dialect/Language	Linguistic Area	Source	Age/Grade
Assessment of Phonological Processes—Spanish	Spanish	Phonology	Hodson (1980)	Ages 3–6
Assessment Instrument for Multicultural Client	Various	Pragmatics	Adler (1991)	
Basic Elementary Skills Test	Spanish, Arabic, Cambodian, Chinese, Farsi, Vietnamese	Math, spelling, reading	Watson, Omark, & Gomez-Huebner (1984)	Grades K–8
Bilingual Language Proficiency Questionnaire	Spanish	Parent interview	Mattes & Santiago (1991)	Grades K–12
Bilingual Syntax Measure I and II	Spanish	Syntax	Burt & Dulog (1978)	Grades 1–2 3–12
Black English Scoring System	African American	Morphology, syntax	Nelson (1993, Appendix C)	Grades 2–7
Boehm Test of Basic Concepts-Revised	Spanish	Semantics	Boehm (1986)	Grades K–2
Chinese Oral Proficiency Test	Chinese	Semantics	National Hispanic University	Grades K–6
Compton Speech and Language Screening Evaluation: Spanish Adaptation	Spanish	All	Compton & Kline (1981)	Ages 3–6
Developmental Assessment of Spanish Grammar	Spanish	Morphology, syntax	Toronto (1976a)	Ages 2–7
Expressive One-Word Picture Vocabulary Test-Revised; also Upper Extension	Spanish	Semantics	Gardner (1983, 1990)	Ages 2–12 Ages 12–15
Language Proficiency Test	Spanish, German, French, Tagalog, Japanese	Various	Garard & Weinstock (1981)	Ages Ad'lsnt Adult
Lindamood Auditory Conceptualization Test-Revised	Spanish	Metaphonology	Lindamood & Lindamood (1979)	Grades K–12
Look, Listen, and Learn	Native American	Lang screening	Southwest Communication Resources (1988)	Ages 3–7
Multicultural Vocabulary Test	Any	Semantics (body parts)	Trudeau (1985)	Ages 3–13
Peabody Picture Vocabulary Test-Revised	Spanish	Semantics	Dunn & Dunn (1981)	Ages 2.6–Adult

continues

Appendix 6–A continued

Name of Instrument	Dialect/Language	Linguistic Area	Source	Age/Grade
Preschool Language Assessment Instrument: The Language of Learning in Practice	Spanish: Cuba, Mexico, Guatemala, Puerto Rico	All, incl. pragmatics	Blank, Rose, & Berlin (1978)	Ages 2.9–5.8
Preschool Language Scale-3	Spanish	Morphology, syntax, semantics	Zimmerman, Steiner, & Pond (1992)	Ages Birth–7
Receptive One-Word Picture Vocabulary Test, Also Upper Extension	Spanish	Semantics	Gardner & Brownell (1985, 1987)	Ages 2–12 12–15
Screening Kit of Language Development	Black English	Morphology, syntax, semantics	Bliss & Allen (1983)	Ages 2–5
Screening Test of Spanish Grammar	Spanish	Morphology, syntax	Toronto (1976b)	
Spotting Language Problems: Pragmatics	Any	Pragmatics	Damico & Oller (1985)	Grades K–12
Structured Photographic Expressive Language Test-Preschool	Black English	Morphology, syntax	Werner & Kresheck (1983a)	Ages 3–6
Structured Photographic Expressive Language Test-2	Black English	Morphology, syntax	Werner & Kresheck (1983b)	Ages 4–9.5
Test for Auditory Comprehension of Language-Revised (English and Spanish Forms)	Spanish	Morphology, syntax, semantics	Carrow-Woolfolk (1981b)	Ages 3–6
Woodcock Language Proficiency Battery (Spanish Form)	Spanish	Semantics: oral and written	Woodcock (1980)	Ages 4–20

Appendix 6–B

Sampling of General Evaluation Instruments for the School-Aged Child Pre-K through Grade 12

In the listing below, an asterisk (*) appears in front of names of instruments used primarily for screening. Rec = receptive language, Exp = expressive language, Ph = phonology, M = morphology, Sx = syntax, Sm = semantics, and Pr = pragmatics.

Name of Instrument	Age	Rec	Exp	Ph	M	Sx	Sm	Pr	Comments	Source
Adolescent Language Screening Test (ALST)	11–17	x	x	x	x	x	x	x	7 subtests, less than 15 minutes	Morgan & Guilford (1984)
Arizona Articulation Proficiency Scale (AAPS)	3–7		x	x					Contains quick screening; black and white; each phoneme listed by age	Fudala & Reynolds (1989)
Assessing Semantic Skills Through Everyday Themes (ASSET)	3–9	x	x				x		Color photos; vocabulary related to themes label, function, definition, category, attribute	Barrett, Zachman, & Huisingh (1988)
Bankson-Bernthal Test of Phonology (BBTOP)	3–9		x	x					Tests directly for 10 phonological processes 80 plates; (I), (F) consonant inventory	Bankson & Bernthal (1990)
Bankson Language Test-2 (BLT-2)	3–7		x		x	x	x	x	Has 20-item screening; 7 subtests; 26 plates	Bankson (1990)
*Bankson Language Screening Test (BLST)	4–8	x	x		x	x	x		19 items plus visual and auditory perception; limited syntax, semantics expressive only	Bankson (1977)
Berry-Talbott Guide to the Comprehension of Grammar	5–8		x		x				Uses nonsense words to assess morphology	Berry (1966)
Boehm Test of Basic Concepts-R	3–7		x				x		26 concepts; individual or group	Boehm (1986)
*Bracken Basic Concept Scale Screening Test	5–7		x				x		Concepts; individual or small group	Bracken (1984)

continues

Appendix 6–B continued

Name of Instrument	Comments	Age	Rec	Exp	Ph	M	Sx	Sm	Pr	Source
Cambridge Kindergarten Screening Test	26 photographs; 8 phonemes; discrimination	4.5–6.2	x	x	x	x	x	x	x	Shahzade et al. (1984)
Carrow Elicited Language Inventory (CELI)	Sentence repetition task; 52 items, no pictures	3–7	x	x		x	x	x		Carrows Woolfolk (1981a)
*Classroom Communication Screening Procedures for Early Adolescents	Metalinguistics, oral/written directions; synonyms, definitions; classroom focus	9–14	x	x	x	x	x	x	x	Simon (1987)
Clinical Evaluation of Language Fundamentals-Preschool (CELF-Pre)	6 subtests; Quick Test of 2 subtests; pictures, colorful plates	3–7	x	x	x	x	x			Wiig et al. (1992)
Clinical Evaluation of Language Fundamentals-Revised (CELF-R)	Standard scores on each of 11 subtests plus recep., exp. and total language composite scores; scoring software available	5–17	x	x	x	x	x			Semel et al. (1987a)
Clinical Evaluation of Language Fundamentals Screening Test	Criterion scores on four or six subtests; includes storytelling and written skills	5–16	x	x	x	x	x			Semel et al. (1989)
Communication Abilities Diagnostic Test (CADeT)	Naturalistic based: stories, game, conversation normative and criterion referenced	3–9	x	x	x	x	x	x		Johnston & Johnston (1990)
Comprehensive Receptive and Expressive Vocabulary Test (CREVT)	10 color photos; series of increasingly difficult words (recep.); definitions (exp.)	4–17	x	x			x			Wallace & Hammill (1994)
Deep Test of Articulation	To determine facilitation contexts: not for initial diagnosis; pictures or sentences	3–12			x	x				McDonald (1968)
Evaluating Acquired Skills in Communication	Verbal, sign, alternative/augmentative communication: for severely impaired	3 mo–8 yr	x	x		x	x	x	x	Riley (1991)

continues

continues

Name of Instrument	Comments	Age	Rec	Exp	Ph	M	Sx	Sm	Pr	Source
Evaluating Communicative Competence	Metalinguistic skills, functional use of school language	9–17	x	x	x	x	x		x	Simon (1986)
Expressive One-Word Picture Vocabulary Test-Revised (EOWPVT-R) and Upper Extension	Single-word vocabulary; 100 items	2–12 12–15		x			x			Gardner (1983, 1990)
Fisher-Logemann Test of Articulation Competence	Word and sentence forms; table on dialects; has screening form; 35 plates	3–Adult		x	x					Fisher & Logemann (1971)
*Fluharty Preschool Speech and Language Screening Test	Uses objects	2–6	x	x	x	x	x	x		Fluharty (1978)
Goldman-Fristoe Test of Articulation	Single words, words in sentences; stimulability; 35 color plates	2–16		x	x					Goldman & Fristoe (1986)
Khan-Lewis Phonological Analysis	Use after Goldman-Fristoe to identify 15 phonological processes	2.5–11		x						Khan & Lewis (1986)
Language Processing Test (LPT)	6 subtests; school related	5–11		x				x		Richard & Hanner (1985)
Lindamood Auditory Conceptualization Test-Revised	Used to determine metaphonology	Pre-K–Adult		x	x					Lindamood & Lindamood (1979)
The Listening Test	5 subtests relating to school function	6–11	x	x				x		Barrett et al.
Multilevel Informal Language Inventory (MILI)	Starts with spontaneous expressive, then elicited, then receptive; can be used to elicit structures after language sampling	4–12		x		x	x	x		Goldworthy & Secord (1982)
*Northwest Syntax Screening Test (NSST)	Picture pointing and sentence repetition	3–8	x	x		x	x			Lee (1971)
Patterned Elicitation of Syntax Test (Revised) with Morphophonemic Analysis (PEST-R)	Delayed imitation format	3–7.6		x		x	x			Young & Perachio (1993)

Appendix 6–B continued

Name of Instrument	Comments	Age	Rec	Exp	Ph	M	Sx	Sm	Pr	Source
Peabody Picture Vocabulary Test Revised (PPVT-R)	Black/white pictures; 2 forms, single words	2.6–Adult	x					x		Dunn & Dunn (1981)
Preschool Language Assessment Instrument (PLAI)	Based on discourse model; designed for school language demands; 60 questions	2.9–5.8		x			x	x		Blank et al. (1978)
Preschool Language Scale-3 (PLS-3)	Concepts, cloze, sentence repetitio; includes articulation screen and language sample check list; family interview	Birth–7	x	x	x	x	x	x		Zimmerman, Steiner, & Pond (1992)
Receptive One-Word Picture Vocabulary Test (ROWPVT) Also Upper Extension	Single word vocabulary	2–12 12–15	x						x	Gardner & Brownell (1985)
*Screening Kit of Language Development (SKOLD)	Black/white pictures for vocabulary; color plates for story completion; sentence repetition 37–55 plates depending on age	2–5	x		x	x	x	x		Bliss & Allen (1983)
*Speech & Language Evaluation Scale	Uses *teacher* rating scale; includes fluency & voice	Adolescent			x	x	x	x		Fressola & Hoerchler (1989)
Structured Photographic Expressive Language Test (SPELT-P)	Earlier developing morphemes & synta; color photos; cloze procedure	3–6		x	x	x				Werner & Kresheck (1983a)
Structured Photographic Expressive Language Test II (SPELT-II)	Age guidelines for individual morpheme; color photos; cloze procedure; 22 phone articulation screening	4–9:5		x	x	x				Werner & Kresheck (1983b)
Test for Auditory Comprehension of Language-Revised (TACL-R)	Can be used with older children with syntax problems using embedding	3–11	x			x	x	x		Carrow-Woolfolk (1981b)

continues

Name of Instrument	Comments	Age	Rec	Exp	Ph	M	Sx	Sm	Pr	Source
Test of Awareness of Language Segments (TALS)	Metaphonology and metalinguistics; 46 item; can also be used with older students w/ LLD	4.6–7	x		x					Sawyer (1987)
Test of Early Language Development-2 (TELD-2)	38 items; tests variety of language areas	2–8	x	x	x	x	x	x		Hresko, Reid, & Hammill (1991)
Test for Examining Expressive Morphology (TEEM)	Cloze format; score sheet separates irregular forms	3–8		x		x				Shipley, Stone, & Sue (1983)
Test of Adolescent Language-3 (TOAL-3)	Includes 10 areas including reading, writing, and oral language; scoring software available	12–Adult	x	x			x	x		Hammill et al. (1994)
Test of Language Development 2–Intermediate (TOLD-I:2)	6 subtests plus composite scores	8.6–13	x	x		x	x	x		Newcomer & Hammill (1991a)
Test of Language Development 2–Primary: (TOLD-P:2)	7 subtests plus composite scores	4–9	x	x	x	x	x	x		Newcomer & Hammill (1991b)
Test of Problem Solving (TOPS) Adolescent & Elementary	5 subtests of aspects of critical thinking	12–17		x					x	Zachman et al. (1991, 1984)
Test of Relational Concepts-Revised (TRC)	Assesses concept knowledge	3–8	x				x			Edmonston & Thane (1993)
Test of Word Finding	Diagnostic for anomia; difficult to administer without practice	6.6–13		x				x		German (1991)
Test of Word Knowledge	2 levels, each w/core battery plus subtests definitions, synonyms, antonyms, multiple meanings	1.5–8 / 2.8–18	x	x					x	Wiig & Semel (1992)
Test of Written Language-2 (TOWL-2)	Individual or small-group administration; essay and multiple-answer formats; 2 forms	grades 2–12		x			x	x		Hamill et al. (1988)
Token Test for Children	Auditory comprehension; manipulation of colored circles/squares: spatial/temporal concepts; requires practice to administer	3–12.5	x					x		DeSimoni (1978)

continues

Appendix 6–B continued

Name of Instrument	Comments	Age	Rec	Exp	Ph	M	Sx	Sm	Pr	Source
Weiss Comprehensive Articulation Test (WCAT)	82 pictures; stimulability test; language sample elicitation pictures; blends phonemes listed by freq. of occurrence	3–7	x		x					Weiss (1980)
The Word Test-Adolescent	Brand names, definitions, synonyms	12–17	x						x	Zachman et al. (1989)
The Word Test-Revised Elementary	Critical semantic features: associations, synonyms, antonyms, absurdities, multiple-meaning words, definitions	7–11	x						x	Huisingh et al. (1990)

Appendix 6-C

Sampling of Metalinguistic Measures for the School-aged Child, Pre-kindergarten through Grade 12

Title	Author	Publisher	Date
Analysis of the Language of Learning	Blodgett & Cooper	LinguiSystems	1987
Evaluating Communicative Competence	Simon	Communication Skill Builders	1986
Lindamood Auditory Conceptualization Test-R	Lindamood & Lindamood	Riverside	1979
Test of Language Competence-Expanded Ed.	Wiig & Secord	Psychological Corporation	1989
Writing Process Test	Warden & Hutchinson	Riverside	1992

Chapter 7

Individualized Educational Program*

Eileen H. Gravani

WHAT IS AN IEP?

An Individualized Educational Program (or IEP) is essentially an outline of a child's special educational needs and the means to meet these needs. It is the basic building block for a specially designed program for a child with special education needs. According to the federal government, an IEP is a "written statement for a handicapped child that is developed and implemented in accordance with 300.341-349" (P.L. 102-119 §05, Stat. 587).

Practically speaking, an IEP is a written planning tool for a child's special education that is developed by school personnel and parents together. This document is developed to meet the special needs of a child with disabilities that affect education. Every student from 3 to 21 years of age who has a disability significantly affecting education

should have an IEP. It does not outline the regular education program unless there are classroom modifications or testing modifications. In other words, if a child is in a regular education classroom without any changes due to his or her special needs and receives only speech services, the classroom program and goals will not be outlined on the IEP.

A key phrase in the paragraph above is that the IEP outlines special needs that affect education. If a communication problem is mild in severity and/or does not affect the child's educational performance, then that child may not have an IEP. An example of this would be a first-grade child with a frontal production of /s/ and /z/. The child is doing well academically and has appropriate social relations with his or her peers. This distortion of /s/ and /z/ is an example of a mild problem that does not affect educational performance. So you might ask, "When is a problem educationally significant? Exactly what is 'educationally significant'?"

Typically, stating that a problem is educationally significant indicates that the problem affects the child's performance in the educational setting— the classroom. It might affect the child in academic subjects, social development, or self-esteem. Federal and state legislation have not specifically indi-

---

*The following booklets from New York State were used in the preparation of this chapter. New York State Dept. of Health (1992); New York State Education Dept. (1992, 1994); and Tompkins-Seneca-Tioga (1995). You may obtain similar information from the Office of Education in your state or from a regional resource center. Each state is required to prepare information and have it available for parents.

cated what constitutes an educationally significant problem. This allows some flexibility in making decisions and allows for differences between children. For example, two children may have similar problems and somewhat similar test scores and have different needs because of the way their classroom performance is affected.

In an effort to determine eligibility for special education and related services, some school districts have developed specific guidelines. These guidelines vary among school districts. Some require that diagnostic testing indicate a deficit of −1.5 standard deviations below the mean. This would place a child in the moderate range for severity. Refer to Chapter 6 for a full discussion of test score interpretation.

Children who do not qualify for an IEP may still receive speech-language services—for example, through speech improvement groups. This will be discussed later when we talk about the IEP meeting and eligibility for services.

Now that we have discussed very generally *what* an IEP is, we will cover what occurs *before* an IEP is developed, *who* develops it, and *when* it is developed. Later we will talk about each of the parts or components of the IEP and work on some practice cases.

EVENTS THAT OCCUR PRIOR TO THE IEP

The typical sequence of events in developing an IEP is that the child is referred (by a teacher, a parent, a doctor, a school nurse, oneself, or another professional) or has demonstrated difficulty on a screening test. Federal law allows the school district either (a) 40 days from the initial referral date or (b) 30 days from the parents' consent for evaluation

to conduct an IEP meeting. The school district is required to use whichever date is earlier. So if a child fails a screening test on September 10, the building administrator or principal is notified, and a letter is sent to the parents. This letter informs the parents that the child has demonstrated some difficulties and will require further testing. The letter also includes a consent form that the parents or guardians need to sign for the school district to begin testing. If the parents send this back by September 25, then the school district will arrange an IEP meeting on or before October 25.

To illustrate, we will follow a 6-year-old (6 years, 0 months) boy, Martin Greene (Marty), through the IEP process. Marty is a first grader who moved into a new school district and demonstrated difficulty with the speech section of the screening test on October 1. His teacher reported that she has difficulty understanding him and often asks him to repeat comments or answers. She indicated to the speech-language pathologist that typically she can understand children's speech patterns after they have been in her class for 2 weeks but that she still has trouble understanding Marty and often relies on the context of the situation. A letter was sent to the parents on October 7, indicating the need for testing and requesting permission. The parents returned the signed consent for testing on October 8, and the arrangements were made for diagnostic testing. The IEP meeting had to be set for November 7 at the latest.

Evaluation Procedures

Federal regulations outline some considerations for testing children to determine if an IEP is needed and to identify the areas of strength and weakness.

Tests and diagnostic materials must

- be given in the student's native language (e.g., Spanish, Korean) or mode of communication (e.g., sign language) so that the child's actual abilities in his or her native language are assessed
- be validated for a specific purpose. This is true for tests in our field.
- be administered by trained personnel
- reflect the student's actual ability rather than the influence of a sensory or motor disability. For example, you might want to be sure that the student has the motor ability to point to a choice of four pictures, as in the Peabody Picture Vocabulary Test (PPVT)-Revised (Dunn & Dunn, 1981) or the visual ability to scan several black-and-white outline pictures, as in the PPVT or the Test of Auditory Comprehension of Language-Revised (TACL-R) (Carrow-Woolfolk, 1981)
- assess in all areas of disability

Therefore, if a child had suspected problems in phonology and in receptive and expressive syntax and morphology, you would need to assess each of these areas. If during your testing you noted any other possible areas of difficulty, these would also need to be assessed.

A minimum of two tests per area of suspected disability is required. A single test is not sufficient to document a disability. This is to verify that a child actually does demonstrate a problem so that a diagnosis is not based on a single assessment measure. Additionally, the results need to be evaluated by a multidisciplinary team. This consists of a minimum of one teacher and one specialist in the area of the suspected disability.

Marty's testing was completed by October 9, and the IEP meeting was set for October

17. Next, we will discuss the people who need to be present at the IEP meeting.

Individuals Involved in the IEP Preparation

Typically, people at the IEP meeting include

- a representative of the public educational agency who is qualified to provide, administer, or supervise the specially designed instruction. This person needs to have the authority to ensure that services outlined in the IEP will actually be provided.
- the child's teacher
- the parent or guardian
- the child (if appropriate)
- for the initial evaluation, a member of the evaluation team or a person who is knowledgeable about the evaluation procedures used
- other appropriate individuals

This list may vary from state to state, depending upon state law or policy, but states are responsible for compliance with federal IEP requirements.

A typical IEP meeting for a child receiving only speech-language services might include only

- a district administrator (the principal or director of student services)
- the speech-language pathologist
- the parent or guardian
- the child (particularly if the student is an adolescent or young adult)
- the classroom teacher (present but not required by federal law for students who demonstrate speech-language problems only)

A child who has more special needs, has had an initial evaluation, or is changing placements might have more people in attendance. In addition to the individuals listed above, these might include

- a psychologist
- an occupational and/or physical therapist
- the school nurse
- a social worker
- evaluation team members
- the classroom teacher, whose presence is in such cases required
- a vocational counselor
- other appropriate individuals, such as representatives from community agencies

Educational agencies (typically school districts) need to document who is present at these meetings. This is done by listing the people attending or having individuals' signatures on the IEP form. This type of documentation is important if later questions arise about a decision made at the IEP meeting.

In Marty's case, a school district administrator, his parents, the classroom teacher, the speech-language pathologist, and a psychologist planned to attend the IEP meeting.

When Is the IEP Developed?

The IEP is developed at a meeting with the participants listed above (agency representative, teacher, parent, and possibly the child) *before* special education and related services are provided. It makes sense that the most appropriate placement for a child with disabilities cannot be determined without first knowing what that child's needs are. Having this as law is actually a safeguard against placing a child in an inappropriate placement without knowledge of the child's abilities and needs. This does not mean that a child cannot be served to some extent by special education before the development of the IEP. It is possible for a child to be placed in a temporary placement as part of the evaluation process. This actually becomes part of the diagnostic information, and the child's performance in the program is considered at the IEP meeting.

Now that we have answered who attends the IEP meeting and when it is, we can turn to the components included in an IEP.

COMPONENTS OF THE IEP

Each IEP must include

- present levels of performance
- annual goals
- short-term instructional objectives
- specific special education and related services to be provided
- projected dates for initiation of services and duration of services
- participation in regular education
- appropriate objective criteria and evaluation

We will discuss each one of these components and also some recommended items that should be included in a good IEP.

Present Levels of Performance

This section may include a variety of information, depending upon the child and his or her needs, such as academic or educational achievement (i.e., preacademic or academic levels), intellectual functioning, functioning in other areas such as speech/language, and possibly level or type of pacing for the effective acquisition of a skill (e.g., reinforcement, repetition, and learning style).

For a child who demonstrates a specific problem in phonology, as Marty does, this information might include

- IQ score (performance and verbal)
- classroom performance: either scores on standardized tests (i.e., Stanford Achievement Test) or information from the teacher on the child's academic levels
- information on the child's speech and language abilities, stimulability, etc.
- information on any other areas of suspected deficits

Information concerning social development—interactions with peers and adults, self-perception, adjustment to the environment—is also included. Information regarding physical health and development is also included in the amount of detail that is appropriate. This would cover general health: vision and hearing abilities, medications, injuries, motor development, and so forth.

Information regarding the amount of adult supervision or support needed might also be included. Obviously, this would be related to the academic, social, and physical areas.

For Marty, this information, is contained in Exhibit 7-1. (Citations to tests are added to these IEP exhibits for your reference only.)

Annual Goals

There are statements that include behaviors in specific areas that reflect the child's needs and can reasonably be achieved within an academic year. Typically, there is an annual goal for each *general* area of need. Therefore a child with a very specific speech-language need may have only one or two annual

goals on his or her IEP. However, a child with multiple needs will have more goals. These annual goals provide a framework or guidelines for the educational plan designed for a specific child.

Some children have special needs that on a severity scale would be termed severe. These children might also demonstrate regression over summer vacation and not retain what had been learned during the academic year. These children have IEPs that extend for 12 months and will be labeled as such.

Some school districts have annual goals and short-term instructional objectives available on computer. There are also programs available commercially. One source is IEPs Unlimited, Inc., 3293 Buckhorn Drive, Lexington, KY 40515. This does make IEP preparation easier. However, as a speech-language pathologist, you should be certain that you are not choosing goals simply because they are printed and missing a goal that an individual child might need.

For Marty, there is only one area of need, so there is only one annual goal: "Improve intelligibility of conversational speech, focusing on decreasing stopping, depalatization, and weak syllable deletion."

Short-Term Instructional Objectives

Short-term instructional objectives are measurable steps or benchmarks between the present levels of performance and the annual goals. Short-term instructional objectives are not session or weekly goals; they cover a period of several weeks to months. Some school districts have advised teachers to plan on writing five to six short-term instructional objectives for an annual goal. Obviously, children do not learn at the same rate, and we can observe uneven learning rates within a single child. So five to six short-term instruc-

Exhibit 7–1 Sample "Present Levels of Performance" Section of IEP for Marty

---

Present Levels of Performance

a. Academic

Reading: Prereading/readiness level: recognizes upper and lower case letters; reads one-syllable words from the following word families: *at* (*bat, cat, mat,* etc.), *an* (*man, fan, can,* etc.), and *en* (*hen, pen, ten,* etc.)

Math: Counts to 100 by 1s and 10s; matches concrete pictures of items to numbers 1 to 12; does well with sequences/patterns.

Written Language: Writes the appropriate letter when sounding out a word 75% of the time.

Other: Interested and attentive during science activities.

Speech/Language

Articulation

Weiss Comprehensive Articulation Test (Weiss, 1980). Articulation Age 4 years, 8 months; Intelligibility 70%; Stimulability 80%; Stopping /f,v/ Depalatization /.

Conversational speech sample: intelligibility 65% to 70%; stopping and depalatization errors consistent, along with weak syllable deletion 70% of the time and final consonant deletion of /k,g/ 60% of the time.

Language (Receptive and Expressive)

Test of Language Development-2 Primary (*TOLD-2 Primary;* Newcomer & Hammill, 1991)

	Raw Score	Scale Score	Percentile
Picture Vocabulary	27	13	84
Grammatic Understanding	10	9	37
Oral Vocabulary	20	9	37
Sentence Imitation	17	11	63
Grammatic Completion	18	9	37

Receptive Language

Peabody Picture Vocabulary Test-R (*PPVT-R;* Dunn & Dunn, 1981): Form L; Raw Score 60; Standard Score 90; Stanine 4

Intelligence/Adaptive Behavior Data: *Weschler Preschool and Primary Scale of Intelligence* (*WPPSI*) revealed above-average intelligence, with verbal and performance abilities similar.

Learning Characteristics: Seems to learn best with visual cues.

b. Social Development

Self: Takes pride in his work; makes comments to peers and adults, "I don't talk very good."

Peers: Liked by classmates; aware of others' feelings; frustrated when others do not understand him, and sometimes ignores children when they do not understand him.

Adults: Does not initiate conversation but does answer questions; angry when not understood after the second attempt; has kicked the wall and table when not understood; refused to talk in music and gym since the teachers have difficulty understanding him; cried and wanted to go home when there was a substitute teacher and she did not understand him.

Family/Community: Parents report that Marty is a helpful child. They understand him but realize that he rarely talks with neighbors or relatives since "They don't know my words."

continues

Exhibit 7–1 continued

c. Physical Development

Pertinent Health Information: History of middle-ear infections; PE tubes inserted in August; otherwise health history is unremarkable.

Vision: normal acuity

Hearing: normal

Gross Motor: good—can hop, skip, catch ball.

Fine Motor/Manual/Dexterity: right-handed; copying of designs very detailed; printing of alphabet is adequate for age.

d. Management Needs

Instructional Characteristics: no significant management problems

Environmental Adaptation: (i.e., equipment): none.

Support: Minimal assistance needed from teacher.

---

tional objectives would be a general recommendation. These short-term instructional objectives should reflect the sequence necessary for learning the targeted skills and should build upon each other.

For Marty, the short-term instructional objectives clearly relate to the annual goal of improving intelligibility:

1. Decrease stopping of /f,v,s,z/ in single words to 20%.

2. Decrease stopping of /f,v,s,z/ in short sentences to 20%.

3. Increase use of /ʃ/ in words to 80%. (Note: Marty was highly stimulable for this sound.)

4. Decrease weak syllable deletion to 20% in sentences.

5. Decrease weak syllable deletion in conversational speech to 20%.

6. Decrease stopping of /f,v,s,z/ in conversational speech to 30%.

Other examples of the relationship between the annual goal and short-term instructional objectives follow below. Samples for phonology, semantics, and syntax/morphology are included.

For the annual goal "Decrease phonological processes in sentences," short-term instructional objectives might be:

1. R. (the child) will decrease regressive alveolar assimilation to 15% in sentences of five to six words.

2. R. will decrease stopping of /f,v,s,z/ to 10% in single words.

3. R. will decrease stopping of /f,v,s,z/ to 15% in short sentences.

4. R. will decrease stopping of /f,v,s,z/ to 20% in sentences with two clauses.

5. R. will decrease weak syllable deletion to 10% in words at the short-sentence level.

6. R. will decrease weak syllable deletion to 15% in words in sentences with two clauses.

For the annual goal "Increase semantic skills," short-term instructional objectives might be:

1. R. will demonstrate understanding of common categories by grouping objects according to categories, such as type of animal (*forest, farm, jungle, pet*), food

group, or furniture (according to rooms of the house), for 9 out of 10 items.

2. R. will demonstrate understanding of spatial concepts (*top, bottom, beside, behind*) during stories and play activities 80% of the time.

3. R. will use the spatial concepts (*top, bottom, beside, behind*) in short sentences during play or classroom activities 80% of the time.

4. R. will demonstrate understanding of shape names (*circle, oval, square, rectangle*) during play, art, and classroom activities 80% of the time.

5. R. will demonstrate correct use of shape names (*circle, oval, square, rectangle*) in response to questions 80% of the time.

For the annual goal "Increase syntactic and morphological skills," short-term instructional objectives might be:

1. R. will demonstrate understanding of personal pronouns in sentences by pointing or manipulation of figures 80% of the time.

2. R. will use personal pronouns in sentences when retelling stories 75% of the time.

3. R. will use complete sentences when appropriate while relating an event/story for 90% of her utterances.

4. R. will indicate comprehension of the regular past tense marker and the "s" verb marker in sentences by pointing 90% of the time.

5. R. will use the regular past tense marker and "s" verb marker appropriately at the story level 75% of the time.

Specific Special Education and Related Services to Be Provided

Each educational agency or school district is required to offer a variety of educational programs and services to meet the needs of students with disabilities. Obviously, children with different needs are going to require different types of services. This variety is often referred to as a *continuum of services*. The educational agencies are required to provide the *least restrictive environment* (LRE) to the maximum extent that is appropriate. This means that handicapped children should be educated with children who are not handicapped as much as possible.

Educational programs can include classroom services and related services, such as speech-language therapy, audiology, psychological services, physical therapy, occupational therapy, and counseling. These services are necessary for the student to benefit from classroom instruction, but the goals and objectives for these services may not directly relate to the classroom curriculum. An example of this might be a physical therapy goal for increasing trunk control. Although this goal does not directly relate to specific classroom curricula, it does relate to the student's daily life and will relate generally to the student's educational performance.

This continuum of services can include the following:

1. *Regular education classroom with consultant teacher services.* This type of placement provides either direct or indirect services to students with disabilities in full-time regular education. *Indirect* consultant services provide consultant services to the classroom teacher to assist in modifying materials or the presentation to meet the needs of students with disabilities. The times for these consultant services need to be regular so that as the curriculum changes throughout the year and the child's needs change, there is continued assistance. With *direct* service, the specialist works with individual

students or provides group instruction. This may be done within the classroom so that the student can benefit from the regular education program. Students may also be taken out of the regular education classroom for services.

2. *Resource room:* This provides specialized supplemental instruction in an individual or small-group setting. Resource room programs typically supplement classroom instruction. Resource room teachers work in cooperation with the classroom teachers to maintain or improve academic performance. Students may be in a resource room setting for up to 50% of the instructional day. Groups are composed of students with similar academic, social, physical, and management needs.

3. *Special classroom:* The guidelines for these classrooms vary from state to state and typically are concerned with teacher–student ratio and student instructional needs. Students in these classrooms may spend a part of this day with nonhandicapped peers, but their primary placement is in a special education classroom. This placement may be necessary to provide the adult attention and direction that the student needs to learn.

4. *Special schools:* Special schools, in separate buildings, are also used in order to supply intensive services for students with severe or multiple problems. School districts and states vary in the usage of these special school placements. A survey by Hasazi, Johnston, Liggett, and Schattman (1994) compared programs using a high percentage of separate classrooms or schools for special education placements versus programs that use separate placements less frequently. Factors that were cited as important were finances, organization of special education, parent advocacy, implementors (e.g., at the state level), and knowledge and values of the site implementors.

5. *Private schools:* Students whose needs cannot be appropriately met in public school programs may be served in programs provided by private schools. These schools may have day school or residential components and may be in state or out of state.

6. *State schools:* These schools have a specialized focus and are available for students who have specific educational needs. These programs may have day school or residential components. An example would be a school for deaf or severely hearing-impaired students or a school for deaf–blind students.

7. *Home or hospital instruction:* At times, students require temporary instruction at home due to severe illness or special circumstances. These students are still entitled to services. State laws indicate guidelines for serving these students. Because these are very restrictive placements and allow limited social interaction, they should be reevaluated frequently.

All special education and related services necessary to meet the child's special education needs must be listed. The amount of time also needs to be listed and clearly stated for the development of the IEP and its implementation. The total amount of service cannot be changed without another IEP meeting. A sample statement would be "Speech/language services three times per week for 30 minutes per session. One time per week will be in the classroom. Services to begin September 15 and continue until annual review."

Projected Dates for Initiation of Services

This includes the date(s) that the recommended program is to begin and the duration of the services. Typically, the services are provided as soon as possible after the IEP is finalized. Some exceptions can occur and include when the meeting occurs over the summer or other vacation time or if transportation needs to be arranged.

This section also needs to include whether the IEP is to be in effect for 12 months or the academic year.

Participation in Regular Education

This section needs to be specific and may give the percentage of time spent in regular education or list specific regular education classes that the child will attend. The grade level, curriculum, support, and learning outcomes should be listed. Examples might be

- *Art*, second grade, with assistance from a teaching assistant, same general outcomes as class
- *Math*, fifth grade, use calculator, key words underlined in directions and word problems, same learning outcomes as class

Students with severe disabilities may be in special classes most of the day, and their IEPs may list noncurricular activities with nondisabled peers, such as lunch, school assemblies, and club activities.

Physical Education

The physical education program needs to be documented. The student will receive either a regular or an adapted physical education program. If the student receives an adapted program, goals must be written for physical education.

Classroom Modifications

For the student to be successful in the classroom, there must often be modifications in the classroom program. These modifications need to be documented so that they can be implemented appropriately.

Modifications may include

- specialized equipment such as a computer or word processor, communication board, Braille writer/books, large-print books, auditory training equipment, or, for students with physical disabilities, a prone board or a transfer board for moving from a wheelchair
- modified directions
- increased time to respond verbally
- taped texts
- highlighted texts
- note-taking assistance
- shortened assignments
- peer tutoring
- study sheets
- reduced paper/pencil tasks
- use of a calculator
- preferential seating
- interpreter
- frequent breaks
- behavior management system

Keep in mind that this list, though fairly thorough, is not all-inclusive; you may see an IEP with other classroom modifications noted.

It is important to note that Public Law No. 102-119, the Individuals with Disabilities Education Act Amendments of 1990, added definitions to two terms that affect classrooms and equipment available for special needs. These are *assistive technology device* and *assistive technology service*. An *assistive technol-*

ogy device is defined as "any item, piece of equipment, or product system, whether acquired commercially off the shelf, modified, or customized, that is used to increase, maintain, or improve the functional capabilities of children with disabilities" (34 CFR 300.5). Technological devices and assistive services should be available to a student if they are listed on the IEP and found to be required for the student to receive a free, appropriate public education. These devices and services would be listed under "related services on the IEP" and then noted in the section on classroom modifications. It should also be noted that hearing aids fit the definitions of an assistive technology device and that if these are listed on the IEP, the school district is obligated to supply them (Peters-Johnson, 1994).

Testing Modifications

Modifications in testing or assessment also need to be noted. Some of the frequent modifications include

- Time limit—extended or waived
- Special location of exam
- Method of recording answers
- Type of questions asked or omitted
- Presentation of questions (signed, read aloud, use of Braille, large type)

Thus a student with a severe hearing loss who signs might have parts of an exam signed rather than given orally, or a student who has difficulty with written expression might be allowed to give test answers orally or in written phrases.

Appropriate Objective Criteria and Evaluation

On the IEP, there must be clear ways to document whether a student has achieved or made progress toward annual goals and short-term instructional objectives. These may be standardized testing or less formal means of assessment, such as pre/post testing, classroom observation, and assignments for class.

Some questions that may be helpful to ask in reviewing IEPs are:

1. Does the information concerning the student's present level of performance clearly describe the impact of the disability on the student's educational performance?
2. Does the IEP reflect the student's needs?
3. Is there a clear relationship between the present level of performance, recommended program, annual goals, and short-term objectives?
4. Do the goals and objectives focus on the *special* education needs of the student?
5. Do the current goals and objectives relate to goals and objectives from previous IEPs?
6. Does the IEP list all the services that the child needs, and are the frequency and duration of services clearly documented?
7. Are the individuals who will provide the services clearly specified in the IEP?
8. Is there contact with nondisabled peers?
9. Are the IEP goals and objectives functional? Will they assist the child in his or her present environment or an anticipated environment?

IMPROVING IEPs

In an article reviewing IEPs, Lynch and Beare (1990) found the following areas of weakness in the IEP documents:

- limited parental involvement

- vague objectives and criteria for successful performance
- prepared programs or activities listed not age appropriate

Additionally, only 4% of the objectives were related to skills outside of the classroom.

The authors suggested several ways that IEPs can improve.

- using age-appropriate content and materials (within a grade level)
- choosing functional objectives to make more of an impact in other settings
- focusing on generalization (teaching in a natural setting with a variety of materials, people, and situations)
- using specific objectives and criteria
- increasing parental involvement (e.g., setting home-related objectives or formulating some jointly monitored objectives)

IEPs are sometimes challenged on the basis of procedural violations. An example might be the people in attendance at the IEP meeting. The required parties are a school district representative, a teacher (or speech-language pathologist if speech/language is the only area of concern), the parent, and possibly the evaluator. A meeting between a parent and a teacher or speech-language pathologist is not a legal IEP meeting. Another reason that an IEP may be challenged is a possible violation of parental rights, such as lack of notification concerning the IEP meeting, insufficient time allowed for notification, or a notification sent not in the parents' native language.

IEP REVIEW

After it is written, how useful is the IEP? How often is it checked? A survey by the Illi-nois State Board of Education (1995) indicated that for the 1991–1992 school year, approximately 35% of the reviews of IEPs were done monthly or more frequently. An additional 37% of the reviews were quarterly or more frequently. Slightly less than 18% of the reviews were semiannually or more frequently.

Annual Review

IEPs must be reviewed at least every 12 months. This process is called an annual review. The purpose of the annual review is to evaluate whether the program described in the IEP is still appropriate and meeting the student's needs. Progress made throughout the time that the IEP has been in effect is reviewed, and recommendations are made. The individuals involved in this process are essentially the same as those present at the initial meeting:

- a representative of the school district
- the parents
- the classroom teacher (not required if the child receives only speech-language services)
- speech-language pathologist (if the student is on the caseload)
- other professionals who are responsible for implementing goals on the student's IEP
- the student (if appropriate)
- other individuals/representatives (e.g., community agencies)

The LRE is considered, and a recommendation is made to continue, modify, or discontinue the student's special education program. This may mean a change in classification, placement, or the way that the services are delivered. If the student will continue to have an IEP, new annual goals and short-term instructional objectives are written.

Triennial Evaluation

Every 3 years, many of the areas initially tested are reevaluated in comprehensive detail. Procedures for evaluation are similar to the initial evaluation. The purpose of this evaluation is to determine whether there are any changes in needs and whether the student continues to be eligible for special education. The parents are notified prior to the evaluation. After the evaluation is complete, there is a meeting to review the information. This may be arranged to coincide with the annual review meeting.

PROCEDURES IF A STUDENT IS NOT ELIGIBLE FOR AN IEP

We have discussed the scenario of a child who is referred, is evaluated, and receives an IEP. In other words, the student is found to have a problem that is educationally significant. But at times, testing indicates that a child's problem is mild or mild to moderate. Additionally, there appears to be no impact on classroom activities. In this case, there would be an IEP meeting, and after the findings were reviewed, the student would be ruled ineligible to have an IEP. However, the student might still receive some services. Many school districts have speech improvement programs and would enroll a child who has misarticulations that are not affecting his or her education. Additionally, the speech-language pathologist might consult with the classroom teacher and set up a classroom program for that child. Another possibility might be to place that child on a "watch" list and monitor his or her progress.

If a student is found to be ineligible for an IEP, the parents receive a letter from the school district. The letter outlines reasons for the decision, citing specific testing. The letter also outlines the parents' rights to appeal and the due-process procedure.

DUE PROCESS

At times in the IEP process, the parents/guardians of the child and the school district are not in agreement. Typically, these differences are discussed informally. However, a set of procedures called *due process* is designed to protect the right of students with special needs, parents of these students, and school districts. These are ensured by federal and state law.

Typically, informal resolution is attempted first. If this is not successful, formal procedures may be requested by the parents or guardians or the school district.

Parents may request due-process procedures for a variety of reasons:

- failure to follow the time-line requirements for an IEP (e.g., meeting 30 days after the parents' consent for evaluation)
- failure of the school district to implement the IEP recommendations
- failure of the school district to consider an independent evaluation when making IEP recommendations
- disagreement with the IEP recommendations
- failure of the school district to review the student's program on an annual basis
- failure of the school district to reevaluate the student every 3 years

Due-process procedures may also be initiated by the school district. The local educational agency (typically a school district) is responsible for ensuring that students with special needs receive a free appropriate public education. Some reasons that a school district may initiate due process are:

- Parents do not consent to the initial evaluation.
- Parents do not consent to the initial recommendation in special education.
- Parents withdraw consent for a proposed placement.
- The school district wants to establish that its evaluation is appropriate and avoid paying for an independent evaluation.

The hearing is conducted by an impartial hearing officer. This individual should not have a personal or professional interest in the case that would interfere with his or her impartial decisions and may not be an employee of the school district. Hearing officers need to have familiarity with special populations, education, and legal issues.

Parental rights prior to the hearing include that the parents or someone they delegate may have access to the student's educational records relating to the identification, evaluation, educational placement, and provision of a free, appropriate public education. Copies of records must be supplied at a reasonable cost. A right of both the parents and school district is that information to be presented at the hearing must be available to both parties at least 5 days before the hearing. This is to allow both parties access to the same information. Remember, the goal of this hearing is not "to win" but to supply the student with the most appropriate educational program to meet his or her needs.

A notice is sent to both parties concerning the date, time, and place of the hearing. Ad-

ditionally, a list of rights for both parties is supplied. These rights for parents and the school district at the hearing include the following:

- Counsel (a lawyer) may be present to give advice.
- Experts in the field may be present to give advice.
- Evidence is presented by both parties.
- Cross-examination is allowed for the witnesses.
- Witnesses (e.g., school district employees) may be required to attend.
- Written or taped recordings of the hearing must be available.

Rights available to the parents also include the decision about whether the hearing may be open to the public and whether the child may be present. An interpreter for the deaf or a translator must be available to the parents at the hearing if needed.

The time line for these hearings is fairly quick. This is to ensure that the student receives the most appropriate services. Federal law requires that the final decision from the hearing must be reached and copies mailed to each party within 45 days from the request for the hearing. In the interim, the student remains in the original placement (the one that he or she was in initially).

If either the parents or the school district wish to appeal the decision of the hearing officer, they may appeal to the State Educational Agency. A designated official will review the entire set of records related to the hearing, ensure that the procedures followed federal and state laws, and request additional evidence if necessary. Both parties are given the opportunity to present written or oral arguments. The State Educational Agency official makes the decision concerning the presentation of the arguments. A final decision is made within 30 days of the request, and copies of the decision are mailed to both parties.

If either party is not satisfied with the decision, they may bring civil action in either a state court or a federal district court. Issues that deal with federal law and may affect decisions in other states are typically brought to federal district courts.

Common Issues in Due Process

Some recent decisions dealt with the LRE, testing modifications integration into regular education. Summaries of these cases are included below.

Need for Integration

Parents of a 6-year-old student with autism wanted their child to be placed in regular education on a full-time basis. The school district recommended placement in a special education classroom. The parents then requested homebound placement with supportive services. A due-process hearing was requested.

One conclusion of the hearing was that the student did not have an absolute right to be placed in a regular education classroom but did have a right to be placed in regular education to the greatest extent possible, with appropriate support. The hearing officer ordered that a new IEP be developed that would consider the student's need for integration into a regular education class. The officer ordered the parents and school district to work together to develop a plan that would establish ways for keeping data on the student's performance and would include involvement in regular and special education classrooms (Detroit Public School, 1993).

Least Restrictive Environment

Parents of an 8-year-old with a hearing impairment were not in agreement with the school district regarding the placement. The school district had placed the student at a regional day school for the deaf, 17 miles from her home. At the school, the student was mainstreamed into a regular education classroom with an interpreter. She received instruction in total communication from the speech-language therapist and auditory training, language reinforcement, and tutoring from the deaf education teacher. The parents wanted their child placed at her local school. The parents requested a due-process hearing.

The hearing officer found that the district's placement on the IEP was appropriate for that student and that the IEP was being implemented in the LRE. The hearing officer based this on the fact that the student's academic abilities were significantly behind grade level and that she needed the comprehensive services offered at the regional school. There was no evidence that the program offered at the student's local school would be appropriate for her educational needs. Additionally, services for students with hearing impairments were centralized at the regional school, and the availability of services at other locations was limited (China Springs Independent School District, 1994).

Classroom/Testing Modifications

Parents of a student who was eligible for special education services requested a due-process hearing to change their child's IEP. The school district used a special education aide to record the student's oral responses to essay questions. The parents wanted to limit the personnel who could record the oral answers and maintained that the district's use of the aide violated federal law (IDEA).

The hearing officer concluded that a trained special education aide was an appropriate person to record answers and that the IEP should not be changed. The hearing officer also concluded that IDEA requires that IEPs be developed to provide educational benefit for the student and includes special instruction and related services. However, federal law does not require IEPs to include every service or modification that might possibly be of some value (Child with Disabilities, 1993).

Preparing Yourself for Due-Process Challenges

These are only a few of the cases that deal with common issues in due process. Although due-process hearings are not common and many disputes between parents and school districts are resolved informally, you should be prepared. During the 1990s, the number of due-process cases has increased. If you conduct yourself professionally and are accountable, you can protect yourself in case of due process. Some things that you can do are:

- Administer the test according to the way that it is standardized.
- Note any modifications you may have made.
- Be aware of the population used for standardization of the tests that you use— both number and whether it is representative of the U.S. population.
- Be aware that all testing must follow the federal guidelines stated earlier in the chapter (e.g., tests administered in the child's native language).
- Take care that there are two tests for each area of disability.

- Be sure that the annual goals and short-term instructional objectives clearly relate to the identified needs.
- Keep attendance, noting the reason for any missed sessions.
- Keep brief notes on each session, including the goal, general activity, and performance.
- Document any conversations or correspondence with parents.
- Keep in contact with the classroom teacher to learn about communication behaviors and generalization in the classroom.

SERVICES FOR YOUNGER CHILDREN

Services for Children Ages 3 to 5 Years

Many children entering elementary school may be identified and receive special services prior to entry into kindergarten. As you are reviewing children's folders or reading reports, this will become increasingly evident. The procedure for evaluating and providing services to preschool children with special needs is strikingly similar to that for children in public schools.

A referral for evaluation is made to the appropriate agency. In many states, services for preschool children are administered through the school districts. When a district receives a referral, a letter is sent to the parents. This letter includes a list of evaluators and requests the parents' consent for the evaluation. The letter also informs the parents of their due-process rights. After the parents give written consent for the evaluation, it is scheduled. The evaluation includes a physical examination, psychological examination, social history, parent interview, observation of the child, and assessment in all areas that are related to the possible disability/disabilities. While the evaluation process is occurring, the meeting to determine recommendations (IEP meeting) is arranged. This meeting needs to occur within 30 days of the referral.

At the meeting, the evaluation results and other information are reviewed. At the meeting, the child will be found either eligible or ineligible for special education services. If the child is found to be ineligible, there needs to be clear documentation of the reasons. This explanation should include specific tests or reports that led to the recommendation and the rationale for the decision. Also included are a list of due-process rights to be used if the parents wish to appeal. If the child is determined to be eligible for special education services, an IEP is developed. The IEP for a preschool child is very similar to an IEP for school-age children. It includes a statement of the recommended program, a list of current levels of functioning, annual goals, short-term instructional goals, criteria, and whether the placement is the least restrictive alternative. Also included are descriptions of the program/placement options and the rationale for rejection of any option not selected. The program or related service provider is notified, and arrangements for services are made. The parents need to give written consent for the placement. Transportation may be arranged unless the child is to receive the services at home or in a day care setting. The IEP needs to be implemented within 30 days of the IEP meeting. As with school-age children, the IEP needs to be reviewed after 12 months. At this time, the child's progress and present levels of functioning are reevaluated, and if the child continues to be eligible for services, a new IEP is

developed. Before the child begins kindergarten, a meeting is arranged to discuss the types of services for which he or she may be eligible. This meeting will help plan the transition from preschool to a school-age program and will ensure that the child continues to receive services during the transition.

Early Intervention

Federal laws require states to provide services to infants and toddlers with disabilities. In many states, these services for children from birth to their third birthday are overseen by the State Department of Health. For some states, the managing agency is the state Department of Education, and a few states use other state agencies.

These infants or toddlers must have a developmental delay or a diagnosed physical or mental condition that has a high probability of resulting in a developmental delay in physical development, cognition, communication, social/emotional development, or adaptive development.

Developmental delay means that a child has not achieved developmental milestones in the areas listed above that are expected for the child's age after any adjustments for prematurity have been made (New York Early Intervention Program—Revisions, Appendix A, Sec. 69-4.1 g). New York State's Early Intervention Program uses the following criteria to document developmental delays:

- a 12-month delay in one functional area;

- a 33% delay in one functional area or a 25% delay in each of two areas;

- a score of at least 2 standard deviations below the mean in one functional area or 1.5 standard deviations below the mean in each of two functional areas if standardized instruments are individually administered; or

- the clinical opinion of a multidisciplinary team if a standardized score is inappropriate or cannot be determined.

The diagnosed medical or physical conditions include:

- low birth weight (less than 1,501 grams)
- gestational age of less than 33 weeks
- central nervous system insult or abnormality
- congenital malformations
- asphyxia (Apgar score of 3 or less at 5 minutes)
- abnormalities in muscle tone
- hyperbilirubinemia
- hypoglycemia
- growth deficiency/nutritional problems
- inborn metabolic disorder (IMD)
- perinatally or congenitally transmitted infection
- maternal prenatal alcohol abuse
- maternal prenatal abuse of illicit substances
- prenatal exposure to therapeutic drugs with known potential developmental implications
- maternal PKU
- suspected vision or hearing impairment
- serious illness or traumatic injury with implications for the central nervous system
- elevated venous blood levels
- chronic serious otitis media (continuous for a 3-month minimum)

The general procedure is similar to the development of the IEP for school-age children. The time line follows:

- Identification (by health care providers, hospitals, child care providers, local school districts, qualified personnel)
- Referral (within 2 days of identification)
- Family is informed of rights
- Parents give consent for testing
- Evaluation is completed
- Individualized Family Service Plan (IFSP) meeting—within 45 days of referral
  The IFSP is developed.
- A review of the IFSP is conducted every 6 months

The IFSP is a written plan for services and includes

- the child's present level of functioning
- information concerning the family (some of this information is included only with parental consent)
- expected outcomes
- early intervention services to be provided
- dates, duration, and frequency of services
- location of services
- transition plan for preschool (upon reaching the age of 3 years)

The primary difference between the IEP and the IFSP is the emphasis on family involvement both in the IFSP and in the delivery of services.

If parents have concerns about the IFSP, procedures are available that are similar to the due-process procedures for school-age children and their parents.

It is evident that when services to children with special needs are provided, there should be a strong commitment toward meeting the child's needs and dealing with family concerns. Additionally, there is a strong emphasis on accountability and documentation. The emphasis on accountability and documentation result in a significant amount of paperwork. As you can see in the IFSPs and IEPs for younger children and IEPs for older students, there also is an emphasis on assist-

ing these individuals as they make transitions from early intervention programs to preschool services to school and later to the community.

CASE STUDIES

Exhibits 7–2, 7–3, and 7–4 give IEPs for the first three cases whose assessment you followed in Chapter 6: Steven, James, and Christine.

Exhibit 7–2 IEP for Case 1: Steven

Individualized Educational Program

Student Name: Steven

Address:

Dominant Language: English

Telephone:

Current Teacher: Ms. Rose

Current Program: Regular classroom—1st grade

Classification: Speech Impaired

D.O.B.

C.A. 6 yrs., 6 mos.

Referral Received: 2/25

Consent for Eval: 3/10

Consent for Place. _____

Actual Placement _____

Present Level of Performance

a. **Academic**

Reading: Difficulty in sounding out words (decoding); comprehension of stories read by teacher is adequate; cannot decode stories well enough to judge comprehension of material he has read.

Math: At appropriate level; can do addition and subtraction that does not involve carrying; recognizes number patterns; can count by 1s, 2s, 5s, and 10s.

Written Language: Uses only the initial sound for inventive spelling of words; other letters may be listed but bear no resemblance to the sounds in the word or to the actual letters used in the word.

Other: Very interested in social studies and science.

Speech/Language

Articulation

Goldman-Fristoe Test of Articulation (Goldman & Fristoe, 1986)—overall 11th percentile; Stimulability score of 35; errors consist of /l/ and /r/ in all positions and blends.

continues

Exhibit 7–2 continued

Receptive Language

Peabody Picture Vocabulary Test-Revised (Dunn & Dunn, 1981) Age Equivalent 6-0; Stanine = 4; Standard Score = 90; 26th percentile.
Clinical Evaluation of Language Fundamentals-Preschool (*CELF-Preschool;* Wiig, Secord, and Semel, 1992)

	Standard Score	*Percentile*
Linguistic Concepts	9	37
Basic Concepts	12	75
Sentence Structure	8	25
Receptive Total	98	45

Expressive Language

CELF-Preschool	*Standard Score*	*Percentile*
Recalling Sentences in Context	4	2
Formulating Labels	9	37
Word Structure	7	16
Expressive Total	83	13
Total (Receptive and Expressive)	90	25

SPELT-2: 76% correct; 6th percentile rank
Expressive One-Word Picture Vocabulary Test (*EOWPVT;* Gardner, 1990) Age Equivalent 5-9; Stanine = 4; Standard Score = 92; 30th percentile

Intelligence/Adaptive Behavior Data: *Wechsler Preschool and Primary Scale of Intelligence* (*WPPSI*) revealed intelligence within normal limits, with performance slightly better than verbal.

Learning Characteristics: Has difficulty with tasks involving speech sounds and sound-letter associations.

b. Social Development

Self: Easygoing, cooperative; sometimes comments, "This is easy for me" or "This is hard for me, but other kids know it."

Peers: Well liked by peers; cooperative and willing to help others on the playground and in block building; others seem willing to help him with reading.

Adults: Cooperative; tries hard to please.
Family/Community: easygoing; plays by self or with neighbors; good attention span for building tasks (e.g., Legos).

c. Physical Development

Pertinent Health Information: General health is good; no allergies.

Vision: normal

Hearing: normal

continues

Exhibit 7–2 continued

Gross Motor: Good for age.

Final Motor/Manual/Dexterity: Good for manipulation of small objects and for paper-and-pencil tasks

d. **Management Needs**

Instructional Characteristics: No management problems

Environmental Adaptation (i.e., equipment): none

Support: Additional assistance needed in reading and writing tasks.

Annual Goals

I.   Improve articulation, particularly in multisyllabic words in conversational speech
II. Improve phonemic awareness in the following areas
    A. Rhyme
    B. Grouping by sounds
    C. Syllable segmentation
    D. Phoneme segmentation for one-syllable words
    E. Phoneme blending for single words
    F. Association of sounds and letters
    G. Spelling (inventive)

Short-Term Instructional Objectives

For Annual Goal I:

Note: Syllable segmentation for Goal II would be emphasized in conjunction with objectives for weak syllable deletion.

1. Decrease weak syllable deletion for familiar words to 10%.
2. Decrease weak syllable deletion in three- to four-sentence short stories to 20%.
3. Decrease weak syllable deletion in conversational speech to 20.
4. (Note: Steven was stimulable for /l/ in the initial position.) Increase use of /l/ in the initial position of words to 80%.
5. Increase use of /l/ in the initial position of words in two-clause sentences to 80%.

For Annual Goal II:

1a. Identify the word that does not rhyme out of a choice of four words (phonological oddity task, e.g., *man, tan, feet,* and *can*) 80% of the time (Bradley & Bryant, 1983).
1b. Identify the word that rhymes out of a choice of two (rhyme judgment task, e.g., *man, feet, can*) 80% of the time.
2. List a word that rhymes when given two sample words (e.g., *cat, bat,* _____) 75% of the time
3. Identify two words that have the same initial sound out of a choice of three words (e.g., *hen, chick, hand*) 80% of the time.
4. List a word with the same initial sound when given a list of three words (e.g., *bug, bed, build,* _____) 75% of the time.

continues

Exhibit 7–2 continued

5. Identify two words that have the same final sound out of a choice of three words (e.g., *leaf, roof, pop*) 80% of the time.

6. List a word with the same final sound when given a list of three words (e.g., *bus, ice, dress,* _____) 75% of the time. A choice of picture cards will be used initially.

7. Segment the number of syllables correctly 80% of the time for the following progression:
   a. compound words (e.g., *cowboy, rainbow*)
   b. two-syllable words that are not compound (e.g., *baboon*)
   c. familiar three-syllable words (e.g., *elephant, telephone*)

8. Segment phonemes for one-syllable words 80% of the time, progressing from continuants to stops:
   a. Two-phoneme words (e.g., *off, on, zoo, so, in, us, up, out*)
   b. CVC words (e.g., *sun, man, fan, fish, roof, mat*)

9. Blend phonemes 80% of the time, using the following progression:
   a. the initial phoneme segmented from the rest of the word (e.g., *s un*)
   b. The final phoneme segmented from the rest of the word (e.g., *fa n*)
   c. Three-phoneme words with a continuant in the initial position (e.g., *f a t*) (Ball, 1993)
   d. Three-phoneme words with stops as the initial sounds (e.g., *b a t*) (Ball, 1993)

10. Associate sounds and letters 80% of the time in the following progression:
    a. 10 consonant sounds—first pointing to the letter when he hears the sound and later saying the sound when he sees the letter
    b. same as above with five short vowel sounds
    c. same as above with the remaining consonant sounds
    d. same as above with five long vowel sounds

11. Spell word, using inventive spelling with two appropriate sounds, 80% of the time. Emphasis will be placed on using the initial and final sounds, but any appropriate sounds will be accepted.

Recommended Program

Placement: Continue in regular education first-grade classroom.
Speech-language services: Five times per week, 30-minute sessions; two of these sessions will be in the classroom.

Projected Dates for Initiation of Services

Speech-language services for Steven will begin on April 15.

Time in Regular Education

Steven is placed in a regular education first-grade classroom.

Objective Criteria

1. Pretest and posttest for short-term instructional objectives
2. Classroom performance for reading decoding and spelling strategies
3. Readministration of the CELF

Exhibit 7–3 IEP for Case 2: James

Individualized Educational Program

Student Name: James

Address:

Dominant Language: English

Telephone:

Current Teacher: Ms. Dwyer

Current Program: regular ed., third grade

Classification: Speech Impaired

D.O.B.

C.A. 8 yrs., 2 mos.

Referral Received: 9/15

Consent for Eval: 9/30 _____

Consent for Place. _____

Actual Placement _____

Present Level of Performance

a. **Academic**

Reading: Reading comprehension and decoding are at grade level; end of second-grade scores for reading comprehension were 1 S.D. below the mean.

Math: At grade level; does addition and subtraction for two places easily, some difficulty with three places; beginning multiplication of the 2s and 3s tables.

Written Language: Spelling is at age level; writing is grammatically correct; sometimes the content is unclear because there is a lack of specific vocabulary.

Other: Does well in reasoning tasks in science.

Speech/Language

Articulation

Test of Language Development-2 Primary (Newcomer & Hammill, 1991)
Word Articulation subtest—Scale Score 7; 16th percentile; speech patterns consistent with Black English.
Word Discrimination subtest—Scale Score 12; 75th percentile. *Goldman-Fristoe Test of Articulation* (Goldman & Fristoe, 1986)—speech patterns typical of Black English.

Language (Receptive and Expressive)

Test of Language Development-2 Primary (*TOLD-2 Primary;* Newcomer & Hammill, 1991)

	Raw Score	Scale Score	Percentile
Picture Vocabulary	22	9	37
Grammatic Understanding	22	9	37
Oral Vocabulary	7	5	5
Sentence Imitation	16	7	16
Grammatic Completion	21	7	16

(Productions for the last two subtests were consistent with Black English.)

continues

Exhibit 7–3 continued

Comprehensive Receptive and Expressive Vocabulary Test (CREVT; Wallace & Hammill, 1994)

	Raw Score	Scale Score	Percentile	Age Equiv.
Receptive	29	92	30	7-6
Expressive	2	75	5	4-9
Total		80	9	

Clinical Evaluation of Language Fundamentals-3 (CELF-3; Semel, Wiig, & Secord, 1987)
Rapid Naming subtest
151 seconds—just below the norms for age 6 years
16 errors—between the norms for ages 6 and 7
Test of Word Finding (German, 1991)

	Raw Score	Scale Score	Percentile
Picture Naming—Nouns	16		
Sentence Completion	8		
Description Naming	9		
Picture Naming—Verbs	16		
Picture Naming—Categories	12		
Total	61	76	15

Intelligence/Adaptive Behavior Data: *WISC-III* indicates normal intelligence, with performance subtests higher than verbal.

Learning Characteristics: Does best when learning if has visual, auditory, and haptic information.

b. **Social Development**

Self: Self-confident, quiet; seems aware of his strengths and weaknesses

Peers: Interacts well with peers; has made friends easily in the short time he has been in the school.

Adults: Cooperates; friendly to adults; respects authority.

Family/Community: Relates well to family and family friends; relates well to older brother; sometimes James relies on his brother to express ideas, "talk for both of them."

c. **Physical Development**

Pertinent Health Information: Good health; unremarkable health history.

Vision: normal

Hearing: normal

Gross Motor: Average for age

Fine Motor/Manual/Dexterity: Average for age

d. **Management Needs**

Instructional Characteristics: No significant management problems

continues

Exhibit 7–3 continued

Environmental Adaptation (i.e., equipment): none

Support: Minimal assistance for strategies to learn/organize vocabulary.

Annual Goals

I.   Improve receptive concepts for space and time
II. Improve expressive vocabulary
  A.   Increase use of concepts
    1. Spatial
    2. Temporal
  B.   Increase metalinguistic strategies for classroom vocabulary use
    1. Phonemic
    2. Categorization
    3. Associations
III. Decrease use of proforms and increase use of alternative descriptions

Short-Term Instructional Objectives

For Annual Goal I:
1. Demonstrate understanding of the spatial concepts *left* and *right* by following simple directions, 80% of the time.
2. Demonstrate understanding of *left* and *right* by following classroom directions, 80% of the time.
3. Demonstrate understanding of ordinal numbers in following simple directions with manipulatives or paper-and-pencil tasks.
4. Demonstrate understanding of temporal concepts *before* and *after* by following simple directions, 80% of the time.
5. Demonstrate understanding of temporal concepts *before* and *after* when answering questions on worksheets after reading a paragraph, 80% of the time.
6. Demonstrate understanding of time concepts (days of the week and months of the year) when answering questions during calendar activities, 80% of the time.

For Annual Goal II.A:
1. Use spatial concepts when giving directions or explanations 80% of the time correctly.
   a. Left/right
   b. Ordinal numbers
2. Use spatial terms (listed above) correctly when writing short sentences, in 8 out of 10 sentences.
3. Use temporal concepts correctly when giving instructions or explanations 80% of the time.
   a. Before/after
   b. Days and months
4. Use temporal terms correctly (listed above) when writing brief entries in a journal, 8 out of 10 times.

For Annual Goal II.B:
1. Group words with similar beginnings when given a list of classroom vocabulary an average of three out of four possible times.
2. Group words with similar endings when given a list of classroom vocabulary an average of three out of four possible times.

continues

Exhibit 7–3 continued

3. Organize classroom vocabulary into categories, discussing similarities and differences. James will correctly categorize three out of every four items and list two similarities and two differences. (An example from his Social Studies Unit on the Inuit would be animals of the Arctic, e.g., *whale, seal, walrus, sardine.*)
4. For more abstract classroom concepts, list one similarity and one difference. An example from the Inuit unit would be *hibernation* and *migration.*

For Annual Goal II.C:

1. Use diagrams and visual cues to illustrate classroom vocabulary and associations (e.g., insect drawings with six legs vs. spiders with eight legs). James will construct the diagrams/cues and explain three important characteristics.
2. Construct and use a time line to explain changes (e.g., for life cycles) and explain each change clearly.

For Annual Goal III:

1. Describe a minimum of three features about each object (color, shape, size, texture, other striking perceptual features, function, person who typically uses it, etc.) for 8 out of 10 common household, grocery, or classroom objects.
2. Provide definitions of objects, listing at least two pieces of critical information for an average of 7 out of 10 objects. Activities will progress from having the objects actually present to completing the activity without physical objects.
3. During sessions, when unable to easily retrieve a word, James will be prompted to use descriptions, definitions, category names, etc. He will use at least one strategy after a prompt 7 out of 10 times.

Recommended Program

James will continue in a regular education third-grade classroom.
Speech-language services: three 30-minute sessions per week, one or two of them in the classroom

Projected Dates for Initiation of Services

Speech-language services will begin on Nov. 1.

Extent of Time in Regular Education

James is placed in a regular education classroom.

Objective Criteria

1. Pretest and posttest for short-term instructional objectives.
2. Classroom performance for use of spatial and temporal terms and classroom vocabulary. Oral and written work will be reviewed.
3. Readministration of standardized testing (e.g., *Test of Word Finding*).
4. Analysis of language sample from spontaneous conversation to evaluate Annual Goal III.

Exhibit 7–4 IEP for Case 3: Christine

Individualized Educational Program

Student Name: Christine

Address:

Dominant Language: English

Telephone:

Current Teacher:

Current Program: Ninth grade

Classification: Learning Disabled—language comprehension problems

D.O.B.

C.A. 14-0

Referral Received: 3/25

Consent for Eval.: 4/5

Consent for Place.: _____

Actual Placement _____

Present Level of Performance

a. **Academic**

English/Literature: Attentive, hard worker, turns in assignments promptly; writing uses single or conjoined clauses with little variety; often papers have part of the theme correct but miss major points.

Math: Adequate with help from teacher and tutoring; does equations after seeing similar ones; new ideas from text seem difficult.

Social Studies: Has difficult time relating ideas; essays have not been satisfactory.

Science: Difficulty relating information; tests and lab reports have not been satisfactory; conclusions for lab reports are weak.

Foreign Language: Passing; does satisfactorily learning vocabulary and verb tenses.

Speech/Language

Articulation: not a concern; voice, fluency, and pragmatics are appropriate.

Language—Expressive and Receptive

Peabody Picture Vocabulary Test-Revised (*PPVT*-R; Dunn & Dunn, 1981)

Standard Score 87; 20th percentile

Evaluating Communicative Competence (*ECC;* Simon, 1986; criterion-based measure)

Receptive: Generally low to average; low in Inference.

Expressive: Causal Connectors—low; Opinion—no elaboration; 20 Questions—no logical progression; Barrier games—lack of detail.

Clinical Evaluation of Language Fundamentals-3 (*CELF-3;* Semel et al., 1987)

	Scale Score	Percentile
Concepts and Directions	4	2
Word Classes	8	25
Semantic Relations	7	16
Receptive Total	78	7
Formulated Sentences	6	9
Recalling Sentences	10	50
Sentence Assembly	9	37
Expressive Total	90	25
Total (Exp. and Recep.)	83	13

Intelligence/Adaptive Behavior Data: *WISC-III*—low average range.

continues

Exhibit 7–4 continued

Learning Characteristics:

b. **Social Development**

Self: At this time, Christine has low self-esteem; often makes remarks like "I just can't get it."

Peers: Relates well to peers; has fewer friends now because she is so busy with schoolwork and is often "down."

Adults: Courteous; relates well to adults.

Family/Community: Has a good relationship with parents; parents report that she is somewhat withdrawn now.

c. **Physical Development**

Pertinent Health Information: unremarkable health history; in good health

Vision: normal

Hearing: normal

Gross Motor: average—in P.E. class

Fine Motor/Manual/Dexterity: average

d. **Management Needs**

Instructional Characteristics: Does best with explanations and multiple examples.

Environmental Adaptation (i.e., equipment): none

Support: tutoring

Annual Goals

I. Improve comprehension and use of clausal connectors
    - A.   Logical
    - B.   Disjunctive
    - C.   Temporal
    - D.   Conditional

II. Improve organization of information
    - A. Receptive
        1. Note taking from texts
        2. Note taking from lecture
        3. Other situations—movies, stories, computer
    - B. Expressive: use of the following frameworks
        1. Main idea with supporting information
        2. Temporal sequencing
        3. Logical sequencing
    - C. Improve higher levels of learning
        1. Inference
        2. Synthesis

continues

Exhibit 7–4 continued

Short-Term Instructional Objectives

For Annual Goal I:

1. Comprehension of logical connectors (*because, since, so*) in short paragraphs, 9 out of 10 times.
2. Expressive use of logical connectors in short paragraphs, 9 out of 10 opportunities.
3. Comprehension of disjunctive connectors (*but, except, however, although*) in short paragraphs, 9 out of 10 times.
4. Expressive use of disjunctive connectors in short paragraphs, 9 out of 10 opportunities.
5. Comprehension of temporal connectors (*before, after, when, while*) in short paragraphs, 9 out of 10 times.
6. Expressive use of temporal connectors in short paragraphs, 9 out of 10 opportunities.
7. Comprehension of conditional connectors (*if, when, then*) in short paragraphs, 9 out of 10 times.
8. Expressive use of conditional connectors in short paragraphs, 9 out of 10 opportunities.

For Annual Goal II.A:

1. Use of headings, topic sentence, and logical ordering for a short section (four to five paragraphs) from a text. Eight out of 10 pieces of information will be related appropriately.
2. Use of headings, topic sentences, and logical and/or temporal ordering for three pages from a text. An average of 8 out of 10 pieces of information will be related appropriately.
3. Use of introduction and logical ordering for a 5-minute segment of a course lecture. Eight out of 10 pieces of information will be related appropriately.
4. Use of introduction statement and logical and/or temporal ordering for a 20-minute segment of a course lecture. An average of 8 out of 10 pieces of information will be related appropriately.
5. Use of titles/headings and logical and temporal ordering cues when watching movies, reading short stories or newspaper articles, etc. An average of 8 out of 10 pieces of information will be used appropriately.

For Annual Goal II.B:

1. Write a paragraph of five to six sentences in length, using logical sequencing and connectives throughout. This will be done for three consecutive attempts to complete the objective successfully.
2. Write a one-page paper, using logical sequencing and connectives throughout. This will be done for two consecutive attempts to complete the objective successfully.
3. Use of logical sequencing and connectives in a short (2-minute) summary of class material. At least four logical relationships will be included, with appropriate clausal connectors.
4. Write a paragraph of five to six sentences in length, using temporal sequencing and connectives throughout. This will be done for three consecutive attempts to complete the objective successfully.
5. Write a one-page paper, using temporal sequencing and connectives throughout. This will be done for two consecutive attempts to complete the objectives successfully.
6. Use of temporal sequencing and connectives in a short (2-minute) summary of class material. At least four logical relationships will be included, with appropriate clausal connectors.
7. a. Concept maps or diagrams will be used to illustrate the relationship of a main idea and at least five supporting pieces of information.
   b. An explanation of the concept map and the relation of the ideas to the main idea will be clear and use a minimum of three appropriate clausal connectors.

continues

Exhibit 7–4 continued

For Annual Goal III.C:

1. After reading a short paragraph, Christine will answer questions concerning the paragraph. Questions will deal with information not directly stated. Inference will be used appropriately for 8 out of 10 responses.

2. After reading a page of a course text, Christine will answer questions concerning the section read. Questions will deal with information not directly stated. Inference will be used appropriately for an average of 8 out of 10 responses.

3. After reading several paragraphs of a story or a newspaper article, Christine will synthesize the information into a clear statement or conclusion. This will be done at least three consecutive times to meet the objective successfully.

4. After reading one to two pages of a course text, Christine will synthesize the information into a clear statement or conclusion. This will be done at least three consecutive times to meet the objective successfully.

Recommended Program

Resource room: one class period per day.
Speech-language services: three periods (45 min.) per week; one out of the three sessions may be in conjunction with a classroom teacher or resource room teacher.
Classroom modifications: give outline of material to be covered in class or for the unit. (This applies to all classes except Art, Music, and P.E.)
Testing modifications: time limit for testing waived; written directions should be simplified, with key words in bold.

Projected Dates for Initiation of Services

Resource room and speech-language services will begin on May 1.

Extent of Time in Regular Education

Christine will be in regular education for 80% of the academic day.

Objective Criteria

1. Pretests and posttests will be used for all objectives.
2. Written work for courses will be reviewed and evaluated.
3. Classroom performance (use of outlining, etc.) will be evaluated to determine generalization.
4. Standardized testing will be readministered.

After examining the IEPs for Cases 1, 2, and 3, write an IEP for Case 4, Megan, using feedback from your instructor. You will need to include the assessment information that you prepared at the end of Chapter 6. Remember to include all the components of the IEP. You need to consider Megan's strengths and weaknesses in preparing her IEP. You may want to consider speech and language goals that will have an impact on her performance within the classroom curriculum and socialization.

REFERENCES

Ball, E. (1993). Assessing phoneme awareness. *Language, Speech, and Hearing Services in the Schools, 24*, 130–139.

Bradley, L., & Bryant, P. (1983). Categorizing sounds and learning to read: A causal connection. *Nature, 301*, 419–421.

Carrow-Woolfolk, E. (1981). *Test for Auditory Comprehension of Language-Revised*. Chicago: Riverside.

Child with Disabilities, 20 Individuals With Disabilities Education Law Report 314 (SEA Vermont 1993), 11/4/93, XIV 44. (1993). *Language, Speech, and Hearing Services in the Schools, 25*, 125.

China Springs Independent School District, 21 Individuals With Disabilities Law Report 468 (SEA TX 1994), 10/06/94, 21 (6), XIV 52. (1994). *Language, Speech, and Hearing Services in the Schools, 26*, 207.

Detroit Public School, 20 Individuals With Disabilities Law Report 406 (SEA MI 1993), 11/18/93, XIV 54. (1993). *Language, Speech, and Hearing Services in the Schools, 25* , 125.

Dunn, L., & Dunn, L.M. (1981). *Peabody Picture Vocabulary Test-Revised*. Circle Pines, MN: American Guidance Service.

Gardner, M. (1990). *Expressive One-Word Picture Vocabulary Test-Revised*. Novato, CA: Academic Interventions.

German, D. (1991). *Test of Word Finding*. Chicago: Riverside.

Goldman, R., & Fristoe, M. (1986). *Goldman-Fristoe Test of Articulation*. Circle Pines, MN: American Guidance Service.

Hasazi, S.B., Johnston, A.P., Liggett, A.M., & Schattman, R.A. (1994). A qualitative policy study of the least restrictive environment provisions of the Individuals With Disabilities Education Act. *Exceptional Children, 61*, 491–507.

Illinois State Board of Education. (1995). *Report on the evaluations of effectiveness of special education programs for 1991–92 and 1992–93*. Springfield, IL: Illinois State Board of Education.

Individuals With Disabilities Education Act of 1990, Pub. Law No. 101-407.

Individuals With Disabilities Act amendments of 1990, Pub. L. No. 102-119, Sec. 3 et seq., 105 Stat. 587.

Lynch, E., & Beare, P. (1990). The quality of IEP objectives and their relevance to instruction for students with mental retardation and behavioral disorders. *Remedial and Special Education, 11*, 48–55.

New York State Department of Health and New York State Commission on the Quality of Care for the Mentally Disabled. (1992). *Your family rights: A family guide for the New York State early intervention program for infants and toddlers with disabilities*. Albany, NY: Author.

New York State Education Department and University of the State of New York. (1992). *A parent's guide to special education for children ages 5–21: Your child's right to an education in New York State*. Albany, NY: Author.

New York State Education Department and University of the State of New York. (1994). *Transition services: A planning and implementation guide*. Albany, NY: Author.

Newcomer, P., & Hammill, D. (1991). *Test of Language Development-2 Primary*. Austin, TX: Pro-Ed.

Peters-Johnson, C. (1994). School services. *Language, Speech, and Hearing Services in the Schools, 25*, 275.

Semel, E., Wiig, E., & Secord, W. (1987). *Clinical Evaluation of Language Fundamentals-3*. San Antonio, TX: Psychological Corporation.

Simon, C. (1986). *Evaluating Communicative Competence*. Tucson, AZ: Communication Skill Builders.

Tompkins-Seneca-Tioga BOCES Continuing Education. (1995). *Your child: Your rights—Parents' guide to education for all, 0 to 5 years*. Ithaca, NY: Author.

Wallace, G., & Hammill, D. (1994). *Comprehensive Receptive and Expressive Vocabulary Test*. East Aurora, NY: Slosson.

Weiss, C. (1980). *Weiss Comprehensive Articulation Test*. Chicago: Riverside.

Werner, E., & Kresheck, J. (1983). *Structured Photographic Expressive Language-2*. Sandwich, IL: Janelle.

Wiig, E., Secord, W., & Semel, E. (1992). *Clinical Evaluation of Language Fundamentals-Preschool*. San Antonio, TX: Psychological Corporation.

New York State Public Health law 2500-a, 2500-e, Article 25, Title IIA, Sec. 69-4.1 and 4.4, 1994 revisions.

Chapter 8

Models of Service Delivery

Jacqueline Meyer

As an introduction to this chapter on intervention, I present three quotations. The first is from Stark & Wallach (1980): "The single most significant deterrent to educational growth [of students] remains the inability to use oral and written language, to speak and to read" (p. 6).

The second quote comes from critic Jack Beatty (1985) in an *Atlantic Monthly* review of a work by author Studs Terkel. Beatty describes Terkel this way:

His social perceptions flow from his literary and musical culture. . . . Style, language, story, rhythm, voice, tone, laughter: these aesthetic qualities, these properties of language and music, have made him feel more. Feeling more, he sees more. Seeing more, he cares more. The arts and humanities, his example suggests, are the proper stuff of character education. (p. 100)

The third one occurred during a class discussion in a course that included both speech pathology and education majors. The second day of class, a social studies teacher looked at several speech pathology students and said, "What is it that you people do?"

The long answer to that question is the subject of this chapter; the short one is that speech-language specialists attempt to decrease speech and language deficits so that the students who have been placed in our care can access the glorious stuff of language, the foundation of lifelong education.

You may remember that in the very early days of our field, "speech correctionists" trained teachers how to help students in their classrooms who had "speech problems," most commonly either articulation or fluency deficits. Gradually, however, school speech-language specialists removed students from their classrooms, and the years of our providing itinerant service and/or "pull-out" intervention became decades. Since the 1980s, however, new and markedly different ways to deliver intervention have been introduced under a bewildering variety of names, such as *collaboration, team teaching, consultation, push-in, pull-aside, inclusion, multiskilling,* and *curriculum-based instruction.* Professionals in our field have been hard pressed to understand the changes inherent in these service delivery models, let alone to keep up with them.

My personal experience has led me to adopt two premises regarding service delivery: (a) flexibility is one of the most powerful clinical attributes in providing effective intervention, and (b) the appropriate delivery system is the one that most benefits the student at a specific time. No longer do most school clinicians say that they "consult" or "use pull-out" exclusively. This means that although the pull-out model can be the most efficient type for a student at a particular juncture, a combination of two or even three others may best serve another pupil. To understand the strengths and weaknesses of individual models we will look at each type in some detail. This chapter will conclude with four cases begun in Chapter 6 and continued in Chapter 7. By the end of this chapter, then, we will have determined alternate ways to address the Individual Educational Programs (IEP) goals of the first three students. What will be missing, however, are lengthy descriptions of general intervention techniques, such as how to use minimal pairs in articulation intervention, because I am assuming that you have already completed course work in clinical treatment. The specific techniques that are listed were chosen only to illustrate how different service models can affect your choice of approach and vice versa. The chapter will also include a representative sample of the explosion of intervention ideas current in the literature.

DEFINITIONS OF INTERVENTION TYPES

The list below is not exhaustive, nor do all professionals agree on the definitions; I have narrowed the number of categories to make the differentiations between them clearer than they probably are in actual practice. My intent is to encourage you to understand/consider the choices you have when you implement IEP goals. You should be aware that in addition to our services, many of these models are also used in the schools by physical and occupational therapists, school psychologists, and learning disabilities and reading specialists.

- *Consultative* (indirect) intervention provides information to regular education teachers to assist in adjusting the learning environment and/or modifying their instructional methods to meet the individual needs of a pupil with a handicapping condition who attends their classes (New York Board of Regents, 1988).

- *Collaboration:* The definition most widely accepted is from Idol Paolucci-Whitcomb and Nevin (1986). "Collaboration is an interactive process that enables people with diverse expertise to generate creative solutions to mutually defined problems. It enhances the outcome and produces solutions that are different from those that the individual team members would produce independently. It provides effective programs for students with needs within the most appropriate context, thereby enabling them to achieve maximum constructive interaction with their nonhandicapped peers" (Idol Paolucci-Whitcomb & Nevin, p. 1).

- *Pull-out* intervention provides intermittent direct services. Speech and language services are provided as a supplementary service to regular or special education programs. Intervention may be aimed at an individual student or a group of students. Typically, the students scheduled into a group session exhibit similar communication disorders (e.g., language, articulation, fluency, and voice; Neidecker & Blosser, 1993, p. 187).

- *Team teaching* can be defined as a synonym for collaboration, but it can also refer to a system in which two teachers share students. They prepare lessons independently, often divided along subject lines: for example, one instructor teaches math and the other language arts. In the case in which the speech-language pathologist team-teaches with a classroom teacher, he or she may "take over" the whole class for an assignment or they may both be involved in teaching a single lesson at the same time. In either case, team teaching "emphasizes the use of naturalistic environments and meaningful contexts" (Miller, 1989, p. 155).

- *Self-Contained Language Class:* In this case, the speech-language pathologist is the primary teacher and offers intense intervention on a continual basis within the context of the curricula. At the younger level, the classrooms are often developmentally based, as in a "prefirst" transitional class. Other students may be served in a special language course for hearing-impaired students at the high school level. Self-contained classes may also include "cross-categorical" groups, such as a mixture of students whose conditions all require language intervention (e.g., autism or a cognitive impairment).

- *Multiskilling:* This term, more commonly applied to the health care field, refers to a single professional who is cross-trained to "provide more than one function, often in more than one discipline" (Pietranton & Lynch, 1995, p. 38). What is different about this model compared with others we have discussed is that a person so designated could replace another professional: for example, a "'rehab specialist' could practice across multiple scopes of practice, [including] speech-language pathology, occupational therapy and physical therapy" (Pietranton & Lynch, 1995, p. 40).

Multiskilling is often suggested as a means of saving money. The American Speech-Language-Hearing Association (ASHA) appointed an ad hoc committee to examine the implications of this mode of service on current and future audiologists and speech-language specialists. How this model might be applied to the schools was not clear at the time this text was published.

- *Inclusion* represents a philosophy of valuing diversity by educating students who have disabilities within the regular education program; this includes their having access not only to the classroom but to other facilities and extracurricular activities as well. The disabilities may be severe, and the children who are included under this model are challenged in ways that heretofore have rarely been seen in the typical classroom.

Remember that intervention is an integral part of the concept of dynamic assessment discussed in Chapter 6. Many of the service delivery models described above can include dynamic assessment/intervention, although it may not be mentioned specifically in the examples.

RATIONALES FOR NEW INTERVENTION TYPES

Why have all of these service delivery models appeared? Has something changed to make the pull-out mode not as desirable? In a word, yes. Pressure for change has come from a number of sources and for a number of reasons. Let us look first at some general reasons for altering the ways in which intervention is being provided in the school environment (Eger, 1992; Huffman, 1992).

- Changing school populations have resulted in a far more varied caseload.

Consider first just the number and variety of cultures in the schools compared with 20 years ago. In addition to the likelihood that more students will be at risk, ponder the other stresses on family life that a changing economy can produce. Think about the possible speech and language implications of autism or cerebral palsy for students who are now part of the regular classroom for the first time. Be careful, however, that you do not ascribe results to reasons without research to substantiate your conclusions. Often it is not easy to sort out cause and effect in language disorders. Let us suppose that Jason watches TV nonstop and rarely engages in conversation. Does he not talk because he was so entranced by television that he did not practice enough, or did he turn to TV because he had language deficits? Both? Neither?

- The diminishment of economic resources for many sectors of our society has had one sure effect: less funding. Taxpayers are demanding results, and specialists' services have become suspect. The people who pay the bills, and their school board member representatives, are demanding a person who can wear more than one hat.

- As the general field of education has undergone changes, new buzz words have appeared in a climate of "out with the old, in with the new." How members of our profession deal with such trends as site-based, total quality, or outcome-based management, the whole-language movement, curriculum-based learning, and high-tech equipment will determine whether we will have a real role in the larger educational community.

Pressure for changes has also specifically affected our profession:

- The knowledge base that speech-language pathologists are expected to have has exploded. We are still a field that educates our newest members as generalists, but clearly there is too much to absorb and remember. Consequently we must learn to rely on other professionals to share some of our "load," and that usually means working in teams of one sort or another.

- We are required to *prove* the connection between language deficits and problems in school, plus demonstrate how intervention can both improve academic performance and enhance "our" students' ability to function productively in society.

- As we work with other professionals, we must be willing either to translate our terms into ones used in the educational world or to adopt theirs. *Syntax* may have precise meaning for us, but not necessarily for the art teacher. Formal in-service presentations and informal sharing of information will be an increasing, regular part of our academic year.

- The ability to work effectively with colleagues from different backgrounds is no longer just desirable, it is absolutely necessary; this means learning curriculum and instructional techniques aimed at larger groups of students.

- We must acknowledge and accept the responsibility that continual postgraduate education is a necessity in cutting-edge areas like assistive technology.

- Because the law requires that students with handicapping conditions must receive services in the least restrictive environment, we must be prepared to develop alternate modes of service delivery rather than to rely routinely on the pull-out model.

- Research within our field has sensitized us to the needs of children who may not appear obviously at risk for a speech-language disorder. These include children who do not seem to have language problems but who score poorly on reading tasks (Hill & Haynes, 1992), as well as some students Launer (qtd. in Paul, 1995, p. 478) refers to as "porpoise kids": Children who can compensate in earlier grades, but whose language deficits come to the surface when the amount and complexity of work markedly increases in upper level classes.

- Increasing numbers of students qualify for speech-language services, and there is a chronic shortage of speech-language pathologists in many areas.

- Research has shown that early language problems, translated into later learning problems, follow students through adolescence and into adulthood (Hall & Tomblin, 1978).

Let us see how these factors affect the choice of service delivery models.

CONSULTATION

I have listed this category first, because I think that all models include consultation to some degree. I concur with Zins et al. (qtd. in Curtis & Meyers, 1985, p. 35), who stated, "Consultation represents the foundation on which alternative services delivery systems are based. It is the problem-solving process through which students' needs are clarified and appropriate strategies for intervention are developed and implemented." Although the authors of this article are school psychologists, all specialists now concur that consultation enhances the effectiveness of any type of intervention in the schools. It does so by improving classroom teachers' un-derstanding of the serious educational implications of different conditions as well as increasing their skills in addressing them within the regular class. In our particular field, generalization of consultation benefits to nonlabeled students has led to improved long-term academic performance (Roller, Rodriquez, Warner, & Lindahl, 1992).

The term *consultation* is used so loosely, however, that you should always look carefully at what authors mean when they are encouraging its use in our field. It can include everything from giving information to a teacher while providing no direct intervention, to the fully collaborative model explained under the heading "Collaboration." It can also vary from a situation in which one specialist assumes the role of expert (i.e., the advice giver) to one in which consultant and consultee roles shift back and forth depending on the situation.

In one of my earliest attempts at consulting, I assumed that I was the "expert." With a number of children on my caseload in her first grade class, I planned to give Karen, their teacher, the benefit of my training in language diagnosis and intervention, and often I did. One day, however, I was presenting a language enrichment lesson to the entire class using an "art" component requiring scissors, glue sticks, and so on. I carefully handed out the materials and began giving directions, but because the children were horsing around with all the neat stuff I had given them, they barely heard my instructions. In the most tactful of tones, Karen commented later, "Jackie, with first graders it's usually better to give directions *before* you hand out materials." As the months passed, I learned from Karen and Marie and Ann (first grade) and Cindy and Michelle (second grade) how to handle groups of 25 or more children with vastly varying abilities; what first-, second-, and third-grade children were expected to learn during those critical years; and the importance of providing "seat work" so that class members not involved in my group could continue learning. In short, I learned what Montgomery (1992) meant when she said, "The practice setting for a school-based speech-language specialist is the world of education" (p. 364).

Based on this insight, here are two examples of information from our professional background that I shared with these same elementary school teachers:

1. The reason some of their students were spelling the word *train* as *chrain* was that /ch/ is a combination of /t/ + /sh/; therefore, when second graders sound words out, the two blends (*t* + *r* and *ch* + *r*) are actually quite close. How to deal with it? First, by teaching the students that in English, *chr* is always pronounced *kr* as in *Christmas* or *chrysalis*, and, second, by having them practice by dividing a group of mixed *chr* and *tr* pictures into two separate piles.

2. The reason some students were not completing spelling assignments correctly was that the directions in their spelling books were too syntactically complex. How to deal with it? By explaining to the teacher what constitutes syntactic complexity and then demonstrating how to simplify unintentionally difficult classroom material.

I have included these two examples because if I had not been present in their classrooms, I would never have considered addressing these issues, nor would the teachers have thought to ask me. Nelson and Kinnucan-Welsch (1992) presented verbatim comments transcribed from audiotaped interviews with school speech-language pathologists that abound with descriptions of

their experiences and their personal reactions to collaboration. I recommend them to your reading because they so clearly represent the real world you are entering.

In addition to learning specific information about the classroom, I discovered that effective consulting depends not only on learning new skills but also on accepting certain suppositions. The assumptions that follow are not listed in order of importance because they are all equally valuable.

- The consultee must feel free to accept, reject, or adjust any of the consultant's ideas. With shifting roles, this is particularly important; for consultation to work, coercion cannot be part of the mix.

- Both the consultant's and the consultee's ideas should receive equal consideration.

- Partners (or team members) must really listen to each other, not just wait for a pause in the dialogue to insert their own ideas. If the members of the team are from different sociocultural backgrounds, potential differences in interpersonal style may complicate interchanges. Because you are the professional who has had training in the effect of multicultural differences on communication, expect to take the lead in dealing with this issue.

- Confidentiality must be an accepted part of any planning meeting. The teachers' lunchroom is no place to air the details of a conference. All team members must feel free to throw out ideas spontaneously without worrying about being quoted in an unflattering light later.

- Consider both short- and long-term goals. Although the primary intent of collaboration is an agreement on goals/techniques to address a specific student's deficits, a secondary consideration is improving the ability of both colleagues to respond more effectively to a similar situation at some future time—our old friend generalization, or in the new parlance, *dynamic assessment/intervention.*

- Schedule regular meetings to review progress and to adjust goals/techniques as necessary. According to Curtis and Zins (1981), initially a specialist's role is often determined more by what others *expect* than by what they desire. This is very important when you consider the third quotation at the beginning of this chapter: "What is it that you people do?" Many teachers and administrators have a very fuzzy idea indeed of our job as speech-language specialists, often equating our field exclusively with articulation deficits.

- Implementing the results of consultation implies that administrators have agreed to abide by them. It is usually the case that the "specialist" bears the brunt of explaining the concept of consultation to the people in charge, so be prepared to do so, particularly if this is a new program in your school.

- If consultation is a new concept, do not emphasize how dissimilar it is from the present program; comparing its similarities to familiar procedures will help speed acceptance. Change is more likely to occur if manageable objectives are chosen that allow participants to blend new ideas with existing practices (Crais, 1992).

- As goals are discussed, but before they are implemented, you should clarify the problem and the objectives, explore the resources available, and evaluate and choose among alternatives (Curtis & Meyers, 1985).

- After implementation, evaluating approach effectiveness is necessary. Regardless of the delivery system, accountability still means *proving* that intervention using these new procedures leads to superior results.

Exhibit 8–1 is based on the work of Nancy Huffman; duplicating this as a handout would be a good introduction of the collaborative model for teachers and administrators.

Elksnin and Capilouto (1994) described other ways that collaboration can work in the classroom:

1. one teaching and one observing

2. one teaching while the other "drifts," (e.g., monitors behavior, corrects assignments, provides brief assistance)

3. each professional using a "station" at which he or she teaches a different part of the lesson to half the class; at some point, the students switch

4. parallel teaching: this also requires stations, but identical information is presented by both professionals

5. remedial teaching: one professional instructs students who have mastered the material while the other reteaches unlearned information

6. supplemental teaching: one professional teaches using a "standard" format, and the other uses a modified one

7. team teaching: described previously

The approaches these authors report as either being used most frequently or designated as being most useful are the teacher/drifter, team-teaching, teacher/observer, and station models.

Exhibit 8–1 Mediating Speech-Language-Hearing Competence: Arenas of Action for the Speech-Language Specialist (SLP)

1. SLP coteaches a subject area with a classroom teacher. This engages both in curriculum analysis, facilitating an increased awareness that all areas have language components.
2. SLP accompanies student or class to physical education, music, or art to work on following directions, positional concepts, and basic concept development.
3. SLP accompanies a student to a work-study site to reinforce communication abilities with less familiar people or strangers.
4. SLP becomes involved with a long-term language arts project, such as a class newspaper, pen pals with another classroom, poll taking, or letter writing for persuasion or information.
5. SLP is in classroom during free play to foster/manage peer communication, turn taking, and social skills for targeted children.
6. SLP can teach/practice WH-concepts with classroom teacher. Students can interview each other practicing WH-questions and publish a "Who's Who" book as a classroom project.
7. SLP can coteach a telephone communication unit, including rules for use, behavior, sequencing, taking messages, appropriate conversation, and so forth.
8. SLP may work with teacher to develop materials to augment classroom instruction, such as experience stories, game boards, picture stories, augmentative communication books, and boards.
9. SLP preteaches social communication skills that would be appropriate at a restaurant, store or museum where a field trip is planned.

Source: Reprinted with permission from N.P. Huffman, *ASHA*, Vol. 34, No.11, © 1992, the American Speech-Language-Hearing Association.

Finally, the following adaptation from Christensen and Luckett (1990) can serve as a checklist of 10 steps for presenting an oral language lesson to the class:

1. careful planning
2. classroom discipline
3. teacher involvement
4. a good lesson plan
5. effective follow-up activities
6. keeping good records of your IEP-targeted student performance
7. being on time for class; most classroom teachers keep very tight schedules
8. providing the classroom teacher with several backup activities in case an emergency causes you to miss the class
9. involving the classroom teacher in active participation during your presentation
10. asking the classroom teacher to critique your presentation, particularly if lessons

involving the whole class are new to you; consultation can also include roles that do not stress the collaboration described above

Exhibit 8–2 features an example of a letter that can introduce the collaborative model to teachers in your school. Providing a written outline can allow your colleagues some time to consider the possibilities of the approach without having to respond immediately to your request.

Service delivery models can also include roles that do not stress the collaboration described above. The following represent only a few of the many hats you may wear.

- If you are a part of a district's diagnostic team, your results may be presented in a report, and although you may meet with teachers, most probably it will not be on a continuing basis; you, personally, may never work directly with the student.

- As a school speech-language pathologist, you may apply your general exper-

Exhibit 8–2 Sample Letter to Teachers Introducing Collaboration Model

---

Date

To: Primary Teachers
From: Your Name
Re: Speech-Language Schedule

Dear

   Within the past month, I have attended two conferences on developing a collaborative language intervention program. Increasingly, research is showing that without a direct application to classroom subjects, traditional "pull-out" language intervention is of limited benefit to students as they work in the classroom.

   In addition, the experts are now saying what you have been telling us for years: removing children from class not only fragments their day but also separates them from the very information that you are teaching. On this Superintendent's Day, I hesitate to suggest another meeting/study/discussion, but with your help, I would like to try some new ways of serving your students who are low in language. Could we meet together or separately to talk about this?

   Some of my ideas for language intervention that I think might fit our situation are

- preteaching vocabulary that will be part of your upcoming lessons
- reviewing difficult vocabulary/directions that most of your class has already mastered
- acting as another teacher following your presentation of a new concept to the whole class
- acting as a teacher to allow your class to be divided into smaller groups to complete an activity
- teaching a "language" lesson to your whole class (e.g., on listening skills, taking notes, vocabulary building)
- reviewing texts or other books to identify what areas of language will be difficult for your lower ability students and suggesting ways to modify them

   One of the most exciting things about this approach is the very close relationship with the whole-language approach. This concept is what Jill, Nancy, and I [special education teachers] have been using for several years, but in my case, it has not always been directly related to your activities. I have a number of handouts that I can share with you that talk about ways that intervention goals can be included as part of your overall whole-language program.

   In the meantime, I would like to try a radically new schedule. One of the messages that you have given me is that it is very difficult for you to schedule *exactly* when you will be doing a particular lesson because you need the flexibility to "teach to the moment." Therefore, for a start, I will be available every Monday and Wednesday morning from 8:30 to 10:39 in the primary wing. On Thursday morning, I will be in the kindergarten area from 8:30 to 9:56. In addition, I can be available most afternoons on request.

   I will still need to "pull" certain kids, particularly for articulation intervention, and I see myself taking kids for follow-up activities based on problems in the classroom, (e.g., a group of kids from Marie's room who need extra work on rhyme). *These students do not have to be on my caseload.* The research has also shown that the students who end up on the speech-language specialist's caseload often do not include students with very similar needs who have not been labeled. This approach allows them to get help too.

   Beginning next week, I will send around a sheet, and if you do know of a time when I can be of assistance, make a note of when I should arrive, about how long I can expect to be there, and any materials I should bring with me. If you haven't signed up, and I am available, I'm all yours. I have talked to David and Gloria [Superintendent and Vice Principal] about this, and they have suggested we give it a try.

continues

Exhibit 8–2 Sample Letter to Teachers Introducing Collaboration Mode *continued*

Attached to this letter are four checklists, just for your information; they outline very nicely classroom activities/abilities that depend on language comprehension or expression. I have activities already prepared for any of these that I can give to you or present in your classroom. Please note below a time when we could meet.

Thank you,

Please see me _____

Name _____

tise to adapting mainstream materials so they are appropriate for a labeled student or adapting intervention materials for classroom use, as in making changes in level, curricular area, material, equipment, input/output mode, or skill/sequence rules (Schuh, Tashie, & Jorgensen, 1981).

- After observing the interaction between student and teacher in the classroom environment, you may make suggestions addressing a mismatch of teaching/learning styles.

- As an "expert" in a specific area, you may consult and teach parents about preschool language or teach organizational skills to middle-school students with language impairments.

- You may present inservice training to teachers or other speech-language professionals on augmentative communication (Haney, 1992; Light & McNaughton, 1993), developing listening skills (Dollaghan & Kaston, 1986; Edwards, 1991), or dysphagia.

- You may demonstrate how computers can be used to implement IEP goals (Cochran & Masterson, 1995; Masterson, 1985; McGuire, 1995).

Conversely, another professional may present *you* with information concerning a new reading series or teach you the basic curricular content of second-grade mathematics and science. It is time again for the reminder that when you begin intervention, you have not left assessment behind. Each time you evaluate the effect of intervention on a student's skills, you make a decision what to do next: continue without change, move "up" or "down," or embark on another goal. These decisions should be reflected in daily notes as part of your accountability procedures.

In sum, then, what are the advantages of language intervention provided within the regular classroom environment? Most commonly cited are cost-effectiveness, extended opportunity for labeled students to practice pragmatic objectives, increased relevance of speech and language goals to the curriculum, enhanced generalization, and heightened teacher understanding of student language goals, the techniques and procedures used by speech-language professionals, and the overall impact of language on learning (Eger, 1992; Masterson, 1993; Nelson & Kinnucan-Welsch, 1992). Goodman (1986) stated that language intervention presented in the classroom is easier to learn because it has a discernible purpose and is inherently more interesting, relevant, "whole," and part of a real event. In a series of articles on collaboration by school speech-language professionals, the practitioners all point to the presence of language learning throughout the day; unexpected, increased gains in student language skills; and the chance to use a writing-process approach as an integrated part of a student's literature, science, and social studies course material (Borsch & Oaks, 1992; Brandel, 1992; Ferguson, 1992; Montgomery, 1992; Roller et al., 1992).

Other authors (Hoskins, 1990a, 1990b; Marvin, 1987; Simon, 1987; Simon & Myrold-Gunyuz, 1990) have cited additional advantages of collaboration: enabling the speech-language specialist and the classroom teacher to identify and teach speech and language skills critical for academic success, preventing future speech and language problems by serving whole classrooms of students, and addressing all students' cognitive and linguistic disabilities, developmental language problems, and social communication skills. Be familiar with these advantages to counter automatic "knee-jerk" arguments against collaboration.

Are there disadvantages to consultation-collaboration? Elksnin and Capilouto (1994) reported that survey results of 31 school speech-language professionals listed these potential negatives: additional hard-to-come-by planning time, increased paperwork, difficulty in scheduling, IEP goals that were hard to incorporate into these models, possible lack of individualization, possible boredom/lower expectation on the part of the "typical" students, addressing difficult behavior problems in large groups of students, and dealing with a different teaching philosophy or an uncooperative teacher. You should be aware that some of these factors were reported by speech-language pathologists who had never actually adopted the new models.

Disadvantages noted *by classroom teachers* may affect your ability to convince them of the advantages and efficacy of new modes of delivery: perceived lack of planning time, decreased instructional time, "invasion" of territory, and the fear that higher level students would become bored. Other sources have reported that parents may have difficulty accepting that individual pull-out sessions are not necessarily more valuable than sessions that take place in the classroom (Eger, 1992). According to Sanger, Hux, and Griess (1995), educational professionals questioned whether speech-language specialists were prepared to deal with problems like behavior management, reading and writing issues, and English as a second language. Other authors have warned that teachers may become uneasy because "good oral language interaction can often be very noisy" (Christensen & Luckett, 1990, p. 111). They have also stressed that if the regular education teacher is not directly involved in "your" language lesson, your presence can serve as an excuse to run an errand or use the Xerox machine.

Some administrators may also prefer to stay with the way things have been done before, particularly when state and federal laws dictate conditions under which intervention should be provided. On the other hand, Guilford (1993), a supervisor of a speech-language hearing program, stated, "In my experience staff know that there is a need for change [in service delivery models] spurred on by the increasing number of students who qualify for speech-language services and the chronic shortage of SLPs. However, they want the changes to occur for other people—not them!" (p. 63). Change is harder for some people than others, but it is a fact of life in our field. If you are just beginning your career as a speech-language specialist, try to accept "Thou shalt not become rigid" as the Eleventh Commandment. Nelson and Kinnucan-

Welsch (1992) stated that "The cycles of unlearning and relearning are uncomfortable, but the discomfort is essential" (p. 47). In a sense, your status as a novice in the field is an advantage; you do not have as much to unlearn as some of the rest of us.

Conoley and Conoley (1982) also have some words of assurance: you do not have to consult in every single classroom. If this concept is unfamiliar or scares you, pick only one or two teachers at first, preferably those with whom you have the best rapport. Encourage them to be honest about what they feel the two of you can realistically accomplish in a collaborative endeavor. At first, be willing to serve in a capacity in which you will be least disruptive to the classroom routine, such as assisting in a writing lesson. Be flexible about scheduling; perhaps you could start by being in the classroom only once a week. Here is an editorial comment from *Word of Mouth* that you may want to hang on your wall:

We . . . need to be kinder with ourselves for not being an expert on everything. That's the reason team intervention exists. There is too much to know these days for everybody to be good at everything. We can rely on others for knowledge that we have not yet obtained. And regardless of the criticism that others may have when we don't know something, it makes people feel good to believe they can teach somebody something. ("Editorial Comments," 1995, p. 10)

Amen and amen.

COLLABORATION

As you have probably deduced by now, collaboration relies heavily on the consultation model described above. In fact, some authors use the term collaborative consultation (Russell & Kaderavek, 1993). I have separated the two terms because while consulta-tion does not necessarily require at least two professionals working closely over an extended period of time, collaboration always does. Russell and Kaderavek stressed that although cooperation is the goal of coordinated service delivery in the schools, in practice this theoretical construct is "not necessarily evident in the actual practice of the model" (p. 76). They suggested that peer coaching and coteaching are possible solutions to the barriers of the hierarchical relationship that often exist between consultants and classroom teachers and the consequent negative attitude that develops because of it. As noted previously, it is not uncommon for teachers to consider their classrooms their kingdoms and resent any interference with their right and obligation to teach as they see fit. Not infrequently, teachers want you to take children, "fix" them, and then return them to their tutelage. Collaborative models are designed to diminish these feelings.

In the peer coaching model, the speech-language professional and the classroom teacher both model techniques for each other; neither is "superior." This model involves (a) a preobservation conference, (b) the actual intervention, and finally (c) the postobservation conference (Schmidt & Rodgers-Rhyme, 1988, cited in Russell & Kaderavek, 1993, p. 76). I hope this reminds you of some of the assessment steps described in Chapter 6. The peer teaching model fits particularly well if the teacher has been the source of the referral because the observation part of the peer coaching process has been started, and a working relationship has already been established. Discussion may focus on possible adaptations of curricular material by the classroom teacher, preteaching of vocabulary/concepts by the speech-language professional or small-group activities in which both are engaged. After therapeutic intervention has taken place, its effectiveness is evaluated, and based on that, further plans are developed. Coteaching differs from team teaching (see below) in that the classroom teacher plans activities addressing curriculum goals, and the speech-language professional incorporates communication objectives *into* those goals. Therefore the two professionals together develop both curricular and language intervention goals, plan the activities, implement them, and then evaluate their students' progress.

TEAM TEACHING

This model can be used as a synonym for *collaboration*, but it can also refer to a system in regular education in which two teachers share students. They prepare lessons independently, usually divided along subject lines: for example, one sixth-grade teacher instructs all math lessons, and the other sixth-grade teacher instructs all language arts activities. In the case in which a speech-language specialist team-teaches with a classroom teacher, he or she may "take over" the whole class for a period or they may both be involved in teaching a single lesson at the same time. In either case, team teaching "emphasizes the use of naturalistic environments and meaningful contexts" (Miller, 1989, p. 155). A speech-language pathologist can also team-teach with a special educator or a learning disabilities specialist to help increase awareness that all subjects have a language component (Eger, 1993). He or she can accompany students to classes in physical education, art, music, computers, or industrial arts to work on following directions, positional concepts, and basic concept development within the context of the subject. An example of this is described in an article by Ellis, Schlaudecker, and Griess (1995). Physical education teachers, the classroom instructor, and the speech-language specialist incorporated the teaching of basic concepts

into a kindergarten PE class that emphasized the 28 most missed concepts on the Boehm Test of Basic Concepts-Revised. The program ran for 8 weeks, and the students received 30 minutes of concept instruction each week by the classroom teacher/and or speech-language pathologist. These activities were often ones suggested by the speech-language pathologist. An additional 30-minute physical education period integrated the concept into the regular P.E. curriculum (e.g., throwing a ball to the "first person in line").

In 1990 I team-taught a class one period a week with Marty, a seventh- and eighth-grade social studies teacher. Our experience illustrates the many, often unanticipated, ways that a single program can address the needs of a group of students. Marty was concerned that "my kids" never expressed any opinions during class discussions. (Please note that teachers will often bestow on you ownership for students whom you see, sometimes giving you credit for their improvement but also holding you at least partly responsible for any behavioral lapses.) When I considered the three students who were in Marty's class, I was not surprised that they did not venture an opinion. First, their language deficits and limited cultural literacy precluded their being aware of current events. One of Marty's questions concerned the demolition of the Berlin wall. None of my students had any idea where Berlin was, let alone the historical significance of the wall that had divided the east and west portions of the city. Typically, language–learning-disabled students do not, or cannot, read *Time* or a newspaper and altogether avoid watching national news on TV.

Marty and I planned a year-long program designed to teach students how to state, substantiate, and defend opinions. Students with limited language skills are usually asked lower level questions, which, as classified in

Bloom's taxonomy (Bloom, Engelhart, Furst, Hill, & Krathwohl, 1956), test only knowledge or comprehension. Consequently labeled students frequently have little opportunity to answer the type of questions that will be increasingly required in middle and high school. The program, called *What's Your Opinion?*, helped students develop and practice the language of evaluation as a natural part of successful communication in the classroom. Several opinion questions were presented weekly, one used as a basis for oral discussion and the other requiring a written response. At first, the questions were general, and students did not need to have read widely or "be smart" to answer them, for example, whether school should be in session year round, or what the best bad-for-you junk food was. Later questions, however, related directly to the seventh-grade social studies syllabus, such as whether we should return land to Native Americans that had been unfairly taken from them in the past. Written answers were graded and counted as a completed assignment, with detailed comments included with every assignment handed back. As the students' skill increased, they were required to use textbooks, the newspaper, *Junior Scholastic*, and similar sources to gather background and supporting arguments. Cooperative learning groups were frequently used, with labeled students placed in heterogeneous, not homogeneous, teams. Class sessions were regularly videotaped. I will discuss how this program related to other modes of delivery in the "Pull-Out" section later in this chapter.

One of the most motivating features of *"What's Your Opinion?"* was the role of the Polaroid camera. Each week after written opinions were completed, six students were chosen by lot. Copies of their opinions were typed, individually framed, mounted, and placed on a bulletin board in the front hall of the school next to their photographs. The camera work was done by three other students who were credited for their photographic talent. During the second semester, the students also created opinion questions for second graders, an opportunity to practice the metalinguistic skill of adjusting language for students younger than themselves.

The program was originally instituted as a way to assist the labeled, mainstreamed student. Almost immediately, however, it became clear that every class member was a beneficiary. This was particularly true for the students who usually "slip through the cracks"—those who were not severely impaired enough to be labeled but whose limited language skills made classroom interchanges difficult for them. Last, the program represented a structured, natural way for the speech-language specialist to introduce IEP goals to the middle-school teachers.

It is instructive to read the following guidelines that Marty and I created for the program because they speak so clearly to the shared nature of our collaborative endeavor. They also reflect the careful planning that is always at the heart of effective teaching/intervention.

- Regardless of ability, all students will contribute opinions during discussions as well as through written assignments.

- Both the speech-language pathologist and the classroom teacher will be supportive and encouraging, even when neither agrees with the students' responses.

- Teachers will restate or clarify opinions as necessary so that all group members can follow the direction of the discussion.

- Conversations should be as free flowing as possible; strict adherence to "raise your hand before speaking" will not be required.

- All groups will be heterogeneous, and only rarely will cooperative learning groups be formed other than at random.

- When background information is given by one of the teachers, written outlines will be used to limit "lecture" time.

- Even when the topic is serious, the tone of the classroom will be as light as possible within the parameters of appropriate classroom behavior.

- Before each completed written assignment is returned, detailed written reactions of the teacher/specialist will be added to it.

- As much as possible, the opinion questions will feature the current week's curriculum topic.

- Each student will be encouraged to use the word-processing program on the classroom computer, the Polaroid camera, and the videotaping equipment.

As a result of this program, students gained skill in thinking up, formulating, and answering questions that required evaluation, the highest level of thought in Bloom's taxonomy. Students also learned to back up their opinions with cogent reasons and to appreciate the ideas of others, even if they did not agree with them. They learned skills in interviewing and use of the word processor and camera as tools. They also discovered ways to find facts as they listened to or read background information, and they gained increased awareness of the larger world around them. Finally, they applied these new skills directly to the seventh-grade social studies curriculum in the presence of their typical classmates. In a pull-out program, they would have had little opportunity to do so.

From my speech-language specialist's point of view, I found myself entering into a new phase of my career. I helped develop a list entitled "14 Steps to Nurture Independent Research" and practiced using "anticipatory set" to gain student attention at the beginning of a lesson. I relearned the Bill of Rights, who first circumnavigated the globe, and the constitutional powers of the governor of New York State. In addition, I discovered how to present this information in an interesting fashion to 28 seventh graders at 8:30 a.m., first period in the morning, something Marty had been doing that period plus six periods more a day for years.

One of the criticisms of the team-teaching model from speech-language pathologists is that they fear losing their sense of identity: they worry that they will become a tutor or a teacher's aide, not the specialist they have worked so hard and for so many years to be. I think that is why the *collaborative* aspect of team teaching is so important. Each professional brings to the discussion the richness of his or her training and experience. We bring background, focus, and training in evaluating and instructing in the area of language development, including the effect of language difficulties on school performance and social behaviors. We have the ability to perform task analyses that will facilitate school performance and a keen understanding of the overlapping roles of listening, speaking, reading, and writing across all content areas. We have an acute awareness of how individual differences can affect learning and the role motivation plays in language learning (Wadle, 1991).

I would add that we also recognize the implication of such concepts as school "scripts" and the role of pragmatics on the nonacademic performance of the student, which, if deficient, can be utterly devastating. You may not consider yourself an expert on the effect of multicultural differences on the school population after you read Chapter 11, but you will probably know more than many educators do. What team teaching and collaboration are all about is how to apply this knowledge to the needs of a particular student, at the same time sharing the information with colleagues whose training is different from our own.

Let us consider these two goals for auditory sequencing: "By April 1991, Benjamin will sequence four items in a logical order without assistance, as measured by a 30% improvement on the _____ test" versus "By April 1991, Benjamin will be able to retell four events in correct order from a story in his fourth-grade literature book so that he can take part in his classroom oral book reports" (Montgomery, 1992, p. 363). Obviously the second goal will assist Benjamin in the classroom in a way that the first one might not. I hope that it is equally clear that speech-language specialists must understand the requirements of the classroom environment before they will be capable of writing pertinent goals.

PULL-OUT INTERVENTION

Usually speech pathology students are familiar with this mode of service because it is the one used in the majority of university speech and hearing clinics; as part of your clinical courses, you have probably written lesson plans for individual clients or members of small groups. Secord (1989) listed these as advantages of the pull-out model: It allows for highly structured training, and you are free to use a variety of approaches to learning without being concerned whether they will fit in with a lesson or be appropriate for other students. You can preteach a topic or vocabulary well in advance of the time it will be used

in the classroom. If you have discovered a basic weakness, you can address it immediately and directly without linking it to the curriculum. Thus the pull-out model allows very focused, intense intervention and may be the mode of choice when your student requires repetition or when the presence of other students would be detrimental.

Criticizing one's own performance is often very difficult for a student who has a language-based learning disability, and therefore the privacy inherent in a pull-out session can be a distinct advantage. When I wrote down errors observed during classroom conversational exchanges and pointed them out to students later, they frequently argued, "I didn't say (or do) that!" During my discussion of team teaching in Marty's seventh-grade social studies class, you may remember that I referred to videotaping the cooperative learning groups. Later, in follow-up pull-out intervention sessions, my students and I reviewed these tapes to identify examples of good/poor topic maintenance, eye contact, body language, and sequencing during classroom discussions. In addition, we often examined how effectively the student used pragmatic "rules" to substantiate an opinion, defend his or her own point of view, and/or identify weakness in his or her own and others' opinion statements. Prior to this program, my students' typical response to a classmate's opinion was "That's (or you're) stupid!"—guaranteed to be fighting words in the seventh grade. It appeared easier for students to identify and criticize their own inappropriate responses when they could point to a videotaped image. In some way it created a necessary buffer: they were criticizing the image, not themselves.

Using pull-out intervention is also preferable when you must teach a student how to produce a phoneme for the first time by employing a mirror or an implement near a student's mouth. An older student may find this procedure humiliating if it is performed in the presence of a classmate. Being embarrassed is one of the chief reasons that older students do not like the pull-aside model in the regular classroom. Adolescence is a time when few students like to be seen as different. The disadvantages of this mode of service were covered under the earlier "Rationales" section as the advantages of models depending on classroom interactions.

SELF-CONTAINED LANGUAGE CLASS

Some speech-language pathologists prefer this model over all others because they can spend hours a day with the same students, continually addressing their deficits as an integral part of every subject. Usually the class is limited in size, so caseloads are often far smaller than the average. If the class represents full-time placement, the speech-language pathologist in most states must also possess elementary (or secondary) classroom certification. In some schools, a speech-language specialist spends a half-day in a kindergarten or prefirst class and the remainder of the day working with additional students, using other service delivery models. Larson, McKinley, and Boley (1993) described a for-credit high school language course that is offered at the same time as other classes; it focuses on remediating deficits in thinking, listening, speaking, reading, and writing skills to enable the student to succeed not only in academic situations but in social and vocational ones as well. The authors stated that assigning academic credit provides motivation and incentive for student participation. Another similar course addresses study and organizational skills; depending on the dis-

trict, speech-language pathologists, special education teachers, or learning disabilities specialists may instruct these classes.

Frequently inclusive preschool programs use the self-contained model: that is, the speech-language pathologist is one of several teachers in the classroom throughout the day. Planning is usually done by a team and general as well as specific goals are set for the students in the class. In 1993, these goals hung on the walls of the preschool class in the Main Street School, North Syracuse, New York:

Play/Cognitive:
  categorization/
    grouping   colors
  matching   counting, number concepts
  spatial relations   role play/pretending
  comparison/
    contrast   order
  shapes

Social:
  problem solving   sharing
  expressing feelings cooperative play
  routine   self-help

Sensory:
  imitating designs cutting
  orientation/
    positioning   representation
  pasting/gluing   grasp/hand dominance
  colors   block play/building/constructing

Language:
  imitating
    communication relaying simple messages
  phrases/word
    combinations answering simple questions
  following
    directions   relating events out of context
  sequencing   making choices
  awareness of
    auditory
    information
  in-context
    imitating/
    producing words/sign

Given the age of the students, the necessity for integrating goals is exceptionally clear. With the possible exception of some small motor tasks, each of the other categories has strong language implications.

MULTISKILLING

As stated previously, how this service delivery model might be applied to the schools is far from clear. Pietranton and Lynch (1995) stated, "At best, [multiskilling is] viewed as a sincere, patient-focused effort to improve efficiency and effectiveness of service delivery. At worst, it can sacrifice clinical standards in the name of lower costs" (p. 37). Questions of professional training, effect on the existing practitioners, quality of services, professional ethics, clinical liability, and risk management would all need to be addressed. Multiskilling as it is now defined is *not* the same as incorporating another discipline's goals into the provision of speech-language services. Collaboration might include this scenario: after consultation with a speech-language specialist, an occupational therapist might integrate exercises involving small muscle control into a language activity; for example, having Sally Student color portions of a cartoon strip in a specific manner as she discusses the sequence of actions in the story. In multiskilling, the occupational therapist would make decisions regarding speech-language goals on her own: no speech-language pathologist would be required at any stage.

INCLUSION

Often specialists and teachers are comfortable having students who have mild to moderate disabilities in the classroom but resist the inclusion of those who are more severely impaired, such as those with serious behavioral problems, multiple handicaps, autism, or severe cognitive impairments. Those professionals who support their presence in the classroom to the greatest degree possible state that it is the civil right of these students to be placed in the least restrictive environment, or to be to the greatest extent possible with their nondisabled peers. They state that inclusion leads to improved learning outcomes in socialization, communication, adaptive behavior, functional skills, and a better quality of life marked by a broader range of choices, self-determination, and richer social connections (McSheehan & Jorgensen, in progress, as presented by Sonnenmeier and McGuire, 1995). Sonnenmeier and McGuire stressed that it is our job as speech-language pathologists to create opportunities for all individuals to demonstrate their skills, using chronologically age-appropriate materials and under conditions of high expectations; our goal should be to support all efforts in this regard, not only to provide intervention. They argued that we should be prepared to explain/interpret to others that the sometimes negative behaviors are the only means of communication open to children to let someone know that they want a change of activity or that they do not understand what is expected of them. Therefore, as part of our planning, we need to identify the routines within the classroom and describe the expectation for participation and communication within each routine, using such tools as picture symbols, schedule books, and modified materials and supports, and identifying the opportunities for communication within each routine and the length of time a child is likely to be able to participate.

One of the most sensitive issues in the schools is the provision of a paraprofessional, often a one-to-one aide, to assist the classroom teacher in the day-to-day implementation of these laudatory goals. With tight budgets, teachers are sometimes expected to manage with part-time help and may resent the time taken away from the "typical" classroom pupil and their already crammed-full teaching schedule. There is no easy answer to these issues other than to try to keep the lines of communication open as we struggle to provide the best service we can to every student in our care. If you have students with severe handicaps on your caseload, be sure to check educational sources for additional information (Giangreco & Meyer, 1988; Schulz & Turnbull, 1984).

THE THEME APPROACH

Integrating goals is also the intent of one of the most popular programs in the schools today, the theme approach. I have listed this topic separately because themes work equally well in collaborative or pull-out situations. They can introduce concepts and vocabulary in a relevant, contextual manner, and they permit flexibility and creativity in meeting individual academic/language needs of students who may have very different academic deficits. Because language-learning deficits can profoundly affect students' ability to read and write, the same students may be seen not only by us but by a reading specialist and a special educator as well. Consequently it is easy for fragmentation to occur as each specialist treats his or her "part" of the student. Using themes as part of an interdisciplinary approach to remediation reduces this artificial separation, and for the speech-language pathologist, units also offer many effective, time-efficient opportunities.

There are two basic ways to use a theme: speech-language specialists can develop a topic that will be motivating to most of the students on their caseloads or can work within schoolwide or individual classroom units, such as those commonly associated with the whole-language approach. If you are choosing a theme, do it in concert with other specialists so that fragmentation can be diminished as much as possible. Your initial step is to examine the following list of language areas and match one or more to a student or student group. Using the selected theme, be it space, animals, scarecrows, or world flags, plan an activity that meets IEP goals but also integrates the vocabulary and books of the students' classrooms. There are a number of advantages in using thematic units:

1. You are indirectly providing in-service training on the complexity of language when you review with teachers the linguistic areas that can be addressed through a thematic unit.

2. When you target one area repeatedly in various themes presented throughout the school year, students become aware that intervention techniques can generalize to new circumstances. For example, if a student has vocabulary limitations, you may choose to address adjectives, adverbs, synonyms, antonyms, associations, and categorization during each thematic unit. This alerts the student that learning new vocabulary is a continuing process that crosses subject lines.

3. By becoming aware of curriculum content, speech-language pathologists can choose themes that have a clear relationship to classroom subjects. Jill, a special education colleague, and I chose space as a theme partly because she knew that the space race of the 1960s was covered in eighth-grade social studies and the planetary system in fourth-

grade science. Similarly, when water was the theme, we covered ocean names because in the seventh-grade social studies unit on explorers, it is assumed that students already have this information. A communication theme was a natural subject to reinforce the names of inventions and their developers.

4. There is often a parent component in thematic units. As part of a theme, students frequently build objects, complete artwork, write stories, or use computers/videotape to generate projects. Among other items, my students have developed and illustrated cookbooks and built spaceships, sports arenas, Native American dwellings, miniatures of their own houses copied from a Polaroid photograph, and mobiles of animals, fish, and characters in fairy tales. It is a rare parent who will not make a trip to school to see something concrete a son or daughter has created. This is particularly helpful with the family of a "labeled" student because parent meetings so frequently deal with problems, not celebrations.

How each language area is related to the educational environment is explained below. In some cases, examples of specific goals are included. Part of the information this list contains had its origins in the work of Catherine Bush (1980a; 1980b). The innumerable books and materials featuring themes that have been published since then can serve as ready resources. Developing your own, however, allows you to target topics of interest to your particular students. In addition, the interaction between colleagues as you plan units usually leads to more activities than you could ever use, as well as creating energy and wonderful rapport.

- *Adjectives/Adverbs:* Most students with language disabilities overuse a few adjectives, such as *neat* or *gross*. Practice not only teaches new vocabulary, it encourages precision. *Example:* Provide two adjectives that go with the noun *blimp*, and two adverbs that go with the word *drive*. Apply this linguistic area directly to written work.

- *Analogy:* Before a student can do proportion or solve many word problems in math, he or she has to learn to complete analogies. They commonly appear on standardized tests and are often used as a teaching technique. Having students explain concepts presented during class by using an analogy is good practice (e.g., moving troops across the ocean is like packing for a long trip when you don't know if any stores will be open).

- *Antonyms/Synonyms:* Both forms appear on most schoolwide standardized tests. Learning antonyms and synonyms (*enormous—minuscule*) as a pair is a vocabulary expanding shortcut. Students also need practice in supplying multiple answers. *Example:* What is the opposite of *horizontal*? Give three synonyms for *walk*. Write a paragraph about walking, using your synonyms.

- *Association:* The ability to associate is necessary for storing information in short- and long-term memory, as well as a means of recalling related subjects. This is particularly important in writing tasks that require organization within a paper. Brainstorming ideas for a project or paper is good practice for this skill. *Example:* Say all the words you can think of as fast as you can that could go with the word *wheelchair* (*motor, ill, sit, strong, disability, hands, basketball, person, ramp, injury, illness, roll, fast, smooth, access,* etc.).

- *Categorization:* Placing items or facts into correct categories is a necessary first step in ordering information so that it can be retained and recalled. This is exceptionally useful for a student with word-finding problems, as well as a good topic for a study skills course.

- *Cloze:* Cloze involves the semantic knowledge of what word would make sense if inserted in a blank space in a sentence. Fill-in-the-blank questions are commonly found on examinations. It is important that students be aware of the differences between convergent types (only one correct answer) and divergent ones (many correct answers). This concept can be taught in a unit on study skills. You can practice cloze orally and then in written form, using sentences from grade-level texts.

- *Fiction/Nonfiction Stories:* Being able to distinguish between fantasy and reality is not always easy for the student with language problems. Telling and writing stories of both types on a single theme topic is a means of internalizing the rules that govern each. Reading examples of both in the classroom can also serve as a basis for discussion.

- *Following Verbal Directions:* Of all the language skills most commonly used in the classroom, this is the one that can cause the most trouble if the student is deficient. It is typical of students with a language-learning disability that they absorb only a portion of the directions and consequently complete only part of the assignment. In a unit on communication, my older, mostly male, students built radios from kits. The more skillful

readers read the directions aloud, and then the members of the small groups took turns completing the action. There was no need to impose "penalties" if they did it incorrectly; they all knew that if every single connection was not finished as it should be, the radio was not going to work. They all did. Hallelujah.

- *Idioms, Proverbs, Metaphors, Similes:* Most students with language deficits have profound difficulty understanding idioms and proverbs, partly because these students tend to interpret language in concrete terms and partly because it requires metalinguistic skill. This is the same reason they have difficulty "getting the joke." Understanding figurative language is also necessary for higher level comprehension. *Example:* older students can locate metaphors and similes in their literature texts or, if this is too difficult, explain the meaning of ones you find.

- *Part/Whole Relationships:* The ability to "see the forest for the trees" is a difficult concept for many students. Often students remember a small piece of information and fail to see how it relates to the whole. Discriminating between the entirety and its components is a first step. *Example:* Name the parts of a ring (stone, setting, prongs, band, diamond, etc.). Now name something a ring can be part of (the planet Saturn, an engine, a jewelry collection, etc.).

- *Question Forms:* Being able to ask a specific question and resolve confusion over something the teacher said is a skill many students with LLD do not have. Playing *Jeopardy* is a fun way to practice formulating questions, but applying the skill to classroom subjects will also require teaching students how to know *when* to ask them.

- *Riddles:* Solving a riddle involves inferential reasoning, common in literature, social studies, and mathematics. Riddles are another good topic to include in a unit on study skills for the older student and are a way to increase the complexity of comprehension questions for younger readers.

- *Rhyme:* Current research has indicated that the ability to rhyme—that is, to create a pattern—is a necessary prerequisite for spelling (encoding) as well as reading (decoding). *Example:* Find five different words in Chapter 4 of your science book that rhyme with *near* (hint: they may not all look alike).

- *Scrambled Sentences:* Proper word order is necessary for coherent communication; practicing unscrambling also encourages a student to break out of the "article + noun + verb" sentence structure common in less complex syntactical forms. Use topics from the theme/curriculum. *Example:* Using the four words *the*, *enormous*, *airport*, and *is*, create two different sentences.

- *Sentence Construction:* Using specific words in a sentence requires a knowledge of both semantics and syntactic relationships. It is a metalinguistic skill. *Example:* Take three vocabulary words from a theme (or any classroom subject) and put them into a single sentence.

- *Sentence Types:* This is an example of a metalinguistic skill: using language to explain, analyze, and manipulate language. Most students with LLD experience great difficulty in identifying and/ or defining grammatical information. Once students can produce different kinds of sentences verbally, you can work on transferring them to written work. *Example:* Using the word *shark*, create declarative, interrogatory, exclamatory, and imperative sentences; now write a paragraph in which you have an example of each sentence type.

- *Sequence of Actions:* Understanding a sequence of actions and placing them in proper order is a necessary skill in narrative, mathematics, history, and science. Using an activity that demonstrates a clear sequence is one of the easiest forms to use if a student must write a paper. *Example:* Using a map, draw Magellan's path around the world. Explain it to a class member.

- *Similarities/Differences:* Although many students can see either differences *or* similarities, it is frequently difficult for them to see both. Another common problem is choosing an insignificant comparison while ignoring the most important. These abilities are the basis of all "compare-and-contrast" questions in many subjects. Use the curriculum as the subject here, as in the example. *Example:* Name one way in which the Revolutionary and Vietnam Wars were alike and one way in which they were different.

- *Vocabulary:* Preteaching vocabulary can be an effective means of making classroom information more relevant and understandable to a student with language deficiencies. Ask to borrow word lists from the teacher, or make a list from the books that are being featured as part of the unit. Be aware that there is no substitute for knowing the curriculum;

when Jill, my special educator colleague and I were planning an animal unit, she, not I, knew that students were expected to understand the words *habitat* and *range*, not "where they live." *Example:* Using a vocabulary list, find a new word that starts with each of the letters of your first and last names; define each.

- *Word Definition:* Although this is a skill generally occurring in written form, doing it verbally gives practice without worrying about spelling, handwriting, and so on. It also encourages precision. It is often very difficult for the student with language deficits, and you will need to scaffold the steps carefully. *Example:* Define *orbit*.

Although not linguistic areas, these additional categories of activities also lend themselves to collaboration:

1. introductory letters to the families explaining the theme and asking them to complete specific home activities with their child

2. written products, often in conjunction with the classroom, special education, or English teacher: spelling words, written vocabulary activities, factual essay, and/or a sequential writing activity

3. reading, as an integral part of any thematic unit, using a variety of reading materials: fictional works, basal readers, magazines, the Internet, biographies, and newspaper articles, plus activities in decoding, comprehension, and library resource skills

4. mathematics applications, such as charting, graphing, and word problems

5. computer applications, such as word processing, developing games, using e-mail, and the World Wide Web

Exhibit 8–3 features one means to plan goals featuring a theme involving several subjects; Exhibit 8–4 is used to plan daily/weekly activities and can indicate which delivery model will be used to accomplish individual objectives.

One important warning in using thematic units: it is very easy to become so wrapped up in the topic and its motivating activities that you neglect the goals on the student's IEP. Make sure when you write your lesson plans that all intervention procedures address the most crucial student weaknesses.

In conclusion, the service delivery models you use to provide intervention will vary from student to student and year to year. As surely as I am typing this, however, someone in our field, or an allied one, is developing a new way. For example, the DeSoto County (Mississippi) schools are using specialization to provide "the most efficient services" to a large and diverse caseload of students. Under this model, speech-language specialists are divided into committees focusing on fluency, voice, language, and articulation; membership in the committees is based on the interest and expertise of the speech-language specialists who work in the district (Zarrella, 1995).

Are you wondering how in the world you can master all of these models? In the past, most speech-language professionals preferred to learn about the principles of collaboration by attending conferences or in-service sessions rather than formal university courses. As you work in the field and opportunities to learn new models present themselves, take advantage of them. Almost always, they feature "hands-on" practical suggestions; if you are fortunate enough to do your student teaching under a speech-language specialist who is engaged in other than pull-out intervention, ask questions, keep a notebook, ob-

Exhibit 8–3 Theme Unit Overall Planning Sheet

Theme: Flags   **Subjects:** Art, Social Studies, Language

Goals: 1. Use appropriate vocabulary to describe flags.
                  2. Explain how flags represent countries.
                  3. Draw a picture of a flag of a Middle Eastern country; describe and label its parts.
                  4. Demonstrate how to locate the country belonging to the flag on a map of the Middle East.
                  5. Plan a Flag Day celebration for June 14.
                  6. Using sequencing terms, describe the development of the American flag from Revolutionary times to the present.
                  7. Recite three rules for displaying the American flag.
                  8. Create a flag representing the class, a family, or an individual.

Vocabulary: field, symbol, staff, halyard, hoist (part nearest the staff), hoist (verb), fly (outer part of flag), fly (verb), banner, etiquette, bar, stripe, fringe, pennant, canton

Ongoing Concepts/Areas

___ Vocabulary	___ Sentence Types	___ Word Definitions
___ Rhyme	___ Scrambled Sentences	___ Association
___ Adjectives/Adverbs	___ Sequence of Actions	___ Part/Whole
___ Similarities/Differences	___Sentence Construction	___ Idioms
___ Proverbs	___ Metaphors	___ Similes
___ Cloze	___ Riddles	___ Analogy
___ Categorization	___ Verbal Directions	___ Question Forms
___ Fiction/Nonfiction Stories	___ Antonyms/Synonyms	_____

---

serve, and learn, learn, learn. And don't forget to pass your good ideas along to others.

CASELOAD SIZE

Part of the process in choosing service delivery models is deciding how many other students, if any, should be included as intervention takes place with that student. Because of new models of service delivery, group size has in some ways become irrelevant; if intervention takes place within the classroom, other children will be present, often in very fluid arrangements. During a portion of a class period, you may work next to the child at his or her desk for 5 or 10 minutes, then include the child in a small group for practice, and later observe the child as part of the entire class applying what he or she has learned. Clearly, however, there remain times when a student must be seen outside the classroom on an individual basis for any number of reasons, such as to provide intensive drill, to protect confidentiality, or to teach a difficult, highly individualized technique. Complications arise when you must describe group size on his or her IEP or in an end-of-the-year report that usually includes designations of group size only up to those that include five members. Throughout the country, speech-language specialists are struggling to fit these new delivery models to an "old" law; I have every

Exhibit 8–4 Daily Planner for Theme Activities

Theme: _Flags_   Day/Date: _Mon 5/22_   Anticipatory Set: _Show "Don't Tread on Me" flag from Revolutionary period_

Teacher: _Meyer_   Goal: _Preteach flag vocabulary_

Location: _Speech Room_   Individual Objective: _The students will demonstrate knowledge of 50% of vocabulary._

Materials: _pictures of old and new flags; "blank" flags_

Activities: _Label different parts of flag; discuss importance of flags in history; introduce concept of symbolism; present blank flag for students to label its parts_

Closure: _Set up meeting time to see flag raised in front of school_

Special Considerations for _Jenny: pre-print part names on stickers_

Theme: _Flags_   Day/Date: _Tues 5/23_   Anticipatory Set: _Pledge of Allegiance_

Teacher: _Smith/Meyer_   Goal: _Introduce flag theme to class (Flag Day)_

Location: _Classroom_   Individual Objective: _Students will learn flag vocabulary; brainstorm activities for celebration on June 14_

Materials: _same as 5/22 plus larger blank flag_

Activities: _Label different parts of flag; discuss importance of flags in Middle Ages, modern times; discuss symbolism in cooperative groups; present large flag to label_

Closure: _List places where students have seen flags_

Special Considerations for _Be sure all students from 5/22 are encouraged to display their knowledge._

confidence that as long as we honor the spirit of the legislation, we will work through these difficulties.

The question of caseload size has been and continues to be one of the most emotionally charged subjects in speech-language pathology in the schools. Cassandra Peters-Johnson (1992) provided a quick historical review of numbers in a recent *Asha* article. She wrote that in the 1960s, speech-language patholo-gists reported serving 111 students per week on the average, with about three quarters of them at second-grade level or below. Approximately 80% of the caseload involved articulation. More fluency cases were seen than those involving any other type of language disorder. After the passage of Public Law 94-142, a dramatic downward shift in numbers occurred. The average fell to 43, and language and articulation cases became equally represented. Numbers of older students on the caseload also increased. By 1992, the upward trend appeared to have stabilized at about 52, but the author cautioned that this is an average and that "some speech-language specialists have caseloads much higher and others much lower than the average, . . . with some . . . caseloads of 70, 80, 90 and even 100!" (p. 12).

Because of the enactment of the Individuals With Disabilities Education Act of 1990 (IDEA), these numbers now include children from birth to age 21, with the proportion of language cases increasing to approximately 60% of total numbers. Speech-language specialists in the schools also report that the severity of impairment has increased and that disorders of hearing and swallowing, brain trauma, and neurological disorders have "increased dramatically." In a continuing trend, more children are now labeled as having a specific learning disability than as being "speech-language impaired." When you accept a position in the schools, you would be well advised to ask what the state/district guidelines are regarding maximum caseload, whether these numbers take into account relative severity, and whether time is provided to complete evaluations, meet with teachers, attend conferences, and so forth. Meeting with 10 groups of children a day, 5 days a week, with no breaks other than a 30-minute lunch is burnout waiting to happen. An exhausted, overworked specialist puts the children he or she serves at risk. Exhibit 8–5 illustrates a typical schedule in an elementary school. Note the inclusion of bus duty and other nonacademic activities.

Choosing groups for scheduling and the mode of delivery is complicated, frustrating, and bound to add a few gray hairs to the head of even a young clinician. Deciding whether to group by disorder, age, grade, degree of severity, personality compatibility, availability at a specific time, or teacher preference requires the wisdom of Solomon and the patience of a saint. One fact is certain; as soon as you arrive at an acceptable schedule, something will happen that will necessitate change. Regardless of the circumstances of their workplace, after their first year, all speech-language professionals write their schedules in pencil—and have a large eraser at the ready.

Another area of trial and error involves choosing the format for weekly lesson plans and/or daily logs. There is no one correct way to accomplish this task. Some professionals prefer quite detailed plans, a somewhat streamlined version of the ones most of you have done in your college programs. Others use a highly abbreviated single page for the week but keep individual or group logs in more detail. Almost none take detailed data every session for every student. Most school districts distribute lesson plan books, but these are not always applicable to intervention in speech and language. I suggest that you use your master teacher's system as a starting place and gradually develop your own. Exhibit 8–6 illustrates one way that lesson plans can appear on the same sheet with data from a session, regardless of the mode of service delivery. They are kept in the student or group folder and filed every month or so. Because the sheet also lists the IEP objective for each activity for each student, it is easy for the speech-language professional to make sure that all goals are being addressed on a regular basis. It also facilitates gathering information for end-of-the-year reports.

SAMPLE PROGRAMS FROM THE LITERATURE

The following section represents a bare sampling of ways in which collaboration is

Exhibit 8–5 Planning a Schedule for the Elementary Grades

Time	Monday	Tuesday	Wednesday	Thursday	Friday
7:45–8:00	Primary Meeting	7-8th grade meeting	K meeting	plan	Child Study Team
8:00–8:15	Jerry	Bus Duty	Jerry	Bus Duty	Jerry
	(& aide)				(& aide)
8:30–9:10	Pat, Sally	3rd grade	Pat, Sally	3rd grade	Pat, Sally
	Jamar	"s" group	Jamar	"s" group	Jamar
9:15–9:55	K-garten	Kim	K-garten	Kim	test
	Smith		O'Hara		
10:00–10:40	Mitch	Brad	Mitch, Andy	Brad	
	Andy, Joe		Joe, Brad		
10:45–11:25	7th grade	8th grade	Kristine	Kristine	
	Soc studies	English	Chris, Joe L.	Chris, Joe L.	↓
11:30–12:00	lunch	————	————	————	→
12:00–12:40	Jake, Ben	Jason	Jake, Ben	Jason	Jake, Ben
	Ann, Abel	Bill	Ann, Abel	Bill	Ann, Abel
12:45–1:25	Lindsay, Beryl	6th grade	Lindsay	5th grade	Lindsay
	Katie, Blake, Carl	reading	et al	reading	et al
1:30–2:10	Jamie, Chris	William	Jamie Chris	William	Jamie Chris
	Kristen, Corey	Mei Rakia	Kristen, Corey	Mei Rakia	Kristen Corey
2:15–2:55	Stephan	2nd grade	Stephan	Patricia Sue	Sue, Patty
	Beth, Gaby	lang arts	Beth, Gaby	Whitney, Bill	Whitney, Bill
3:00–3:30	CSE premeeting	planning	planning	CSE mtg	planning

being used or could be practiced in the school environment. The specific techniques and background information that have been reported in recent texts and journal articles are included to encourage you to build on the work of others. You do not have to, nor should you, rely solely on your own ideas. Choosing the selections was extraordinarily difficult because there are so many talented colleagues working in the schools today. Long before this text reaches your hands, however, this list will be out of date. It is an eternal frustration that there are not enough hours in the day to keep up with the excellent information that exists, let alone implement all the good suggestions. My threefold reason

Exhibit 8–6 Planning/Data Sheet for Groups

Time/Days: _MWF 10:00–10:40_	Goals: _Increase expressive vocab_	
Date 11/05	Date 11/07	Date 11/09
STO The students will use 3rd grade synonyms from lang arts curriculum	STO Demonstrate use of thesaurus to find synonyms	STO Use 6 synonyms in a written paragraph
Mat'l Make definition cards for memory game	Mat'l individual copies of thesaurus	Mat'l vocabulary list from cards (11/05)
Name Amanda		
IEP# IV a	IV c	IV a, III a, b, c
too easy—add antonyms	alphabetizing confuses her— synonyms OK	
Name Charles		
IEP# II b	II b	II b, I a
gave opposite instead of synonym. Review!	having both in thesaurus helped synonym–antonym confusion	
Name Joseph		
IEP# I C	I d	I c II d
all correct except feline v canine	OK—nice job	
Name Susan		
IEP# I a	I c	I a, IV c
couldn't read card information	Salli read for Susan—works well	

Comments

11/07 is in the classroom
11/12 in the computer lab next week

for including the soon-to-be-outdated list, however, goes beyond the information contained in the citations: (a) the selections will provide you with a starting place, (b) they will encourage you to read journal articles for their intervention applications rather than as a source of test questions, and, finally, (c) I hope they will seduce you into the habit of reading the current literature.

Before the list is presented, here are a few tips in using journals to keep current in the field:

1. Do not have your journals sent to your workplace; have them sent to you at home.

2. When a journal arrives, put it beside your bed or in your bathroom, preferably on the back of your toilet with a bright colored marker next to it. (I warned you at the beginning of Chapter 6 that I would get personal, but you will be astonished at how much reading you will accomplish!)

3. After reading a potentially useful article, circle its title with the marker or make a note on the cover of the journal so you can find it later.

4. When you consult any article you find helpful, always check the references at the end of it; they represent a list of related sources and a fund of additional information on the topic.

5. When the next issue comes, take the previous one to work and put it on a bookshelf in numerical order.

6. "Read" catalogues; not only do they abound with excellent materials, but just scanning the titles can often spark an idea for a particular student. Remember, however, that it takes several years for research appearing in the literature

to emerge as a catalogue material; your students may not be able to wait.

Later in this chapter, when you are asked to plan intervention using different service delivery models, consider how you could adapt some of the information presented in my list of sources to address the needs of the student subjects in the three cases. Again, this list is a *sample* only; the literature contains hundreds more for the taking.

- Christensen and Luckett (1990): "Getting Into the Classroom and Making It Work"

  The authors describe the techniques used in providing intervention for selected elementary students using whole-class language experiences. Their steps for an oral language lesson appear earlier in this chapter. They also describe the lesson-planning procedure and include two appendices: one listing commercially available resources and the other providing sample lesson plans. This "how-to" article is very helpful for the beginning clinician.

- Dollaghan and Kaston (1986): "A Comprehension Monitoring Program for Language-Impaired Children"

  A program designed to teach children how to listen and tell themselves when they are or are not understanding the message, it contains four phases: (a) identifying, labeling, and demonstrating the three behaviors associated with listening; (b) detecting and reacting to messages that one did not hear in their entirety and asking for help; (c) detecting and reacting to messages that contain inadequate information and asking for clarification; and (d) identifying and reacting to messages that exceed one's comprehension level. This program is a good example of teaching students how to use language to help understand language (i.e., basic metalinguistic skills).

- Edwards (1991): "Assessment and Management of Listening Skills in School-Aged Children."

Although specifically for use with hearing-impaired children, the ideas presented are useful for any student who has receptive language deficits. The three principles listed are (a) team collaboration is essential; (b) auditory skills should be developed in the student's classroom environment; and (c) the skills should be practiced in conjunction with educational goals, not in isolation. This is a good program to introduce the concept of collaboration to the teachers of classes that contain students with receptive language problems or a hearing impairment.

- Snyder-McLean (1984): "Structuring Joint Action Routines: A Strategy for Facilitating Communication and Language Development in the Classroom."

Joint action routines (JARs) are ritualized interactions between participants in the classroom that follow a logical sequence and have recognizable roles; they are derived from activities that occur in students' everyday lives, such as getting ready to go out to recess, preparing food, role-playing a child's story, and playing games. The authors recommend these for students who have severe disabilities and limited communication skills and need help with daily living skills. They are also useful for practicing language skills with children who come from other cultures, and they can serve as easy-to-copy models for parents. Nice for inclusion.

- "Decontextualized Concept Demystifies Reading/Language Connection" (1989).

This article clearly and succinctly describes the difference between contextualized and decontextualized language and presents this difference as an essential link between oral language and success in reading. It could be the basis of a handout for reading specialists and administrators as well as the classroom teacher.

- Hansen-Krening (1982): "Using Riddles to Teach Metalinguistic Skills."

A presentation of the way students in the elementary grades can use riddles to practice their developing metalinguistic skills by manipulating language, particularly useful at third-grade level and above. It would make a fun, motivating presentation for the entire class as well as an excellent vehicle to explain the concept of metalinguistics to classroom teachers.

- Rubin, Patterson, and Kantor (1991): "Morphological Development and Writing Ability in Children and Adults."

This article contains terrific information on the relationship between writing/spelling skills and basic morphological knowledge. It would be particularly useful at the middle- and high-school level because it gives insights into vocabulary building as well as morphology/syntax. The article also includes a brief test that clearly presents the concept of morphology use at the advanced level.

- Moats and Smith (1992): "Derivational Morphology: Why It Should Be Included in Language Assessment and Instruction."

An additional excellent source of information to use with older students, explaining how deficits in morphology affect reading, vocabulary, spelling, and writing skills. It contains information concerning later development of morphological endings, detailed information about affixes, principles for assessment, and two appendices: (a) goals for instruction, including a proposed score and sequence for morpheme instruction; and (b) suggested steps for teaching morpheme groups. Combined with the Rubin et al (1991) article, it could be the subject of a valuable in-service for English teachers at upper grade levels.

- Norris (1992): "Some Questions and Answers About Whole Language."

A fine source of information for the speech-language pathologist who is not sure what whole language is or its effect on the teaching of reading. The author clearly delineates how the speech-language specialist can suggest special adaptations for the students who have language deficits, for example, the use of small groups, assistance in attending to the most relevant information, high levels of direct feedback, and frequent clarification. This is a good vehicle for discussion when consulting with a teacher who uses whole language, particularly in combination with other information about the role of metaphonology. Another excellent source of information about the whole-language movement as it applies to speech-language pathology is Shapiro (1992), "Debatable Issues Underlying Whole-Language Philosophy: A Speech-Language Specialist's Perspective."

- Bristor (1993): "Enhancing Text Structure Instruction with Video for Improved Reading Comprehension."

This is another example of using newer technology to address language goals. The author suggests that speech-language pathologists and teachers use videos to introduce, discuss, and model story or other text elements. This is particularly desirable in the middle grades, when students encounter lengthier and more complex reading material. In my experience, videos may be the only available means to encourage a discussion of "style, language, story, rhythm, voice, tone, (and) laughter" in age-appropriate materials. When students' reading skills are severely depressed, material they can read easily may be years below their interest level. Using a video, for example, of *To Kill a Mockingbird* or *Where the Red Fern Grows* allows students to learn vocabulary and take part in a classroom discussion about setting and plot that would be denied them otherwise.

- Larson, McKinley, and Boley (1993): "Clinical Forum: Adolescent Language. Service Delivery Models for Adolescents With Language Disorders."

Speech-language pathologists who provide services to students in grades 7 through 12 often complain that compared with the materials available for younger language-impaired children, little is available for the older student. I agree that there is less, but articles like the ones in this series can be very helpful. This particular one outlines, in an easily understood figure, current service delivery options for students at the secondary level, as well as six specific rationales for providing these services. It has an excellent discussion of how to set up a for-credit language course for high school students. The list of references at the close of the article would be very helpful for a speech-language pathologist who is new to this population.

- Perry (1990): "Cooperative Learning = Effective Intervention."

This article explains how the concept of cooperative learning groups can be used to provide language intervention. The author reports that among other positive results, goals were achieved more quickly, and unhealthy competition was diminished. This information could be used to encourage collaboration when you have divided students in the classroom into groups, wanting them to share responsibility.

- Brinton and Fujiki (1989): "Impairment of Conversational Management: What Can Go Wrong?"

In my experience, conversations are often actively discouraged in the classroom; as students reach higher grades, more and more information is presented in lecture format, and teachers want quiet attending behavior. Unfortunately, lack of conversational skill can be devastating when the student tries to interact socially with other students or within a cooperative learning group. The authors present a list of common error patterns, such as faulty turn allocation, poor topic maintenance, and failure to correct oneself. A good source to share with teachers.

- Johnson (1987): "Make the Most of Classroom Discussions."

Johnson's article details why discussions help students think for themselves and gives 11 excellent suggestions for conducting a classroom discussion. This article could be used in conjunction with

the one by Perry (1990) on cooperative learning groups and the Brinton and Fujiki (1989) article to provide a foundation for teaching/encouraging students to use oral language to learn. The information in these three related articles would be excellent to share with middle-school teachers in general and with English, social studies, and history teachers at the upper level in particular.

- Westby and Cutler (1994): "Language and ADHD: Understanding the Bases and Treatment of Self-Regulatory Deficits."

This topic is an example of a condition that has language implications, but the students who are so affected often see many other specialists as well. This article describes the nature of ADHD and suggests specific intervention practices to address pragmatic strategies at the same time that cognitive-behavioral techniques are being employed. The role of language in addressing metacognitive deficits by using verbal mediation, cognitive modeling, and instruction in problem-solving techniques would be another excellent topic for an in-service presentation.

- Buchoff (1990): "Attention Deficit Disorder: Help for the Classroom Teacher."

This article represents similar information to the one by Westby and Cutler (1994), but from the point of view of the classroom teacher. I hesitate to tell you that reading *outside* our field is also necessary, but it is often helpful in understanding where the teacher is coming from. In addition, this article provides excellent practical solutions in getting the student organized, giving effective directions, classroom management, developing self-esteem, and parent–teacher partnerships. It also lists the symptoms of ADD.

- Campbell (1993): "Maintaining the Integrity of Home Linguistic Varieties: Black English Vernacular."

What do you tell an English teacher who complains that an African-American student "doesn't speak correct English"? This article contains a description of the linguistic system and rules of Black English and can serve as a good place to start in consulting with teachers who are concerned about this.

- Hamersky (1993): "Vocabulary Maps: Strategies for Developing Word Meanings."

This material can be used with students in Grades 6 through 12 to improve semantics (vocabulary) skills. It includes five different ways that words can be taught, some using visual formats, such as attribute webs and Venn diagrams. It is particularly useful because vocabulary that is part of academic subjects can be targeted while students are learning techniques that they can use independently at a later date.

- Gregg (1991): "Disorders of Written Expression."

This is a primer for speech-language professionals who have little background in writing theory and practice. It includes a list of skills that writing requires, explains how to test for writing disorders, and describes how deficits in specific areas of language affect writing performance. The concept of text discourse is discussed, including cohesion and coherence. Often (but not always), a student's problems in writing are directly traceable to oral language deficits.

Therefore you need to familiarize yourself with the nature of a writing disorder, determine how it relates to your student's oral language ability, explain the connection to classroom teachers, and, finally, address these writing deficits as part of your intervention plan. If this does not convince you that you need skills others can bring to the collaborative model, nothing will.

- Stevens and Englert (1993): "Making Writing Strategies Work."

Strategy instruction, or teaching students not only content but process, is another hot topic in education. You may recognize this as allied to dynamic assessment, or curriculum-based instruction. The particular strategies the authors use provide an excellent way to help students plan what they will write—for example, by using oral language (self-talk strategies) or by asking themselves questions like "Who am I writing for?" and "Did I include all my categories?" This article would be very useful if you team-teach in upper level grades because it encourages teachers or specialists to ask *all* students, on an individual basis, about their thinking processes, not just those who have deficits.

- Kamhi (1995): "Defining, Developing, and Maintaining Clinical Expertise."

The author discusses a subject not often addressed: the impact of factors such as technical skills, interpersonal skills, and attitudes of speech-language professionals on treatment outcomes. On the basis of over 100 interviews with people in the field, Kamhi discusses the maturation of a professional intimately involved in clinical work. Thought provoking and particularly helpful for the new clinician, it is a wonderful introduction to what really comes to matter as professionals practice the art and craft of speech-language intervention. It also serves as some comfort when you can no longer remember the complete anatomy and physiology of the larynx.

- McCauley (1996): "Familiar Strangers: Criterion-Referenced Measures in Communication Disorders."

This excellent article provides a brief history of criterion-referenced measures, defines and gives examples of them, and then proposes some practical guidelines for their evaluation and selection. Most important for the school professional, however, are the suggestions for developing and using informal criterion-referenced instruments. With curriculum-based assessment, this article provides a starting place for the school practitioner who must be accountable for the quality and efficacy of push-in or collaborative teaching and wants some way to measure progress other than by standardized measures.

- Rasinski (1994): "Developing Syntactic Sensitivity in Reading Through Phrase-Cued Texts."

A summary of this article appears in *Word of Mouth* (March 1994), with additional valuable suggestions by the editors in how to apply the concept of the author's phrase-cued texts to students with language-based learning disabilities. This presents an interesting way to address syntactic deficits during reading instruction.

- Wiig and Wilson (1994): "Is a Question a Question? Passage Understanding by Preadolescents With Learning Disabilities."

When a student cannot answer a question, it could mean problems in listening and reading comprehension, linguistic development, word recognition memory, or basic question–answering ability. This source includes a review of Bloom's taxonomy as it applies to the goal of increasing opportunities for students to answer higher level questions. A necessity for dealing with students in the upper grades.

- Reutzel and Fawson (1989): "Using a Literature Webbing Strategy Lesson With Predictable Books."

Another example of an article from a related discipline; the journals/books I have cited outside our field should be available in any college library. The authors describe the six steps of the literature-webbing strategy lesson (LWSL) to improve both comprehension and decoding. I have included this not only because of the excellent figural representations but because the method allows speech-language pathologists a way to encourage cultural literacy while addressing language goals. If students do not recognize what a "knight in shining armor" or "sour grapes" means, they may miss the whole point of a paragraph in a current book about teenagers.

The following three suggestions are taken from the "Idea Swap" section of *Word of Mouth*, a newsletter that presents article summaries of interest to the school-based speech-language pathologist. The "Idea Swap" section features ideas, materials, activities, and other "practical ideas that work," submitted by speech-language pathologists who work in the trenches:

- Campbell and McCall (1992): "Cinnamon Bear Book."

This is an example of an idea that encourages both parent involvement as well as practice in writing. It comes with complete directions. Often children's magazines and books on crafts for kids can be adapted to language use. These are very helpful if you are not artistically talented or if you have difficulty thinking of intervention ideas. It is not cheating to adapt an idea developed by a talented colleague as long as you give credit—and allow others to copy you!

- Watters (1994): "Using Stories on CD-ROM to Teach Speech and Language."

This activity features a CD-ROM that reproduces the text of a book as it "speaks" it, augmented by animation, music, and other sound effects. Watters, an elementary school speech-language pathologist, states that using this computer program improves listening and observation skills, provides an opportunity for modeling sentence structures, increases memory for details, improves interest level, instills cooperation and turn taking, and encourages specific oral language development, including sequencing, categorizing, and identifying objects. This is an excellent example of an activity that you could demonstrate in the classroom to show how language intervention can be continued without your being present.

- Keith (1990): "Using Computers in School Speech and Language."

Keith's article presents 12 questions you can use to evaluate off-the-shelf software, a discussion of generic versus designer software, and a lesson designed for computer-assisted instruction. As in the Watters (1994) activity, this is in-formation that can be shared, particularly when teachers (or computer curriculum coordinators) are choosing software for the year. With school budgets as tight as they are, you cannot afford to waste money on materials that you will not use or that have only limited applicability.

The following nine articles all address another of the current "hot" topics in speech-language pathology: the impact of deficits in phonological awareness, phonological encoding, and metaphonology on learning to read. With the increased use of the whole-language concept in schools, some elementary teachers may deemphasize phonetic reading approaches. Research in our field indicates that for the child who has problems in phonological encoding or decoding (spelling/sounding out), this may be devastating. The articles below will give you information to develop your IEP as well as valuable insights to share with teachers.

- Swank (1994): "Phonological Coding Ability: Identification of Impairments Related to Phonologically Based Reading Problems."

Defines specific phonological coding impairment (SPCI) in detail and clearly defines how a student's early speech problems may negatively affect later school performance.

- Catts (1991): "Facilitating Phonological Awareness: Role of Speech-Language Specialists."

Provides excellent activities for preschool and kindergarten children to improve phonological awareness, such as rhyming games and incorporating sound play into the classroom curriculum. It also lists commercially available tests to assess deficits.

- Masterson (1993): "Classroom-Based Phonological Intervention."

  Lists a variety of methods that can be used in implementing a classroom-based program, such as Hodson and Paden's cyclic approach and whole-language activities. It also lists cautions.

- Temple and Gillett (1984): "Language Arts Learning Processes and Teaching Practices."

  This earlier reference contains good general information including the stages in spelling development. Whole language activities often feature very early writing during a time when, from the point of view of most speech-language pathologists, spelling skills are not present at all. Therefore this section of the text will alert you to the way phonemic awareness, or the lack of it, can affect a student's early attempts at encoding.

- Hoffman (1990): "Spelling, Phonology, and the Speech-Language Pathologist: A Whole Language Perspective."

  This is a nice companion piece to the one by Masterson (1993) because it presents specific suggestions for remediation if spelling is deficient. An excellent source for collaboration.

- Hodson (1994): "Helping Individuals Become Intelligible, Literate and Articulate: The Role of Phonology."

  A very nice summary of normal phonological development as it affects later school progress and the possible continuing need for speech-language services for children who have been severely impaired. This could also be used for a parent/preschool teacher in-service.

- Haskell, Foorman, and Swank (1992): "Effects of Three Orthographic/Phonological Units on First-Grade Reading."

  For speech-language pathologists who have no background in the teaching of reading, this valuable article describes three approaches: phonics, sight word, and "onset-rime." The authors investigated the effects of instruction using onset-rime, a compromise between individual phoneme instruction and the whole-word approach. Often children who have speech-language deficits need direct instruction in phonics combined with a whole-language approach. Before you can suggest this, however, you need some basic understanding of reading methods.

- Paratore (1995): "Assessing Literacy: Establishing Common Standards in Portfolio Assessment."

  Paratore provides a detailed description of her pilot program featuring portfolio assessment/intervention. She presents specific suggestions in incorporating curriculum materials in the process. It also contains a list of reading and writing benchmarks which would be exceptionally helpful to a speech language professional who does not have much background in teaching writing.

- Venkatagiri, H.S. (1995): "Techniques for Enhancing Communication Productivity: A Review of Research."

  This is a wonderful source of information for the speech language professional who needs a basic overview of augmentative and alternative communication. Using seven different criteria, the article compares six approaches to increasing productivity of novel utterances.

CASE STUDIES

Case 1: Steven

Congratulations! For Case 1, you have planned an evaluation, interpreted it (Chapter 6), and chosen appropriate goals (Chapter 7). Now for the final step: How would you remediate Steven's deficits? Considering his age, his grade, his teachers' styles, and his specific IEP, what service delivery model(s) and short-term objectives would you employ? I hope you recognize that most of the goals of his IEP could be addressed through a number of single- or multiple-service delivery models, such as collaborative, team teaching, and pull-out. Before reading on, list at least four ideas with your reasons for including them.

Here are some of my suggestions. Because it is essential to identify an underlying goal first and then to choose different means of implementing it, the goals designated by Roman numerals in Chapter 7 reflect this process. One of the basic skills Steven needs to develop is increasing his conscious phonological awareness (Goal II). He must recognize that words are composed of syllables and phonemes (II.D, II.G) and that they can rhyme (II.A) or begin/end with the same sound (II.B, II.G). (Hodson, 1994).

Once this has been accomplished, he must learn how to manipulate phonological information with increasing speed—that is, perform mental operations on sounds. Work might include sound blending, letter-sound association, presentation of continuant sounds before noncontinuant ones, sound addition/deletion, and categorizing of word beginnings and endings (Goals II.E, II.F, and II.B). Explaining to Ms. Rose why this process is critical will be part of your consultative/collaborative role. Because Steven likes Legos and color, you could suggest that visual cues be employed, such as color coding of sounds. In words like *pat*, *sit*, and *cut*, "t" could be a red Lego. If sound segmentation proves too advanced, Steven might place blocks in a pattern with one block for each word (*he + is + sad*), the syllables in compound words (*bird + house*), noncompound two-syllable words (*lum + ber*), or a sound plus a "word family" (*p + at*, or *p + in*). If this is too elementary for the whole class, the activity might be accomplished only by the "low" group in an extended reading lesson, or in an individual pull-out or pull-aside session. Either you or Ms. Rose could direct this while the other person teaches another group (collaboration/team teaching).

You may suggest that picture card representations of "popping" or "windy" sounds from Lindamood be posted on a bulletin board, or that any teacher involved in the reading process with Steven adopt the use of hand signals to cue a particular sound in the final position, thus employing visual cues to assist his growing auditory awareness (Masterson, 1993).

Because Steven must be able to match a "new" reading word to one previously stored in his memory, it is important that his new vocabulary words exist in proper phonological form. Therefore choose words from class science lessons or reading books, or "direction" words (*top*, *bottom*, *circle*, *underline*, etc.) to practice the techniques listed above when you or Ms. Rose preteach vocabulary (Catts, 1991). If Steven needs more practice than others in his group, again, you could provide it in pull-out (or pull-aside) intervention. A whole-class activity could feature printing signs for each major object in the first-grade class (*door*, *computer*, *desk*, *sink*, etc.), with

Steven deciding what the *final* sound should be or identifying the number of syllables in the word.

You may also wish to discuss with the reading specialist the possibility of a reading method for Steven that will emphasize phonology rather than a whole-word approach (Haskell et al., 1992). One of the possibilities suggested by Bradley and Bryant (1983) is using onset-rime. In an onset-rime approach to reading, Steven would learn to segment and blend single-syllable words. For example, the initial consonant "f" (the onset) is combined with the vowel and remaining consonants "-in" (the rime) to make "fin." Be careful, however, that you do not appear to dictate any one approach as the only possibility. Remember, Ms. Rose and the reading specialist have many years of experience. Your role is to point out how Steven's apparent deficits in metaphonology may make certain reading approaches easier or more difficult for him. In the meantime, you will share with them how your goals in intervention are designed to address these underlying problems. You may wish to refer to some of the citations in the section "Sample Programs From the Literature" that target metaphonology: those by Swank (1994), Catts (1991), Masterson (1993), Temple and Gillett (1984), Hoffman (1990), Hodson (1994), and Haskell et al. (1992).

For speech-language pathologists who have no background in the teaching of reading, for example, the article by Haskell et al. (1992) describes three approaches: phonics, sight word, and onset-rime. The authors investigated the effects of instruction using onset-rime, a compromise between individual phoneme instruction and the whole-word approach. Often children who have speech-language deficits need direct instruction in phonics combined with a whole-language approach. Before you can suggest this, however,

you need some basic understanding of reading methods.

Consider how the following sequence presented by Catts (1991) could be applied to any of the service delivery models discussed earlier. Using a developmental schema, draw attention to sound structure through nursery rhymes, finger plays, and age-appropriate television jingles. Read poems and stories containing rhyme, alliteration, or nonsense sound activities (*deanut dutter danwich; beanut butter banwich*). Ask the music teacher if the choral curriculum could include selections with alliteration ("The Sneaky Snake") or rhythmic and rhymed repetitions.

Other authors suggest these ways to establish and practice *applied* metaphonological principles: incorporate sound play into the classroom curriculum or theme; create nonsense words for common objects; suggest structured activities like choosing the word in a three-out-of-four series that does not rhyme or has a different initial/final sound; use other visuals (boxes = sounds) or key words (*noisy nose*). Van Kleeck (1990) presented another sequence of acquisition that could serve as a springboard for dialogue among the reading specialist, the classroom teacher, and the speech-language pathologist.

Spelling concerns should be addressed partly by determining what phonological skills Steven is bringing to the task (i.e., what stage of spelling he is in—probably early phonemic) and then moving him into the next stage, even though it may not be grade appropriate (Temple & Gillett, 1984). Most important is giving Steven lots of practice in choosing certain phonemic patterns, particularly rhymes; this shows the clear link between the two areas of deficit. Other experts suggest using meaningful writing activities, such as invitations and signs for the classroom (Hoffman 1990).

Because Steven's listening comprehension, including sequencing, also appears to be strongly affected by whether visual cues are present, the presence of pictures and manipulatives should help him become more successful in following directions. In addition to improving the coding of new words into Steven's memory, it will help him to retain vocabulary if there is increased relevance of linguistic targets—that is, if the teacher makes sure Steven knows how and why he should learn them. Small-group or whole-class activities could include using predictable books to train morphology (past tense, plurals, etc.) as well as more sophisticated syntax based on curricular needs ("Someone *has been sleeping* in my bed").

Using Steven's strengths to compensate for his weaknesses should be another goal of your intervention—for example, providing more opportunities to use his good social skills to increase his ability to ask clarifying questions. If motoric sequencing is part of the problem in /r/ production, it may be advisable to use pull-out intervention, perhaps as part of an existing articulation group. Because Steven's only articulation errors occurred in liquids, these will be addressed within the context of the other phonology goals (Goal I).

Certainly in the initial stages of intervention, a large part of your job is translating your diagnostic findings into activities that will improve classroom competence by exposing all his teachers to both Steven's language goals and your procedures.

Case 2: James

We have now determined that James has pervasive word-finding deficits that directly affect expressive tasks; a receptive and expressive semantic problem involving concepts; and deficits in articulation, morphology, and syntax that can be attributed to a language difference. Let us tackle the language difference issue first. How will you handle this? Will you develop ways to change his language to reflect standard American English pronunciation/forms? Think about this before reading on.

One of the many factors you must take into account is how this difference is affecting his overall classroom performance. Often you need to share with teachers and administrators what the concept of a language difference entails, as well as to delineate the specific Black English forms James is using. After this information was given to Ms. Dwyer, she was able to state that the forms in question were not affecting James either academically or socially. Please note this last comment. It is a fact of life in schools that pragmatics are often ignored in an evaluation unless there is a clear indication of serious deficits. Ms. Dwyer recognized the value that children place on being accepted at school and acknowledged that James, even though shy and new in the school, interacted well and was liked by his classmates. In a case like this, in which dialect is not negatively affecting academic subjects, speech-language professionals often have a conference with the parents and explain that the ability to switch code from the language students use at home to the standard forms valued at school can serve them well both academically and later in the workplace. At no time, however, do they disparage the richness inherent in Black English; instead, they present as an option possible "intervention" in this area. Sadly, it should be noted that if the student is not labeled, many districts do not allow their specialists to work with students who are not on their caseload. Even if this is the case, however, an enterprising SLP could present in-service training to faculty and administrators or develop a unit on dialect that could be team taught at various grade levels.

Goals I, II, and III, developed in Chapter 7, reflect the nondialectical deficits that were identified during testing. James's primary difficulty, word-finding problems, can originate as a result of either inefficient storage or inefficient retrieval strategies. Storage strength is an indication of how well learned words are—that is, how available they are in memory. Retrieval strength reflects the accessibility of that information (Nippold, 1992). It is important to identify which one (or both) of these are implicated because intervention strategies will be different. For discussion purposes, let us assume that you have already determined through extension testing that James needs help in both areas. Given Goals II.B (1, 2, and 3) and III, what kinds of intervention and what service delivery models could you use?

Here are some ways I might address meeting James's goals. The more often a student studies and uses an item of information, the more storage and retrieval strength increase. Nippold (1992) stated that retrieval practice is more powerful for increasing the ability to store and retrieve. Therefore we need to prioritize the specific vocabulary that James needs to succeed in different subjects, particularly those in which the terms are brand-new, such as scientific concepts. One of the most efficient ways to address this need is by "preteaching" vocabulary, done individually in pull-aside or pull-out intervention, in a small group within the class, or by engaging parents or aides as partners. Later, when the teacher presents the lesson using these words, James will be familiar with them.

To increase retrieval strength, it is especially important that James can pronounce each word easily. It is very difficult to retrieve a word you cannot pronounce. Specific phonemic cues can be used when the terms are taught, and those same cues can be employed

again when retrieval is practiced: for example, "*Ants* have *antennae*." You will also want to use categorization, grouping items that have something in common (insects that fly), and associative clues to help aid memory (the sound some insects make, or visualizing six legs). Part of consulting would include teaching Ms. Dwyer cueing techniques to use throughout the class day and encouraging using word boxes for a matching question to test vocabulary, at least initially. To the greatest extent possible, the first words addressed by these techniques should have concrete referents. Because James will need many, many repetitions to put these words into storage and access them easily, you should plan with the teacher or librarian (collaboration, consultation) to have available books, pictures, computer programs, film strips, and posters that can provide many opportunities for continued discussion. Spelling words can also be used. Remember, you are teaching the process of how to store/retrieve words as well as the actual vocabulary. Be very explicit about what you are doing so that in later months and years, James will use these methods to learn new material. Note that learning new vocabulary is required of every student in school and that the means of memorizing effectively is a valuable skill. Others may not need the number of repetitions or the cues that James will, but they would certainly benefit from learning such techniques as word webs, semantic maps, and Venn diagrams presented as part of whole-class instruction.

Goal III, decreasing proforms, can be done partly within the context of teaching the processes just described. It could also be addressed directly by teaching how to define or describe objects, sequences, or events. Consider collaboration with the art and/or physical education teacher in teaching spatial and temporal terms for part of James's Goal I.A (1, 2). Unfortunately, most teachers assume that students have mastered calendar facts by second grade at the latest. For students like James, it can be both confusing and embarrassing not to know in what months holidays come, if spring is a season or a month, if today is Monday the 27th, or what the day/date of the day before yesterday was. Consequently, part of your job will be to review this information until it becomes automatic, using classroom routines as much as possible, such as counting down days on a calendar on his desk until assignments are due. A time line can serve as a visual cue to help James understand temporal concepts, as well as review concept vocabulary (Goal B.3). As you develop these programs, be sure to plan how you will maintain records verifying the effectiveness of intervention; remember, accountability is required for all service models, not just pull-out.

Case 3: Christine

Well, you have moved from first to third and now ninth grade. How will you adapt your intervention procedures to reflect this change in age and situation? On the basis of the goals developed in Chapter 7, list at least two activities using three different service delivery models.

One of the imperatives at the high school level is using curriculum materials and assignments exclusively when you plan intervention. A second consideration should be to teach a process that can be applied to as many different subjects as possible addressing Goal II.A and II.C. An example is teaching the use of verbal organizers. Westby (1994) presented a list of text structures (sequence, comparison–contrast, cause–effect, etc.), including the function of each, key words for

recognizing them, and comprehension questions that Christine could use to create study guides. Paul (1995) compiled a number of visual organizers that could assist Christine in learning the meaning of various clausal connectors (II.B7). Because Christine is in class with a number of other low-average students, teaching these ways to understand a given material's organization schema should be helpful to most of them. This could be accomplished during a resource room period cotaught by you and a special education colleague.

Ms. Williams, Christine's English teacher, could provide you with a list of future writing assignments or oral presentations that would allow you to review the appropriate structure(s) and clausal connectors for the type of assignment (Goals II.B and II.C.2). Push-in, collaborative, team-teaching, or pull-out modes could all be used, depending on the situation at the time. Working on the actual assignment could also give you an opportunity to discuss such topics as transitions between paragraphs, topic sentences, and supporting statements. Graham and Harris (1987) discussed how to teach students self-prompts when they are rereading or editing their own work. Paratore's (1995) pilot program featuring assessment/intervention could prove useful in diminishing Christine's discouragement. It features parent involvement and allows Christine a voice in setting academic goals.

At the same time, Christine will need instruction and practice in how to improve her note-taking skills in lecture. She will need assistance not only in organization but also in decoding the meaning when it is not directly stated. Using her textbook could include, at least initially, simplifying some of the syntactic complexity of certain very difficult sections so that the meaning can be deciphered.

At a later date, the reverse procedure could take place for example, taking the two simple sentences you extracted and reforming them into a longer one. Giving Christine a textbook for her permanent and exclusive use would let her highlight topic sentences or section titles. Clausal connectors could also be highlighted in some sections so Christine could see how they are used in actual grade-appropriate materials. The highlighted text, perhaps with a few margin notes, could also serve as a study guide.

Teachers could provide lecture outlines for Christine to follow, teaching her various ways in which information is organized. These could gradually be faded to include only the main outline with numbers and letters to indicate that information should be filled in (Goal II.A.1, 2). Fry, Polk, and Fountoukidis (1984) provided a list of "signal words," words that authors and lecturers use to tell the reader/class members how to read/listen. These include "continuation signals" (there are more ideas to come: *moreover, furthermore, in addition*) and "change-of-direction signals" (we're doubling back: *despite, rather, conversely, even though*; Fry, Polk, & Fountoukidis, 1984). Finding these terms in different textbooks could provide additional practice.

Case 4: Megan

Consider the goals you developed for Megan at the close of Chapter 7 and discuss how they might be implemented. If you have not used each service delivery model, try the remaining one(s) for at least some of the goals. As you conclude this fourth case, I hope you are feeling more confident in your ability to assess strengths and deficits, interpret your findings, and plan appropriate, motivating intervention for students like Steven, James, Christine, and Megan. These students may not really exist, but every fact about them is based on the experiences of real students with real needs who are counting on all of us to put forth our very best effort. Finally, I trust that if someone asks, "What is it that you speech-language people do?" you will be able to tell them more than they really want to know. Enjoy.

REFERENCES

Beatty, J. (1985, February). A voice for the underdog. *Atlantic Monthly*, p. 100.

Bloom, B., Engelhart, M., Furst, E., Hill, W., & Krathwohl, D. (Eds.). (1956). *Taxonomy of educational objectives: The classification of educational goals. Handbook I: Cognitive domain.* New York: David McKay.

Borsch, J., & Oaks, R. (1992). Clinical forum: Implementing collaborative consultation. Effective collaboration at Central Elementary School. *Language, Speech, and Hearing Services in Schools, 23,* 367–368.

Bradley, L., & Bryant, P. (1983). Categorizing sounds and learning to read: A causal connection. *Nature, 30,* 419–421.

Brandel, D. (1992). Clinical forum: Implementing collaborative consultation. Collaboration: Full steam ahead with no prior experience! *Language, Speech, and Hearing Services in Schools, 23,* 369–370.

Brinton, B., & Fujiki, M. (1989). Impairment of conversational management: What can go wrong? In B. Brinton & M. Fujiki (Eds.), *Conversational management with language-impaired children: Pragmatic assessment and intervention* (pp. 95–111). Rockville, MD: Aspen.

Bristor, V. (1993). Enhancing text structure instruction with video for improved reading comprehension. *Intervention in School and Clinic, 28,* 216–223.

Buchoff, R. (1990, Winter). Attention deficit disorder: Help for the classroom teacher. *Childhood Education,* 86–90.

Bush, C. (1980a). *Language remediation and expansion: School and home program.* Tucson, AZ: Communication Skill Builders.

Bush, C. (1980b). *Language remediation and expansion: 100 skill-building reference lists.* Tucson, AZ: Communication Skill Builders.

Butler, K. (1980). *The path to a concept of language-learning disabilities. Topics in Language Disorders*, 1, 6.

Campbell, C., & McCall, C. (1992). Cinnamon bear book. *Word of Mouth*, 3, 10.

Campbell, L. (1993). Maintaining the integrity of home linguistic varieties: Black English vernacular. *American Journal of Speech-Language Pathology*, 2, 11–12.

Catts, H. (1991). Facilitating phonological awareness: Role of speech-language specialists. *Language, Speech, and Hearing Services in Schools*, 22, 196–203.

Christensen, S., & Luckett, C. (1990). Getting into the classroom and making it work. *Language, Speech, and Hearing Services in Schools*, 21, 110–113.

Cochran, P.S., & Masterson, J.J. (1995). "NOT using a computer in language assessment/intervention: In defense of the reluctant clinicians. *Language, Speech, and Hearing Services in Schools*, 26 (3), 213–222.

Conoley, J., & Conoley, C. (1982). How to enter: When to stay. In J. Conoley & C. Conoley (Eds.), *School consultation: A guide to practice and training* (pp. 106–133). New York: Pergamon.

Crais, E. (1992). *Family-centered assessment and collaborative goal-setting*. New York State Speech-Language-Hearing Association, Annual conference, Kiamesha Lake, New York.

Curtis, M., & Meyers, J. (1985). Consultation: A foundation for alternative services. In A. Thomas & J. Grimes (Eds.). *Best practices in school-based consultation: Guidelines for effective practice* (pp. 35–38). Washington, DC: National Association of School Psychologists.

Curtis, M., & Zins, J. (Eds.). (1981). *The theory and practice of school consultation*. Springfield, IL: Charles C Thomas.

Decontextualized concept demystifies reading/language connection. (1989, March) *Syndactics Bulletin*, 6 (3), (Available from P.O. Box 10004, Phoenix, AZ 85064)

Dollaghan, C., & Kaston, N. (1986). A comprehension monitoring program for language-impaired children. *Journal of Speech and Hearing Disorders*, 51, 263–271.

Editorial Comment. (1995, April). *Word of Mouth*, p. 10.

Education for All Handicapped Children Act. Pub. L. No. 94-142, Sec. 3 et seq., 89 Stat. 774.

Education of the Handicapped Amendments of 1986. Pub. L. No. 99-457. Sec. 101 et seq. 100 Stat. 1145.

Edwards, C. (1991). Assessment and management of listening skills in school-aged children. *Seminars in Hearing*, 12, 389–401.

Eger, D. (1992). Why now? Changing school speech-language service delivery. *Asha*, 34 (11), 40–41.

Elksnin, L., & Capilouto, G. (1994). Speech-language specialists' perceptions of integrated service delivery in school settings. *Language, Speech, and Hearing Services in Schools*, 25, 248–267.

Ellis, L., Schlaudecker, C., & Griess, K. (1995). Effectiveness of a collaborative consultation approach to basic concept instruction. *Language, Speech, and Hearing Services in Schools*, 26, 69–74.

Ferguson, M. (1992). Clinical forum: Implementing collaborative consultation. An introduction. *Language, Speech, and Hearing Services in Schools*, 23, 371–372.

Freilinger, J. (1992). Support personnel. *Asha*, 39 (11), 51–53.

Fry, E., Polk, J., & Fountoukidis, D. (1984). *The reading teacher's book of lists*. Englewood Cliffs, NJ: Prentice-Hall.

Giangreco, M., & Meyer, L. (1988). Expanding service delivery options in regular school and classrooms for students with severe disabilities. In J. Graden, & M. Curtis, (Eds.). *Alternative educational delivery: Enhancing instructional options for all students* (pp. 257). Washington, DC: National Association of School Psychologists.

Goodman, K. (1986). *What's whole in whole language*. Portsmouth, NH: Heinemann.

Graham, S., & Harris, K. (1987). Improving composition skills of inefficient learners with self-instructional strategy training. *Topics in Language Disorders*, 7, 68–77.

Gregg, N. (1991). Disorders of written expression. In A. Bain, L. Bailet, & L. Moats (Eds.). *Written language disorders: Theory into practice* (pp. 66–97). Austin, TX: Pro-Ed.

Guilford, L. (1993). Letter to the editor. *Language, Speech, and Hearing Services in Schools*, 24, 63.

Hall, P., & Tomblin, J. (1978). A follow-up study of children with articulation and language disorders. *Journal of Speech and Hearing Disorders*, 43, 227–241.

Hamersky, J. (1993). Vocabulary maps: Strategies for developing word meanings. Eau Clair, WI: Thinking Publications.

Haney, C. (1992). The place for assistive technology. *Asha*, 39 (11), 47–49.

Hansen-Krening, N. (1982). *Using riddles to teach metalinguistic skills. Language experiences for all students*. Menlo Park, CA: Addison-Wesley.

Haskell, D., Foorman, B., & Swank, P. (1992). Effects of three orthographic/phonological units on first-grade reading. *Remedial and Special Education*, 13 (2), 40–49.

Hill, S., & Haynes, W. (1992). Language performance in low-achieving elementary school students. *Language, Speech, and Hearing Services in Schools*, 23, 169–175.

Hodson, B. (1994). Helping individuals become intelligible, literate and articulate: The role of phonology. *Topics in Language Disorders*, 14 (2), 1–16.

Hoffman, P. (1990). Spelling, phonology, and the speech-language specialist: A whole language perspective. *Language, Speech, and Hearing Services in Schools*, 21, 238–243.

Hoskins, B. (1990a). Collaborative consultation: Designing the role of the speech-language specialist in a new educational context. In W. A. Secord (Ed.), *Best practices in school speech-language pathology* (pp. 29–36). San Antonio, TX: Psychological Corporation.

Hoskins, B. (1990b). Language and literacy: Participating in the conversation. *Topics in Language Disorders, 10* (2), 46–62.

Huffman, N. (1992). Challenges of education reform. *Asha, 39* (11), 41–44.

Idol Paolucci-Whitcomb, P., & Nevin, A. (1986). *Collaborative consultation.* Austin, TX: Pro-Ed.

Johnson, E.W. (1987). Make the most of classroom discussions. In H. Hamilton (Ed.), *Teacher's strategies* (pp. 12–14). Springhouse, PA: Springhouse Corp.

Kamhi, A. (1995). Defining, developing and maintaining clinical expertise. *Language, Speech, and Hearing Services in Schools, 26* (4), 353–356.

Keith, O. (1990). Using computers in school speech and language. *Word of Mouth, 2* (3), 10.

Larson, V., McKinley, N., & Boley, D. (1993). Clinical forum: adolescent language. Service delivery models for adolescents with language disorders. *Language, Speech, and Hearing Services in Schools, 24,* 36–42.

Light, J., & McNaughton, D. (1993). Literacy and augmentative and alternative communication (AAC): The expectations and priorities of parents and teachers. *Topics in Language Disorders, 13* (2), 33–46.

Marvin, C. (1987). Consultation services: Changing roles for speech-language specialists. *Journal of Childhood Communication Disorders, 11,* 1–16.

Masterson, J. (1993). Classroom-based phonological intervention. *American Journal of Speech-Language Pathology, 2,* 5–9.

Masterson, J.J. (1995). Computer application in the schools: What we *can* do—what we *should* do. *Language, Speech, and Hearing Services in Schools, 26* (3), 211–212.

McCauley, R. (1996). Familiar strangers: Criterion-referenced measures in communication disorders. *Language, Speech, and Hearing Services in Schools, 26* (4), 353–356.

McGuire, R.A. (1995). Computer-based instrumentation: Issues in clinical application. *Language, Speech, and Hearing Services in Schools, 26* (3), 223–231.

Miller, L. (1989). Classroom-based language intervention. *Language, Speech, and Hearing Services in Schools, 20,* 153–170.

Moats, L., & Smith, C. (1992). Derivational morphology: Why it should be included in language assessment and instruction. *Language, Speech, and Hearing Services in Schools, 23,* 312–219.

Montgomery, J. (1992). Clinical forum: Implementing collaborative consultation. Perspectives from the field: Language, speech and hearing services in schools. *Lan-*

guage, *Speech, and Hearing Services in Schools, 23,* 363–364.

Muma, J. (1978). *The language handbook: Concepts, assessment, intervention.* Englewood Cliffs, NJ: Prentice-Hall.

Neidecker, E., & Blosser, J. (1993). *School programs in speech-language: Organization and management.* Englewood Cliffs, NJ: Prentice-Hall.

Nelson, N., & Kinnucan-Welsch, K. (1992). Curriculum-based collaboration: What is changing? *Asha, 34* (11), 45–47, 50.

New York Board of Regents. (1988). Amendment to Part 200 Regulations of the Commission. Available from: The University of the State of New York State Education Department, Office for Special Education Services, Division of Program Development and Support Services, Room 1069, Education Building Annex, Albany, New York 12234.

Nippold, M. A. (1992). The nature of normal and disordered word finding in children and adolescents. *Topics in Language Disorders, 13,* 1–14.

Norris, J. (1992). Some questions and answers about whole language. *American Journal of Speech-Language Pathology, 1* (4), 11–14.

Paul, R. (1995). *Language disorders from infancy through adolescence: Assessment and intervention.* St. Louis: Mosby-Year Book.

Perry, T. (1990). Cooperative learning = effective intervention. *Language Speech, and Hearing Services in Schools, 21,* 120.

Peters-Johnson, C. (1992). Professional practices perspective on caseloads in schools. *Asha, 34,* 12.

Pietranton, A., & Lynch, C. (1995). Multiskilling: A renaissance or a dark age? *Asha, 37* (6, 7), 37–40.

Rasinski, T. (1994). Developing syntactic sensitivity in reading through phrase-cued texts. *Intervention in School and Clinic, 29,* 165–168.

Reutzel, D., & Fawson, P. (1989). Using a literature webbing strategy lesson with predictable books. *Reading Teacher, 43,* 208–215.

Riley, A.M. (1991). *Evaluating Acquired Skills in Communication.* (EASIC) Tucson, AZ: Communication Skill Builders.

Roller, E., Rodriquez, T., Warner, J. & Lindahl, P. (1992). Clinical forum: Implementing collaborative consultation. Integration of self-contained children with severe speech-language needs into the regular education classroom. *Language, Speech, and Hearing Services in Schools, 23,* 365–366.

Rubin, H., Patterson, P., & Kantor, M. (1991). Morphological development and writing ability in children and adults. *Language, Speech, and Hearing Services in Schools, 22,* 228–235.

Russell, S., & Kaderavek, J. (1993). Alternative models for collaboration. *Language, Speech, and Hearing Services in Schools, 24*, 76–78.

Sanger, D., Hux, I., & Griess, K. (1995). Educators' opinions about speech-language pathology services in schools. *Language, Speech, and Hearing Services in Schools, 26*, 75–86.

Schuh, M., Tashie, C., & Jorgensen, C. (1981). *Strategies for modifying and expanding curriculum for students with disabilities.* Concord, NH: University of New Hampshire, Institute on Disability.

Schulz, J., & Turnbull, A. (1984). *Mainstreaming handicapped students.* Newton, MA: Allyn & Bacon.

Schmidt, H., & Rodgers-Rhyme, A. (1988). *Strategies: Effective practices for teaching all children (participant guide).* Madison, WI: Wisconsin State Department of Public Instruction, Bureau of Exceptional Children. (ERIC Document Reproduction Service No. ED 304 231)

Secord, W. (1989, November). *Developing a collaborative language program.* Paper presented at Oneida, NY.

Shapiro, H. (1992). Debatable issues underlying whole-language philosophy: A speech-language specialist's perspective. *Language, Speech, and Hearing Services in Schools, 23*, 308–311.

Simon, C. (1987). Out of the broom closet and into the classroom: The emerging speech-language specialist. *Journal of Childhood Communication Disorders, 11*, 41–66.

Simon, C., & Myrold-Gunyuz, P. (1990). *Into the classroom: The speech-language specialist in the collaborative role.* Tucson, AZ: Communication Skill Builders.

Snyder-McLean, L. (1984). Structuring joint action routines: A strategy for facilitating communication and language development in the classroom. *Seminars in Speech and Language, 5*, 213–228.

Sonnenmeier, R., & McGuire, K. (1995, March). *Supporting the communication skills of children's language learning needs in inclusive settings.* Paper presented at the Central New York Speech Language and Hearing Association Spring Conference. Syracuse, N.Y.

Stevens, D., & Englert, C. (1993). Making writing strategies work. *Teaching Exceptional Children, 26* (1), 34–39.

Swank, L. (1994). Phonological coding ability: Identification of impairments related to phonologically based reading problems. *Topics in Language Disorders, 14* (2), 56–71.

Temple, C., & Gillett, J.W. (1984). *Language arts learning processes and teaching practices.* Boston: Little, Brown.

van Kleeck, A. (1990). Emergent literacy: Learning about print before learning to read. *Topics in Language Disorders, 10*, 25–45.

Venkatagiri, H.S. (1995). Techniques for enhancing communication productivity: A review of research. *American Journal of Speech-Language Pathology, 4* (4), 36–45.

Wadle, S. (1991). Clinical exchange: Why speech-language clinicians should be in the classroom. *Language, Speech, and Hearing Services in Schools, 22* (3), 277.

Watters, B.T. (1994). Idea swap: Using CD-ROM to teach speech and language. *Word of Mouth, 6*, 10.

Westby, C. (1994). Advanced communication development. In W. Haynes & B. Shulman (Eds.). *Communication development: Foundations, processes and clinical applications* (pp. 341–384). Englewood Cliffs, NJ: Prentice-Hall.

Westby, C., & Cutler, S. (1994). Language and ADHD: understanding the bases and treatment of self-regulatory deficits. *Topics in Language Disorders, 14* (4), 58–76.

Wiig, E., & Wilson, C. (1994). Is a question a question? Passage understanding by preadolescents with learning disabilities. *Language, Speech, and Hearing Services in Schools, 25*, 241–250.

Zarrella, S. (1995). Specialization facilitates service delivery in schools. *Advance, 5* (29), 3, 15.

Part III

Contemporary Issues

Chapter 9

Augmentative and Alternative Communication in the Schools

Mary Ann Romski, Rose A. Sevcik, and Wendy L. Sundgren

Try to imagine what your world would be like if you could not communicate. Every day school-aged children with severe spoken communication disabilities face social and educational isolation as well as significant levels of frustration because they are unable to express their wants, needs, desires, knowledge, and feelings to other children and adults. Their ability to benefit from educational opportunities is significantly compromised.

Over the last two decades, new approaches (e.g., manual signs, communication boards, and electronic communication devices that speak) have been developed to provide avenues by which children with severe spoken communication disabilities can develop functional communication skills. These approaches are all forms of augmentative and alternative communication (AAC). Exhibit 9–1 recounts one student's success after experience with an augmentative communication approach.

Preparation of this chapter was supported in part by NICHD-06016, which sustains the Language Research Center of Georgia State University. Additional support was provided by a Chancellor's Initiative Grant, the Department of Communication and the College of Arts and Sciences, Georgia State University.

The purpose of this chapter is to provide an overview of how AAC systems are employed in school speech-language pathology programs. Particular attention is given to recommended assessment and intervention practices for children with severe spoken communication disabilities and the roles that speech-language pathologists play in AAC service delivery.

OVERVIEW OF AUGMENTATIVE AND ALTERNATIVE COMMUNICATION

To provide an introduction to the field of augmentative and alternative communication, we present some basic definitions, a bit of history, and discuss the influence of social policy issues on AAC service delivery in the schools.

Definitions

AAC is an area of clinical practice that attempts to compensate (either temporarily or permanently) for the impairment and disability patterns of individuals with severe expressive communication disorders (i.e., the se-

Exhibit 9–1 Example of Student's Success with AAC

TE was a 12-year-old student with a primary diagnosis of severe mental retardation accompanied by mild cerebral palsy and significant behavior problems. He communicated primarily via unintelligible vocalizations and gestures. Although he had a cardboard communication board with a few pictures on it, he was not making progress toward spontaneous functional communication. Initially, our primary goal for TE was to determine if he could benefit from a high-technology device with speech output and learn to use it for spontaneous communicative interaction.

In 1985, TE began to participate in an experimental AAC project and was provided with a speech-output communication system. TE accessed the device by pointing to symbols on a touch-sensitive display. Prior to the introduction of the system, his family and teachers participated in a series of instructional sessions during which they learned how to operate the system and use it for communication.

TE was successful! He quickly learned to use the system to communicate a variety of messages. By the end of the next school year, he had a vocabulary of over 75 symbols that he used singly or in combination to express greetings and basic wants and needs as well as to answer questions and interact with unfamiliar partners. After 2 years of experience with the system, TE was given an opportunity to move into a higher functioning classroom. He interacted and developed friendships with typical peers. At home, TE's behavior improved as well. His family reported increased sociability that permitted them to feel more comfortable with TE's presence in the community and made it easier to live with him on a day-to-day basis. In addition, his attention to educational tasks increased, and his overall speech intelligibility improved significantly so that some words were understandable by strangers. Other educational improvements were also evident. He had made a smooth transition from the elementary to the junior high school setting and now had a sight-reading vocabulary of 25 words.

Source: Reprinted with permission from M.A. Romski & R.A. Sevcik, *Breaking the Speech Barrier: Language Development through Augmented Means*, pp. 172–174, © 1996, Paul H. Brookes, Baltimore, MD 21285-0624.

verely speech-language and writing impaired) (American Speech-Language-Hearing Association [ASHA], 1989, p. 107). Any intervention that uses AAC should incorporate the individual's full communication abilities. These abilities may include any existing speech or vocalizations, gestures, manual signs, and aided communication (ASHA, 1991, p. 10). In this sense, then, AAC is truly multimodal, permitting a student to use every mode possible to communicate information and ideas. AAC abilities may change over time, although sometimes very slowly, and thus the AAC system chosen today may not be the system of tomorrow (Beukelman & Mirenda, 1992).

An AAC system is an integrated group of four components used by an individual to en-hance communication (ASHA, 1991, p. 10). These components are symbols, aids, techniques, and/or strategies.

A *symbol* is a "visual, auditory, and/or tactile representation of conventional concepts" (ASHA, 1991, p. 10). Symbols can be considered aided or unaided. Gestures, manual sign sets, and spoken words are unaided. Aided forms include visual graphic representations such as objects, pictures, photographs, line drawings, written words, and Braille.

An *aid* is "a physical object or device used to transmit or receive messages" (ASHA, 1991, p. 10). AAC aids, for example, are communication books, communication boards, charts, and mechanical or electronic devices, including those that speak and computers. Figures 9–1, 9–2, and 9–3 illustrate

AAC devices being used by students with a range of disabilities.

A *technique* is the method by which an individual transmits messages. Techniques can be divided into two broad categories: direct selection and scanning. Direct selection allows the student to communicate specific messages from a large set of options. Direct-selection techniques include pointing, signing, natural gesturing, and touching (see Figures 9–1 and 9–3). Some students use head pointers, headsticks, or eye gaze (or eye pointing) to select items. Scanning is a technique in which the message elements are presented to the student sequentially (see Figure 9–2). The student specifies a choice by responding to the person or device presenting the elements. Scanning techniques include linear scanning, row-column scanning, and encoding (ASHA, 1991, p. 10). Encoding is a technique whereby the student uses a code to convey messages (e.g., Morse code).

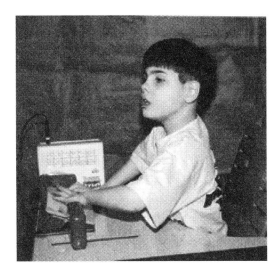

Figure 9–2. Another elementary school student employs a microswitch (here a switch that requires pressure to activate) to access his speech-output communication device. *Source:* Photo courtesy of Maryann Howell.

Strategies are specific ways in which the AAC aids, symbols, and techniques are used to develop and/or enhance communication. A strategy includes the intervention plan for facilitating an individual's performance (ASHA, 1991, p. 10).

History of the AAC Field

AAC is a relatively young field. Its origins date back to the early 1970s, when speech-language pathologists began informally discussing the use of AAC devices and techniques for their clients. The International Society for Augmentative and Alternative Communication (ISAAC) was formed in 1983 at an international gathering in East Lansing, Michigan. *Augmentative and Alternative Communication*, the field's scholarly journal, was established in 1985. Since that time, the field of AAC has seen many developments, including advances in assessment

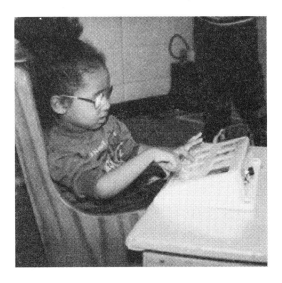

Figure 9–1. A preschool student uses direct selection by pointing to access a six-item display on her AAC device. *Source:* Photo courtesy of Maryann Howell.

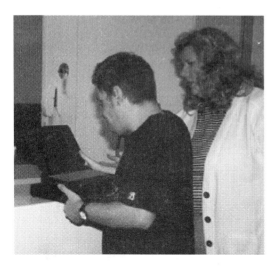

Figure 9–3. Using a laptop computer with communication software, a high-school student uses direct selection to communicate with his teacher at a job training site. *Source:* Photo courtesy of Maryann Howell.

and intervention as well as increases in the number and type of available communication technologies (see Zangari, Lloyd, & Vicker, 1994, for a historical overview of the field). Recently, ASHA has formed a Special Interest Division on AAC (Division 12). This division provides a forum for exchange of information, continuing education, and discussion of issues related to AAC service delivery.

Influence of Social Policy on AAC Service Delivery

Broad changes in social policy have played an important role in increasing the delivery of AAC services in the schools. Federal legislation has addressed issues related to education, assistive technology devices and services, and, most recently, civil rights.

More than 20 years ago, in 1975, the passage of the Education for All Handicapped Children Act (Pub. L. No. 94-142) guaranteed all children from 5 to 21 years of age, regardless of their disability, the right to a free and appropriate public education, including related services (such as speech and language) that they needed to obtain that education. In 1986, the Education of the Handicapped Amendments (Pub. L. No. 99-457) amended this act to include children as young as 3 years of age and, in some states, children at birth. In addition, they included educational planning for young children within the family system. In 1990, the Education for All Handicapped Children Act was reauthorized as the Individuals with Disabilities Education Act (IDEA; Pub. L. No. 101-476). It continues to entitle all children to a free and appropriate education and now includes planning the transition from the educational environment to postschool living environments, including work, community/residence, and leisure and recreation. During 1996, IDEA is undergoing reauthorization by Congress.

In 1988, the Technology-Related Assistance Act (Pub. L. No. 100-407) was passed by Congress and highlighted the role that assistive technology devices and services can play in ensuring that people with disabilities are able to participate fully in society. An assistive technology device is defined as any item, piece of equipment, or product system, whether commercially off the shelf, modified, or customized, that is used to increase, maintain, or improve functional capabilities of individuals with disabilities. AAC devices are assistive technology devices. Under Title I of this act, funding was provided to states through the National Institute for Disability and Rehabilitation Research (NIDRR) for the development of consumer-driven assistive technology programs whose goal is the comprehensive incorporation of assistive technology devices and services into extant public and private service delivery systems (e.g., education, rehabilitation).

Most recently, the Americans with Disabilities Act of 1990 (Pub. L. No. 101-336) was signed into law. This landmark piece of legislation guarantees the basic civil rights of persons with disabilities and addresses the employment and educational access challenges they encounter. The use of AAC devices can facilitate both employment and educational access. The effects of this legislation are now beginning to enhance the participation of people with disabilities in our society.

The impact of two decades of federal legislation is that children with severe spoken communication disabilities now have a basic right to be included in all aspects of our society and be provided with the supports needed for inclusion. A fundamental support for the successful implementation of any and all of this legislation is communication. Without the ability to communicate, often through AAC systems, education, employment, and inclusion in general are clearly compromised.

SCHOOL-AGED CHILDREN WHO USE AAC

A wide range of school-aged children with severe spoken communication disabilities can benefit from the use of AAC systems. These children include those with congenital as well as acquired disabilities. Congenital disabilities include cerebral palsy, cognitive disabilities, dual sensory impairments, developmental apraxia of speech, learning disabilities, multiple disabilities, autism, specific language impairment (SLI), and pervasive developmental disabilities. Acquired disabilities include traumatic brain injury (TBI), aphasia, and a range of physical disabilities (e.g., spinal cord injuries, muscular degeneration).

ROLES AAC CAN PLAY

The roles that AAC systems play in a child's educational program can vary depending on the type and severity of the child's disability. Among these roles are augmenting existing speech, providing an output mode for communication, providing an input and an output mode for language and communication, and serving as a language intervention strategy. For example, Johnny is in middle school and has severely dysarthric speech due to cerebral palsy. His speech is intelligible only to familiar communicative partners. When he goes to the cafeteria to order lunch, the server cannot understand his speech. An AAC system can serve to augment Johnny's existing speech in situations when it is difficult to understand him. AAC serves a very different role for Annie, who is 3 years old and has severe spastic cerebral palsy, almost age-appropriate speech comprehension skills, and a few undifferentiated vocalizations. For Annie, AAC serves as an output mode as well as a language-teaching strategy.

AAC SERVICE DELIVERY

The delivery of AAC services to children with severe spoken communication disabilities requires the collaboration and competence of families, professionals, and paraprofessionals (National Joint Committee, 1992). A broad-based communication assessment and intervention plan is best implemented in *all contexts* of the child's daily life and coordinated by a team of people who can manage the many and varied components of the plan. A collaborative team approach to service delivery incorporates families and a range of professional disciplines including, though not limited to, speech-language pathologists, regular and special educators, physical and occupational therapists, and psychologists (see Catlett, 1993, for a discussion of teams).

To develop and implement an AAC team, a team philosophy is necessary. For example, the National Joint Committee on the Communication Needs of Persons with Severe Disabilities (1992) proposed a set of 12 communication rights that all persons, regardless of the degree or severity of their disabilities, must have. These rights, found in Exhibit 9–2, provide a clear and specific philosophy on which current speech-language AAC service delivery systems, including assessment and intervention, must be founded.

In 1989, ASHA identified nine responsibilities of the speech-language pathologist when providing AAC services: (a) identification of appropriate AAC candidates, (b) determination of appropriate AAC systems for students, (c) development of extensive intervention plans for students to achieve "maximal functional communication," (d) implementation of the intervention plan, (e) evaluation of the intervention outcomes, (f) evaluation and awareness of the new AAC technology and strategies, (g) advocacy in the AAC area, (h) provision of inservices to professionals and consumers and (i) coordination of AAC services.

Conventional "pull-out" therapy approaches, by themselves, have not successfully accommodated the communication de-

Exhibit 9–2 Communication Bill of Rights

1. The right to request desired objects, actions, events, and persons and to express personal preferences or feelings
2. The right to be offered choices and alternatives
3. The right to reject or refuse undesired objects, events, or actions, including the right to decline or reject all proffered choices
4. The right to request, and be given, attention from and interaction with another person
5. The right to request feedback or information about a state, an object, a person, or an event of interest
6. The right to active treatment and intervention efforts to enable people with severe disabilities to communicate messages in whatever modes and as effectively and efficiently as their specific abilities will allow
7. The right to have communication acts acknowledged and responded to, even when the intent of these acts cannot be fulfilled by the responder
8. The right to have access at all times to any needed augmentative and alternative communication devices and other assistive devices and to have those devices in good working order
9. The right to environmental contexts, interactions, and opportunities that expect and encourage persons with disabilities to participate as full communicative partners with other people, including peers
10. The right to be informed about the people, things, and events in one's immediate environment
11. The right to be communicated with in a manner that recognizes and acknowledges the inherent dignity of the person being addressed, including the right to be part of communication exchanges about individuals that are conducted in his or her presence
12. The right to be communicated with in ways that are meaningful, understandable, and culturally and linguistically appropriate

Source: Reprinted with permission from Communication Bill of Rights, *ASHA*, Vol. 34, No. 7, pp. 2–3, © 1992, the American Speech-Language-Hearing Association.

velopment of students who employ AAC systems. Pull-out therapy approaches have failed because they do not facilitate the student's communicative use of AAC in the classroom during daily educational activities. The most effective model for providing AAC services appears to be the transdisciplinary model. This approach involves sharing of information and expertise among team members and requires that all team members have some proficiency in areas in which they ordinarily are not involved. All team members participate in the evaluation, and once the collaborative evaluation has been completed, the team meets to identify the student's needs. At this time, goals and objectives are targeted on the basis of the student's needs, with the entire team responsible for implementation. All team members are equally responsible for carrying out decisions regarding assessment, intervention, and follow-up.

The benefits gained through a transdisciplinary approach include promoting assessment of and intervention with students among a variety of people in different environments, ensuring that the expertise of all team members is shared, making every team member equally responsible, and mandating the coordination of educational services. A more comprehensive view of the student's communication skills is obtained, and this ensures that the student receives communication opportunities across the school day. Team members are more prepared to intervene in all aspects of the student's AAC intervention program. Through the team approach, gaps are eliminated in service, and generalization of communication skills is facilitated.

RECOMMENDED AAC ASSESSMENT PRACTICES

Assessment is an ongoing process. For children with severe spoken communication dis-

abilities, the purpose of assessment is to characterize within a functional context the student's communicative strengths and weaknesses and to determine what type of AAC system can meet these needs. Two outcomes of assessment are (a) to recommend the most appropriate AAC aids and techniques and (b) to set goals for a course of AAC intervention that will permit the child to develop functional communication.

Not surprisingly, standardized speech and language assessment batteries (as well as standardized psychological tests) are difficult to employ with children with severe spoken communication disabilities because of the severity of their oral communication impairments. These assessments may not reveal an accurate picture of the student's abilities because many of them are language based and may be biased against a student who is nonverbal. Often, the children are unable to obtain basal scores on tests, or their scores are so far below those of their chronological age peers that converting a raw score into a standard score is not possible. Some of the factors that may influence these outcomes include unfamiliar examiners, lack of a communication-output mode, difficulty understanding the requirements of the task, stimuli that are too complex (e.g., line drawings), and stimuli that are configured in a difficult manner (e.g., 2 × 2 display on the Peabody Picture Vocabulary Test-Revised; Dunn & Dunn, 1981). It is, therefore, more typical to employ informal measures and systematic behavioral observation within usual environments than to employ standardized tests within isolated settings with children who will use AAC systems (Romski & Sevcik, 1995).

Evaluation of Functional Communication

Functional communication assessment includes three primary components: (a) the child's current communication development (i.e., comprehension skills, communication mode, extant skills), (b) the child's environments (i.e., partners, opportunities; Reichle, Mirenda, Locke, Piche, & Johnson, 1992) and (c) the child's physical abilities to access communication. Relevant assessment begins with systematic behavioral observations in everyday environments and informal measures that inventory and describe these components.

The Child's Current Communication Development

Communication can be defined in the broadest sense as "any act by which one person gives to or receives from another person information about that person's needs, desires, perceptions, knowledge, or affective states" (National Joint Committee, 1992, p. 2). The modes by which children can communicate range along a representational continuum from symbolic (e.g., spoken words, manual signs, arbitrary visual-graphic symbols, printed words) to iconic (e.g., real objects, photographs, line drawings, pictographic visual-graphic symbols) to nonsymbolic (e.g., signals such as crying or physical movement; see Sevcik, Romski, & Wilkinson, 1991, for a discussion of visual-graphic representational systems). Even though some children exhibit conventional modes of communication, such as vocalizations and gestures, these modes may limit the breadth of function that their communications can convey to familiar and unfamiliar partners across multiple environments (Romski, Sevcik, Reumann, & Pate, 1989).

Visual skills are a crucial component of the AAC assessment. These skills directly affect the size and type of symbols a student can use, how these symbols are arranged, and the type of output options available. Children with vi-

sual impairments may require specialized system considerations. For example, it may be necessary to arrange all the symbols in one location to account for visual field loss or to use an electronic speech output device with auditory scanning capabilities for a child with a severe visual impairment but intact auditory abilities.

Young typical children learn to comprehend spoken language before they begin to speak (Golinkoff & Hirsh-Pasek, 1990; Huttenlocher, 1974). For children with severe spoken communication disabilities, it is important to ascertain the level of speech comprehension they currently exhibit. If standardized language comprehension tests, such as the Peabody Picture Vocabulary Test-Revised (Dunn & Dunn, 1981), are not appropriate, informal measures, such as a portion of the Clinical Assessment of Language Comprehension (Miller & Paul, 1995) adapted for use, may provide an indication of the child's receptive abilities in context.

The child's ability to act intentionally on partners in their environments and to affect the behaviors of those partners plays an important role in language and communication development. Communicative intentions vary along a continuum from prelocutionary to locutionary (McLean & Snyder-McLean, 1988). As shown in Table 9–1, the modes children use to make their wants and needs known to their partners and the role partners play in the interaction will vary with children's status along the continuum.

Some children with severe spoken communication disabilities who have no conventional way to communicate may express their communicative wants and needs in socially unacceptable ways, such as through aggressive or destructive means (e.g., Donnellan, Mirenda, Mesaros, & Fassbender, 1984; Doss & Reichle, 1991). The presence of aggres-

Table 9–1 Continuum of Communicative/Linguistic Skills

Communicative Intentionality	Communicative Role		Communicative Form
	Child	Partner	
Perlocutionary			
Reactive	Passive	Active	Cry, eye gaze, laugh, movement, "fussing"
Proactive	Active	Active	Reach
Illocutionary			
Primitive	Active	Active	Physical manipulation
Conventional	Active	Active	Point, vocalization with inflection
Locutionary			
Emerging	Active	Active	Words, signs, graphic symbols combined with gesture and vocalization
Conventional	Active	Active	Words, signs, graphic symbols

Source: Reprinted with permission from M. Romski and R. Sevcik, Communicative Development of Children with Severe Disabilities in *Childhood Language Disorders*, by MD Smith and JS Damico, eds., p. 223, © 1995, Thieme Medical Publishers, Inc.

sive, self-stimulatory, and perseverative behaviors should be addressed during the assessment process. Adaptations may be required for students with extremely challenging behaviors.

The Child's Environments

Second, all of the child's environments may not support communication. What types of opportunities does each environment provide to promote communication? Sometimes the opportunities vary across environments and even across partners within environments. Exhibit 9–3 provides a list of suggested components for an assessment of environments (National Joint Committee, 1992). Third, when no everyday environment appears to provide opportunities for communications, the practitioner can set up a situation in which to elicit intentional communication from the child (see Cirrin & Rowland, 1985, for an example). Finally, the child may be at an earlier point along the continuum of communication development and may not exhibit intentional communication. In this case, the environment should be configured to support communication by, for example, setting up routines (see Siegel-Causey & Guess, 1989, for a detailed discussion of nonsymbolic assessment and treatment strategies).

The Child's Physical Abilities

Motor skills play an important role when determining the most appropriate AAC system for a child. Students who are ambulatory require portable communication systems. For children who are nonambulatory, appropriate seating and positioning are crucial for successful communication.

The child may not have physical access to a mode by which to communicate. If physical access is an issue, an evaluation for alternative forms of access may be appropriate. There are now a range of microswitches and eye-pointing techniques that are available to

Exhibit 9–3 Assessment of the Environment

1. Identify the familiar and unfamiliar partners for communication in each environment.
2. Describe the opportunities (frequency and type) for communication typically observed in each environment.
3. Compare the opportunities for communication among the different environments and partners within each environment.
4. Determine the proportion of communications that are responded to appropriately and inappropriately in each environment.
5. Identify the specific communicative modes and functions that might be useful in each environment.
6. Identify the partners in each environment who have relatively high rates of permitting, accepting, and responding to the communications of the children.

Source: Reprinted with permission from M. Romski and R. Sevcik, Communicative Development of Children with Severe Disabilities in *Childhood Language Disorders*, by MD Smith and JS Damico, eds., p. 224, © 1995, Thieme Medical Publishers, Inc.

interface with computer-based technology so as to permit the child to make a response and access a mode by which to communicate (see Figure 9–2 and Beukelman & Mirenda, 1992; York & Weimann, 1991, for detailed descriptions of alternative access issues).

Another dimension of physical access is seating and positioning. Successful use of a communication system can be a direct result of proper seating and positioning (McEwen & Lloyd, 1990). It is important, for example, for all members of the team to ensure that the student is properly positioned and to be confident in making adjustments when necessary. McEwen and Lloyd (1990) suggested that the position providing the greatest intellectual, social, and functional benefits is the upright, seated position in a wheelchair. Although there are exceptions, the wheelchair should be considered the primary position of choice when using an AAC system in an educational setting (McEwen & Lloyd, 1990).

RECOMMENDED AAC INTERVENTION PRACTICES

Obtaining an AAC device for a child is just the beginning of the intervention proc-

ess. Once an AAC assessment is complete and a specific AAC device is recommended, the AAC team must design and implement an AAC intervention plan to meet the ongoing communication needs of the child. The roles that AAC can play vary depending on the child's chronological age, disability, and individual needs. As previously mentioned, these roles include augmenting existing speech, providing an output mode for communication, providing an input and an output mode for communication, and serving as a language intervention strategy. Although the child's disability may provide some guidance about where to begin along the intervention continuum, it will not dictate the specific intervention. For example, manual signs have been employed with some documented success by children with autism (Carr & Kologinsky, 1983). This success does not mean that manual signs should automatically be employed with every child who has a diagnosis of autism.

Regardless of the role AAC plays for the child, four broad goals, which are often focused on simultaneously, must be at the core of any child's AAC intervention program: (a) acquiring proficiency with the physical operation of the AAC aid/technique, (b) developing language and communication interaction skills, (c) using AAC systems in inclusive settings, and (d) developing natural speech and literacy abilities.

Acquiring Proficiency with the Physical Operation and Use of the AAC Aid/Technique

The first step in using an AAC mode is to access it. If the child is using an unaided mode, like manual signs, access means teaching the physical production of the signs. The speech-language pathologist must ensure that the child's physical productions of the signs are interpretable by familiar and unfamiliar communicative partners. Sometimes, for example, young children with Down syndrome reach a plateau in terms of the number of intelligible manual signs that they produce that are distinguishable one from the other. This plateau is often due to limitations in the child's fine-motor skills and results in familiar partners' having to interpret sign use. Such an outcome may suggest a reassessment of the appropriateness of manual sign for the particular child.

For aided systems, access means that the child and/or his or her familiar communicative partners must be able to operate the electronic device physically. Such operation includes turning it on and off, programming it with a functional vocabulary, ensuring that its battery is always charged, and knowing the procedures to follow for maintenance and repair. If alternative access, such as a microswitch, is required, the child may also need specific practice in operating the device using the switch. Often, a familiar communicative partner must support the child's operation of the device by ensuring that it is in good working order (e.g., battery charged, de-

vice programmed with the appropriate vocabulary).

Developing Language and Communication Interaction Skills

For most children with congenital disabilities, language and communication development is the most important goal of AAC intervention. Depending on the child's current language and communication skills, this goal may range from developing a basic vocabulary of single symbols or signs to express basic wants and needs (see, e.g., Reichle, York, & Sigafoss, 1991; Romski & Sevcik, 1996) to using sentences of symbols and signs to convey complex communicative messages (see, e.g., Beukelman & Mirenda, 1992).

Regardless of the child's current communication skills, vocabulary development is a critical area of emphasis for AAC interventions (Beukelman & Mirenda, 1992). From the time young typical children are 18 months old, they are learning at least two to three new words a day. When they begin elementary school, they have a vocabulary of approximately 6,000 words (Berko-Gleason, 1992). Because vocabulary must be selected and then taught to the children (i.e., manual signs) or programmed into an electronic device, the children often do not have complete control over the choice of their own vocabulary. Thus sometimes what the children can and cannot say is beyond their own power. Including children in vocabulary choice and frequently reflecting on changing vocabulary needs (e.g., transitions from preschool to elementary school, new settings of use) are critical to successful communication.

The issue of grammatical development is also important for children who are beginning to develop grammatical morphemes, word order, and sentence structure. Some recent advances in computer technology permit the child to use one or a few keystrokes to produce an entire sentence. Although these approaches reduce the physical demands of system operation and give the perception that the child is "speaking" in sentences, they do not necessarily facilitate the child's own grammatical development. When the AAC team recommends such an approach, they must be aware of the impact of such a decision on the child's overall language development. Recent technological advances are beginning to address this issue by overtly incorporating grammatical markers in software programs that permit the marking of grammatical morphemes (e.g., past tense, plural, present progressive).

One important reason for developing vocabulary and grammar is to use it for communication and to advance the child's education. In communication interactions, the child must be both sender and receiver of messages to familiar and unfamiliar adult and peer partners. Communicative partners, then, play a critical role in the facilitation of communicative interaction skills. They must be comfortable talking to the child using the AAC device and serving as a communicative model, and they should be aware of strategies they may use that may facilitate or inhibit AAC use.

Using AAC Systems in Inclusive Environments

It is essential that AAC system use take place in inclusive environments. The literature strongly suggests that AAC systems can effectively be embedded within ongoing events of everyday life (Romski & Sevcik, 1988). Using AAC systems in inclusive settings requires that the team work together to

ensure that the child has access to his or her AAC device across the school day and that all adults and children who may interact with the child serve to support the child's communications. Such inclusive use may present a range of challenges. For example, the social studies teacher may have little experience with an AAC device and may need some inservice instruction about AAC. In general, the team may need to provide information about AAC device operation and communicative use to the classroom teacher as well as other students in the classes through a lesson, to set up a peer tutor program, and to troubleshoot any challenges as they arise.

Developing Natural Speech and Literacy Abilities

Developing natural speech and developing literacy abilities are extremely important, though often neglected, goals of AAC intervention. The literature suggests that the use of AAC systems may result in increases in vocalizations and sometimes intelligible speech and literacy (Kopenhaver, Pierce, & Yoder, 1995; Romski & Sevcik, 1996). For example, after 2 years of experience with a speech-output communication device, Jimmy's unintelligible vocalizations for the symbols on his device were transformed into understandable words. His recognition of printed English words improved as well. Unfortunately, speech-language pathologists frequently do not place much emphasis on the development of natural speech and/or literacy skills. When a child begins AAC intervention, the speech-language pathologist must have an estimate of the child's natural speech and literacy abilities. As the AAC intervention proceeds, the speech-language pathologist should monitor and support changes in these abilities by providing specific interventions directed toward the facilitation of these important goals.

CURRENT ISSUES FOR SCHOOL SPEECH-LANGUAGE PATHOLOGISTS

A number of issues related to AAC are currently facing speech-language pathologists who work in the schools. These include, though they are not limited to, funding for AAC devices and services, the rapid development of new technologies, and the use of controversial treatment approaches.

Funding for AAC Devices and Services

There are two types of funding concerns in the schools: funding for individual devices and funding for AAC services. A range of funding sources are available for the purchase of individual AAC devices. These include but are not limited to local or state educational and/or rehabilitation agencies, private medical insurance, public health assistance, and charitable agencies, foundations, and corporations.

Local educational agencies will often fund the cost of AAC devices when these are used for educational purposes and are included in the child's Individualized Education Plan (IEP). Some school systems will permit the child to take the AAC device home for certain periods of time if the parent or guardian is willing to accept responsibility for the AAC device if it is lost, stolen, or damaged. One drawback to this type of funding is that when the child graduates or leaves school, the device remains the property of the local educational agency.

As the child makes the transition to adult life and employment, state rehabilitation agencies may be a source for funding an AAC device. An evaluation detailing how the AAC device will assist the individual in preparing for, getting, or keeping employment is usually required.

Another option for funding an AAC device is the family's private medical insurance. To obtain funding through this source, medical necessity must be demonstrated. A proposal or a justification statement indicating the nature of the need and the exact cost of the AAC device must be written. The justification statement involves submitting information regarding the expected benefits, a physician's order, and a speech-language evaluation report, as well as OT and PT reports as needed, indicating the medical necessity of the purchase (ABLEDATA, 1993). When submitting a claim to a medical insurance company, it is important to review the insurance policy. Insurance companies usually fund AAC devices under the following areas: durable medical equipment, prosthetics, and orthopedics. Determine the specific terminology used in the family's insurance policy, and use it in all correspondence with the company. Sometimes a claim is denied, and an appeal is necessary to obtain AAC device funding.

The second area of funding is for the delivery of AAC services in the schools. AAC services are expensive because they require costly equipment and a large amount of personnel time. Local educational agencies must be creative in how they fund AAC services. For example, speech-language pathology services may combine resources with special education services to fund equipment. As well, informal agreements can be developed with school principals to ensure that the speech-language pathologist can adjust his or her schedule to provide services within appropriate times during the school day (e.g., in the lunchroom, during work training).

Rapid Development of New Technology

One striking characteristic of the AAC field today is the rapid development of new technologies. Changes in the types of devices that are available occur so frequently that it may be difficult for the school speech-language pathologist to keep abreast of every device available. The following five features of AAC devices provide a framework by which to judge new technologies: (a) speech-output capabilities, (b) portability and durability, (c) cost factors (including initial device cost as well as the cost of maintenance and repair), (d) programming capabilities, and (e) the variety of input modes. Recent additions to the AAC device market are able to provide a range of capabilities within one device so that a child may be able to use one piece of equipment for a longer period of time.

Controversial Intervention Approaches

Over the last few years, speech-language pathologists have been faced with ethical issues related to controversial intervention approaches. One such approach, *facilitated communication*, or FC, is defined as a method, or group of methods, for providing assistance to a nonverbal person in typing letters, words, phrases, or sentences using a typewriter, computer keyboard, or alphabet facsimile. Facilitated communication involves a manual prompting procedure, with the intent of supporting a person's hand sufficiently to make it

more feasible to strike the keys he or she wishes to strike, without influencing key selection (Duchan, 1993).

Reports suggest that FC may facilitate literacy skills in the individuals who have used it (Biklin, 1993; Duchan, 1993). Though striking, these reports have created quite a bit of controversy. Results of quantitative research studies question who is actually producing the messages—the child or the facilitator (Wheeler, Jacobson, Paglieri, & Schwartz, 1993).

The speech-language pathologist must consider several important issues before using facilitated communication. First, FC should be considered within the context of a broader AAC intervention plan. Second, literacy should be viewed as continuously developing. It is extremely important to describe thoroughly an individual's written communication abilities during the AAC assessment process so that it is clear what skills the child brings to the intervention. Third, the goal for using FC must be *independent communication*. That is, the intervention must target goals that permit the child to communicate without the physical prompting or assistance of another person.

SUMMARY AND CONCLUSIONS

This chapter provided an overview of issues related to the use of AAC systems in the schools with children with severe spoken communication disabilities. Over the last decade, significant advances have been made in social policy, research, and practice. For children with severe spoken communication disabilities, an AAC assessment includes information about the child's communication development, environments, and physical abilities. It is also important to remember that assessment is an ongoing process that continues throughout the course of intervention. Change must be measured on an ongoing basis, and measurements must serve as a foundation for the reassessment of AAC intervention practices. Children with severe spoken communication disabilities who use AAC systems have indeed demonstrated communication achievements far beyond our clinical expectations. Speech-language pathologists have an ethical responsibility to give children with severe spoken communication disabilities the supports they need to develop functional communication so that they can be educated. Research and recommended practices are continuing to develop, and the communication future is certainly optimistic for children with severe spoken communication disabilities who may use AAC to communicate.

DISCUSSION QUESTIONS

1. What role does the speech-language pathologist play in AAC assessment and intervention? How can speech-language pathologists provide opportunities for parents to use AAC devices at home?

2. What components of a funding packet appear to facilitate obtaining an AAC device?

3. What strategies can you use to keep up with the rapid expansion and development of AAC technology?

REFERENCES

ABLEDATA. (1993). Finding funding for assistive technology. *Exceptional Parent, 23,* 18–28.

American Speech-Language-Hearing Association. (1989). Competencies for speech-language pathologists providing services in augmentative communication. *Asha, 31,* 107–110.

American Speech-Language-Hearing Association. (1991). Report: Augmentative and alternative communication. *Asha, 33* (Suppl. 5), 9–12.

Americans with Disabilities Act of 1990, Pub. L. No. 101-336.

Berko-Gleason, J. (1992). *Language development.* Columbus, OH: Merrill.

Beukelman, D.R., & Mirenda, P. (1992). *Augmentative and alternative communication.* Baltimore: Paul H. Brookes.

Biklin, D. (1993). *Communication unbound: How facilitated communication is challenging traditional views of autism and ability/disability.* New York: Teachers College Press.

Carr, E., & Kologinsky, E. (1983). Acquisition of sign language by autistic children II: Spontaneity and generalization effects. *Journal of Applied Behavior Analysis, 16,* 297–314.

Catlett, C. (1993). Teams and teamwork. *Asha, 35,* 30–31.

Cirrin, F., & Rowland, C. (1985). Communicative assessment of nonverbal youths with severe/profound mental retardation. *Mental Retardation, 23,* 52-62.

Donellan, A., Mirenda, P., Mesaros, R., & Fassbender, L. (1984). Analyzing the communicative functions of aberrant behavior. *Journal of the Association for Persons with Severe Handicaps, 9,* 141–150.

Doss, S., & Reichle, J. (1991). Replacing excess behavior with an initial communicative repertoire. In J. Reichle, J. York, & J. Sigafoos (Eds.), *Implementing augmentative and alternative communication: Strategies for learners with severe disabilities* (pp. 215–238). Baltimore: Paul H. Brookes.

Duchan, J. (1993). Issues raised by facilitated communication for theorizing and research on autism. *Journal of Speech and Hearing Research, 36,* 1108–1119.

Dunn, L., & Dunn, L. (1981). *Peabody Picture Vocabulary Test-Revised.* Circle Pines, MN: American Guidance Service.

Education for All Handicapped Children Act of 1975, Pub. L. No. 94-172.

Education of the Handicapped Amendments of 1986, Pub. L. No. 99-457.

Golinkoff, R., & Hirsh-Pasek, K. (1990). Let the mute speak: What infants can tell us about language acquisition. *Merrill-Palmer Quarterly, 36,* 67–91.

Huttenlocher, J. (1974). The origins of language comprehension. In R.L. Solso (Ed.) *Theories in cognitive psychology: The Loyola symposium* (pp.   ). Hillsdale, NJ: Lawrence Erlbaum.

Individuals with Disabilities Education Act of 1990, Pub. L. No. 101-476.

Koppenhaver, D., Pierce, P., & Yoder, D. (1995). AAC, FC, and the ABCs: Issues and relationships. *American Journal of Speech-Language Pathology, 4,* 5–14.

McEwen, I., & Lloyd, L. (1990). Positioning children with cerebral palsy to use augmentative and alternative communication. *Language, Speech, and Hearing Services in Schools, 21,* 15–21.

McLean, J., & Snyder-McLean, L. (1988). Applications of pragmatics to severely mentally retarded children and youth. In R.L. Schiefelbusch & L.L. Lloyd (Eds.). *Language perspectives: Acquisitions, retardation and intervention* (pp. 255–288). Austin, TX: Pro-Ed.

Miller, J., & Paul, R. (1995). *The clinical assessment of language comprehension.* Baltimore: Paul H. Brookes.

National Joint Committee for the Communicative Needs of Persons with Severe Disabilities (1992). Guidelines for meeting the communication needs of persons with severe disabilities. *Asha, 34* (Suppl. 7), 1–8.

Reichle, J., Mirenda, P., Locke, P., Piche, L., & Johnson, S. (1992). Beginning augmentative communication systems. In S. Warren & J. Reichle (Eds.), *Causes and effects in communication and language intervention* (pp. 131–156). Baltimore: Paul Brookes.

Reichle, J., York, J., & Sigafoos, J. (1991). *Implementing augmentative and alternative communication: Strategies for learners with severe disabilities.* Baltimore: Paul H. Brookes.

Romski, M.A., & Sevcik, R.A. (1988). Augmentative communication system acquisition and use: A model for teaching and assessing progress. *NSSLHA Journal, 16,* 61–75.

Romski, M.A., & Sevcik, R.A. (1995). Communication development of children with severe disabilities. In M.

Smith & J. Damico (Eds.). *Childhood language disorders* (pp. 218–234). New York: Thieme Medical Publishers, Inc.

Romski, M.A., & Sevcik, R.A. (1996). *Breaking the speech barrier: Language development through augmented means.* Baltimore: Paul H. Brookes.

Romski, M.A., Sevcik, R.A., Reumann, R., & Pate, J.L. (1989). Youngsters with moderate or severe retardation and severe spoken language impairments. I: Extant communication patterns. *Journal of Speech and Hearing Disorders, 54,* 366–373.

Sevcik, R. A., Romski, M. A., & Wilkinson, K. (1991). Roles of graphic symbols in the language acquisition process for persons with severe cognitive disabilities. *Augmentative and Alternative Communication, 7,* 161–170.

Siegel-Causey, E., & Guess, D. (1989). *Enhancing nonsymbolic communication interactions among learners with severe disabilities.* Baltimore: Paul H. Brookes.

Technology-Related Assistance Act of 1988, Pub. L. No. 100-407.

Wheeler, D., Jacobson, J., Paglieri, R., & Schwartz, A. (1993). An experimental assessment of facilitated communication. *Mental Retardation, 31,* 49–60.

York, J., & Weimann, G. (1991). Accommodating severe physical disabilities. In J. Reichle, J. York, & J. Sigafoos (Eds.). *Implementing augmentative and alternative communication: Strategies for learners with severe disabilities* (pp. 239–256). Baltimore: Paul H. Brookes.

Zangari, C., Lloyd, L., & Vicker, B. (1994). Augmentative and alternative communication: An historical perspective. *Augmentative and Alternative Communication, 10,* 27–59.

Chapter 10

Third-Party Payments, Supervision, and Support Personnel

Mary Ann O'Brien

The purpose of this chapter is to acquaint the reader with several key areas of current concern. The three topics of third-party payments, supervision, and support personnel share a core of administrative involvement. They are also important for the school practitioner. Each one provides evidence of the increasing complexity of the school environment as a service delivery site as well as the concomitant demands on the school speech-language pathologist to be a broadly educated and well-informed professional.

The appendices to this chapter provide additional depth in several areas, along with useful forms for various aspects of professional development and evaluation.

THIRD-PARTY REIMBURSEMENT

Although the intent of the laws that enable government-supported education to children with disabilities is noble, the reality is that Congress has never adequately provided the needed level of funding to support services and programs. This has created financial difficulty for local school districts. Out of need, schools have had to seek alternative methods of funding programs to help defray expenses for providing education and services to students with disabilities. Billing third-party payers for speech-language pathology and audiology services has long been an accepted practice in health care agencies and in private practice. In 1976, the federal government legislated access to third-party money for these same services delivered in schools. Although the possibility of bringing in additional funding for overburdened educational systems was enticing, it took several years for schools to understand the law and to undertake the complicated processes involved in collection and billing.

History

In 1975, Public Law No. 94-142, the Education for All Handicapped Children Act, was passed. It ensured the provision of a free and appropriate public education for all children at no cost to parents. The key phrase is "at no cost to parents." In 1977, the regulations interpreting the act were published. They indicated that states could use whatever state, local, federal, and private monies were available to meet the requirement of providing a free and appropriate public education. In spite of this clearly articulated intent, many third-party payers interpreted the law and regulations to mean that provision and funding of services were the responsibility of the schools and responded by discontinuing payment for services for children. Medicaid specifically denied payment for any services required in a child's Individualized Education Program (IEP), even if the child was eligible for Medicaid services (Wolf, 1991). This refusal to reimburse extended to the hospital and private practice settings, where it was Medicaid's position that speech-language pathology and audiology services for school-aged children were automatically educational and thus should be funded by education rather than health care funds.

In 1980, the Office of Special Education and the Office of Civil Rights, both in the U.S. Department of Education, jointly published a Notice of Interpretation saying that private insurance could be used by an educational agency only if parents incurred no financial loss and if their participation was voluntary. The inference was that private insurance *could* be used with parents' consent if they suffered no financial loss. Using this interpretation, a private agency in Illinois, the Trans-Allied Medical Educational Services, Inc. (TAMES), was established and worked very successfully with school districts in the state to obtain reimbursement for speech-language and audiology services provided in an education setting. The use of private insurance, however, can be hazardous. We will discuss this later in this section.

In 1986, Congress passed Public Law No. 99-457, the Education of the Handicapped Act Amendments (title changed in 1991 to Individuals With Disabilities Act—IDEA). It addressed the Medicaid funding issue and expanded special education and related services to children aged 3 to 5 years. It also added a new part, the Handicapped Infants and Toddlers Early Intervention Program (Part H), that encouraged states to provide early intervention services for handicapped

infants and toddlers at no cost. Congress indicated that with the passage of Public Law No. 99-457, it was the policy of the United States to provide financial assistance to states to facilitate the coordination of payment for early intervention services from federal, state, local, and private sources, including public and private insurance coverage (American Speech-Language-Hearing Association [ASHA], 1991). Part H also indicated that Part H funds were to be used as the "payer of last resort." No one was volunteering to be the payer of first resort!

In 1988, Public Law No. 100-360, the Medicare Catastrophic Coverage Act, was passed. Its purpose was to establish catastrophic coverage to pay for extended hospital stays and prescription drugs for older people. Unfortunately, the cost was prohibitive, and the act was eventually repealed. However, that act contained a Medicaid technical provision that was not overturned when the act was repealed. It notes that state education agencies are financially responsible for educational services. In the case of a Medicaid-eligible handicapped child, state Medicaid agencies remain responsible for the "related services" identified in the child's IEP if those services are covered under the state's Medicaid plan. Clearly, Congress is saying that Medicaid has to pay.

The last barrier to payment of Medicaid money for provision of certain related services in schools was eliminated in 1990, when the Health Care Financing Administration (HCFA) reversed its 1984 stance and proposed regulations that would cover services that are medical and remedial in nature. It still held that educational services are not reimbursable but defined educational services as pertaining to traditional academic subjects, such as science, history, literature, foreign language, and mathematics, and also talked about vocational services. This change in position was triggered by both the passage of Public Law No. 99-457 and a lost lawsuit in Massachusetts, in which the court ruled that determination of whether a service is educational should rest on the nature of the service and not on the state's method of administering the service (ASHA, 1992c).

Informed Consent

In its 1990 report to the Legislative Council, ASHA's Governmental Affairs Committee recommended that speech-language pathologists and audiologists know about informed-consent procedures and promote the use of the following guidelines by school administrators for informing parents:

- The IEP must be developed and signed *before* the family is requested to authorize third-party payments.

- The parent must grant informed, written consent to allow the school to bill medical insurance.

- The family should be informed in writing of the following facts:
  1. There is a risk to their lifetime health insurance cap if their insurance is used to pay for services in the schools.
  2. Consent to bill third-party payers is purely voluntary.
  3. Consent or lack of consent to bill third-party payers will not alter the quality, type, duration, or manner of speech-language pathology or audiology services that the child needs and receives.
  4. The child will receive all necessary speech-language pathology or audiology services even if the parents

deny consent to bill third-party payers.

- Speech-language pathologists and audiologists should recommend that as part of the informed-consent process, schools provide families with a written projection of the amount expected to be billed to the family insurance. In addition, the amount actually billed to the insurance company must be disclosed to the family.

Private Third-Party Payers

Initially, there was confusion about whether and when schools could access private insurance money, but in 1980, through a Notice of Interpretation, the U.S. Department of Education notified states that Part B of IDEA and Section 504 of the Rehabilitation Act of 1973, and their implementing regulations, allow use of private insurance when parents incur no financial loss and when the use of that insurance is voluntary.

Wolf (1991) wrote that private health insurance carriers will not allow their potential liabilities to increase and that the billing of private third-party payers for "related services" in the schools has had negative repercussions. He noted that health insurance plans that do provide coverage designate limits on the amount of treatment. Insurance plans also have a lifetime cap specifying the total dollar amount that the plan will cover over an individual's lifetime. If payments for "related services" in the schools reach the lifetime cap, a child may be left without health care coverage for the rest of his or her life. Wolf was concerned that billing the third-party payer for services in the schools may either deplete the specific coverage or exhaust the lifetime cap. He and others argued that risking the lifetime cap in this manner violates the child's right to free public education. Accessing private health insurance remains voluntary for the parents and a risk to future insurance benefits.

Inasmuch as federal law allows the billing of private insurance companies, and inasmuch as Medicaid is the payer of last resort, many schools are investigating the use of private insurance before accessing Medicaid monies. Speech-language pathologists and audiologists must be aware of coinsurance and deductible insurance requirements. School districts must absorb these costs for children aged 3 through 21 years, on the basis of the "free and appropriate public education" language in Public Law No. 94-142 (ASHA, 1991). Speech-language pathologists and audiologists must also know individual state requirements for students from birth to 2 years, 11 months (Early Intervention). If insurance problems occur for an individual family, that family may have to bring suit against the school district to attempt to recoup damages. Employees of that district should be as aware of the requirements of the law in these cases as is the administration. Ignorance is never an excuse.

Issues

No radical change of national proportions flows smoothly at its onset. Third-party billing for certain related services in schools is no exception. Speech-language pathologists and audiologists have become competitors for third-party funds. Members of the professions "took sides," depending upon their work site. Those in *favor* of schools' billing said that the possible benefits included

- additional money for an overburdened educational system

- money for schools and programs in need
- more favorable budgetary consideration for speech-language pathologists and audiologists because of the funds resulting from their work
- increased number of qualified providers, triggered by the incentive to raise the requirements for school speech-language pathologists in states that do not require a master's degree
- more service for rural and other underserved populations
- a new market for practitioners who can bill directly and serve as consultants—a new career track for school speech-language pathologists and audiologists
- increased attention to the parameters of informed consent
- better accountability practices

Those *opposed* to schools' billing said the most negative issues were

- increased insurance claims and private insurance companies' dropping coverage of speech-language and audiology services
- haphazard policies and procedures established by states and resulting ethical problems
- paucity of supervisors and monitors
- professional liability involving physician referral, credentials, and service
- increased documentation; decreased child contact time
- the possible bankruptcy of two underfunded and overextended systems (education and Medicaid)
- caseload management: needs versus available time
- parents not fully informed

- the money generated flowing into the general fund and not into the speech-language pathology and audiology program
- different standards for determining service needs in private practice and public school settings

One of the issues mentioned above, that of qualified providers, continues to cause heated debate in several states. Public Law No. 99-457, the Education of the Handicapped Act Amendments of 1986, included a "Qualified Personnel" section requiring states to ensure that school personnel meet the highest education and training standards applicable to a particular profession. Those standards are as different as the states themselves. In some states, it is a master's degree; in some it is a bachelor's degree; in still others, it is a state license or ASHA certification. To be an eligible provider—that is, one whose services are eligible for Medicaid reimbursement—the speech-language pathologist and audiologist must usually hold the highest required credential in the state. Where there is conflict between or among a given state's agencies, confusion proliferates.

As the enrolled provider, the school district must ensure that services are provided by staff who meet state licensure and other payer credential requirements. If these requirements are not met, the school district will not be reimbursed. This fact has both positive and negative aspects. The positive is that states may look to a master's entry requirement for speech-language pathologists who choose to work in the schools. The negative aspect is that licensed or ASHA-certified speech-language pathologists will be asked to direct or supervise practitioners who do not meet minimum requirements. This is an ethical problem with possible legal implications

that must be challenged at both local and state levels (O'Brien, 1991).

In its 1990 report to the Legislative Council, the ASHA Governmental Affairs Committee outlined 16 issues and guidelines that covered the pros and cons, and responded effectively to the many questions raised by the committee and by members. These were broken into two topic areas: (a) child and family issues and (b) professional issues.

Child and Family Issues and Guidelines

Issue 1: Eligibility Criteria Used by Education Agencies May Cause Services in Noneducational Settings to Be Disallowed by Third-Party Payers. The guidelines state that although a student may not be eligible to receive special education or related services in the school, that student may be eligible to receive services outside the school from a private provider or in an agency or hospital clinic. When writing the evaluation report, the speech-language pathologist/audiologist should indicate the nature of the student's disability and the reason that student was ineligible for service in the school. Furthermore, the parents must be informed of their rights to pursue services elsewhere, services possibly covered by third-party payers.

Issue 2: Parents' Rights to Informed Consent Is Unclear to Many Service Providers and Parents. According to the guidelines, speech-language pathologists and audiologists must know about informed-consent procedures and promote the use of the guidelines outlined previously in this chapter.

Issue 3: Parents May Have Insufficient Information About Third-Party Reimbursement Processes. According to the guidelines, the responsibility for acquiring the necessary information to provide parent education rests squarely on the speech-language pathologist/audiologist. ASHA suggests use of its summary of relevant federal regulations and details the necessity of obtaining state-specific information on third-party billing for speech-language pathology and audiology in the schools.

Issue 4: Children Should Receive Uniform Speech-Language Pathology and Audiology Services From Qualified Personnel, Regardless of Funding Source. The guidelines stress the necessity for providers to maintain at least minimum qualifications for practice as defined by federal and state regulations. They state that no child should be denied services or have services reduced in any form or manner because of the funding source and state that speech-language pathologists should use available resources to ensure consistency of care within all settings.

Issue 5: Confidentiality of School Records May Be Compromised by Allowing Third-Parties to See All Information in the Educational Record When They Make Coverage Judgments. According to the guidelines, providers must know the confidentiality requirements of the state in which they practice, and parents should be informed of those requirements.

Professional Issues and Guidelines

Issue 1: There Is Confusion About the Documentation Procedures Required for Special-Education-Related Services and Health Insurance. According to the guidelines, the documentation must meet the requirements of the payer. Administrators and providers should collaborate to avoid duplication of effort and paperwork.

Issue 2: Speech-Language Pathologists and Audiologists May be Unaware of Billing Collection Results, Especially Denials and Appeals. The guidelines state that providers should have a right to obtain feedback on denials and unpaid claims. (Note: that "right" can probably be accessed by collaborating

with administrators and suggesting that good feedback will result in fewer rejected claims.)

Issue 3: Schools, as Providers of Health-Insurance-Reimbursable Services, Must Meet Certain Requirements. The guidelines state that schools must secure and meet personnel and organization requirements before submitting any claims.

Issue 4: Third-Party Reimbursement May Influence the Need for Qualified Personnel in the Schools. The guidelines state that providers must meet the requirements of the payer. (Note: if the private insurer or the state Medicaid authority requires the provider of services to have a state license or ASHA certification, the school must meet those requirements.)

Issue 5: Federal Regulations Require Providers to Access Other Third-Party Payers Prior to Billing Medicaid. According to the guidelines the Medicaid statute requires that Medicaid be the payer of last resort. (Note: providers should investigate the requirements of the state in which they are practicing. Some states require districts to pursue private monies; others discourage it.)

Issue 6: Health Insurance Policies Generally Include Limitations on the Number of Hours, Units of Service, or Maximum Benefits Paid (i.e., Yearly or Lifetime). According to the guidelines, speech-language pathologists and audiologists should have knowledge of Public Law No. 94-142 regulations and the requirement that schools ensure that there will be no reduction in a child's or family's health insurance coverage, whether measured in hours, units of service, or lifetime caps.

Issue 7: The Establishment of Fees and Billing Procedures May Be Unfamiliar to Speech-Language Pathologists and Audiologists in the Schools. The guidelines state that speech-language pathologists and audiologists should know about proper methods for determining fees. Interested members should contact Publication Sales at the ASHA national office. Professionals also should know that Medicaid is not mandated by law to cover the usual and customary charges of providers. (Note: in the schools, the business officer and immediate supervisor usually oversee the specific processes and procedures involved with data collection. Fees are most often regulated by the state Medicaid authority.)

Issue 8: An Additional Source of Funds May Influence the Level of Service in the Schools. According to the guidelines, the level of service is determined by the child's IEP or Individual Family Service Plan (IFSP); for children from birth to 2 years, 11 months, regardless of funding source.

Issue 9: Services Will Be Subject to Deductibles and Coinsurance. The guidelines state that speech-language pathologists and audiologists should be aware of coinsurance and deductible insurance requirements. The school districts must absorb these costs for children aged 3 through 21 years on the basis of the "free and appropriate public education" language in Public Law No. 94-142. Speech-language pathologists and audiologists should also be knowledgeable about individual state differences for children from birth to 2 years, 11 months, regarding practices or coinsurance and deductibles.

Issue 10: Schools May Appear to Be Double-Billing or Even Multiple-Billing—That Is, Using Education and Health Funds for the Same Service. The guidelines state that although schools may receive funding from multiple sources to pay for services, this is legal financing and is not considered "double-billing." Federal statutes allow schools to seek funding from all public and private sources to provide a free, appropriate public education. Some schools may use private billing services to obtain third-party funds. Such billing practices should be used only when they are cost-effective and reflect actual services provided.

Issue 11: Some School Districts Will Be Required to Bill Health Maintenance Organizations (HMOs), Preferred Provider Organizations (PPOs), and Self-Insured Plans. The guidelines state that speech-language pathologists and audiologists should be familiar with all forms of health insurance and managed care. Cornett (1988), ASHA's (1986), and *Governmental Affairs Review* are excellent resources for information on these systems for financing services. (Note: in most schools, speech-language pathologists and audiologists are charged with quality service provision and accurate data collection. Business officials work with payers.)

Issue 12: When There Is a Third-Party Billing for Speech-Language Pathology and Audiology Services in the Schools, Supervision Requirements Exist for Supportive Personnel. According to the guidelines, speech-language pathologists and audiologists should read and be familiar with the articles "Guidelines for the Employment and Utilization of Supportive Personnel" (ASHA, 1981), and "Position Statement on Training, Credentialing, Use, and Supervision of Support Personnel in Speech-Language Pathology" (ASHA, 1995).

Issue 13: The Sale of Products May Become an Issue for School-Based Speech-Language Pathologists and Audiologists. The guidelines state that the federal regulations for special education and related services do not include the sale of products. Assistive technology used in the schools is not for sale to children through third-party payers. (Note: school districts often exercise the option of purchasing assistive technology equipment for students. Speech-language pathologists and audiologists should become familiar with procedures in their assignment.)

Issue 14: Third-Party Reimbursement May Bring Additional Professional Liability to Speech-Language Pathologists and Audiologists. The guidelines state that speech-language pathologists and audiologists providing service should obtain adequate and appropriate professional liability insurance *in addition* to the general liability insurance coverage carried by their employer.

Issue 15: The Provider, for Reimbursement Purposes, Can Be the Speech-Language Pathologist or Audiologist or the Educational Agency Itself. According to the guidelines, speech-language pathologists and audiologists should know about the ramifications of being the enrolled provider. The enrolled provider *should* be the school district because it is the school district that receives the reimbursement.

Issue 16: There May be an Impact on Other Service Providers as a Result of Health Insurance Coverage of Services Provided in Schools. According to the guidelines, eligibility of schools to receive third-party reimbursement does not change the mission of school-based services—that is, to provide appropriate special education and related services. Availability of funding should not be interpreted as an incentive to expand services to children who are not eligible for special education and related services and whose services are not otherwise covered by other education funds.

ASHA Policy

In November 1990, the ASHA Legislative Council approved the following five points as ASHA's official policy on third-party reimbursement:

1. That necessary services shall be provided regardless of funding source, location, or parental authorization.

2. That services shall be provided at no cost to individuals or families.

3. That providers must be clinically competent.

4. That treatment standards must be equal and treatment may be appropriately delivered in both educational and health care settings.

5. That a family's refusal to authorize use of private insurance does not relieve public agencies of their responsibility to provide appropriate services. (p. 54)

Getting Started in an Assignment in a School That Bills Medicaid

If assigned to a school district that bills Medicaid or other third-party payers, a speech-language pathologist/audiologist should do some groundwork to ensure professional and personal integrity:

- Immediately look into personal liability insurance above that carried by the agency.

- Know the interpretations of federal, state, and local laws and regulations that govern the practice of speech-language pathology and audiology in the schools.

- Know the scope of practice of the state license and the definition of the state certification.

- Understand the ASHA Code of Ethics and its application to the performance of responsibilities.

- Research third-party reimbursement options in your state and in your area.

- Research the differences in documentation needed for related services provided under special education regulations and those provided under Medicaid regulations.

- Be certain that the school district, not the individual, registers as the service provider when third-party money is claimed.
- Be familiar with various forms of health insurance and managed care.
- Know your administrator/supervisor, and collaborate on implementation processes and on streamlining paperwork.

School districts that decide to bill Medicaid for speech-language pathology and audiology must adapt their documentation to include Medicaid requirements. The basic requirements, at least for the Federal Medicaid reimbursement process (ASHA, 1992c), are:

1. The IEP must require the service.
2. Parental consent must be obtained.
3. There must be some form of physician authorization (required by Medicaid, but not always by other third-party payers).
4. Services provided must be documented in some way.
5. There must be some form of progress summary completed at set intervals—monthly or quarterly, for example.
6. There must be some form of daily documentation. School attendance records for providers and students can be used, but personal documentation gives the provider an excellent grasp of time and progress. A daily note or some form of documentation about what was done with the child not only enhances professional performance but serves the purposes of accountability and protection from liability. The information accumulated serves the basis for district billing and must be totally accurate.

Third-party billing in schools has created an acute awareness of the importance of accurate, meaningful documentation. Long, beautifully written reports may make the provider appear erudite but may not document change and growth in a measurable fashion. Evaluation reports may be comprehensive but may not sufficiently document the medical need for service. The focus is now on accuracy and outcomes, not length and excessive narrative. This focus must change the way record keeping is taught in colleges and universities. It must change the way school providers think about therapy and record keeping. At the onset, it was predicted that third-party billing in schools would increase paperwork and decrease time with students. But if third-party billing is analyzed positively, it can reduce irrelevant paperwork and increase quality time with students.

SUPERVISION

Supervision can be broadly defined as any activity or process intended to improve an individual's skills, attitudes, comprehension, and performance as related to employment roles and responsibilities. It is part of professional preparation and practice. It is an important factor in facilitating a growth process that should continue throughout an individual's education and professional career (ASHA, 1993). ASHA requires it for acquisition of the Certificate of Clinical Competence (CCC). State licensure boards require it for practicum and initial work experience. Most national regulatory bodies require a mechanism for ongoing supervision throughout professional careers. And education agencies usually base continued employment and often pay increases on supervision reports. A good supervision process validates and supports the changing, expanding roles and responsibilities necessarily assumed by speech-language pathologists and audiologists who choose to work in the school setting. These professionals are no longer just making decisions about the mouth and the ear. They are involved in making decisions about a student's total educational program. They are essential members of an educational team.

One of the most widely used supervisory models in speech-language pathology and audiology today is the Anderson model (Papir-Bernstein, 1995). It identifies a continuum of three stages of supervision based on the professional development of the supervisee:

1. The *evaluation-feedback stage* gives the supervisor a more dominant role. It is effective with individuals who are just starting their careers or with those who have more experience but who may be undergoing burnout and need some direct clinical input.

2. The *transitional stage* is used effectively with experienced, competent individuals who are becoming more personally involved in their own professional growth. The supervisor must be careful not to move too quickly to this stage and cause frustration and discouragement.

3. The *self-supervision stage* is used with individuals who are searching for personal mastery, and who have the ability to self-analyze and truly alter their clinical attitudes and behaviors. (Not everyone reaches this stage.)

None of the stages is time bound or evolves through natural progression. Individuals can be at any stage and can move between stages at any time in their careers. Their position depends on a variety of situational and personal variables.

There are almost as many supervisory styles as there are supervisors. Anderson identified three that include most of them. They can all facilitate growth if matched effectively with the development of the supervisee.

1. The *direct-active* style is often called the *traditional supervision style* and is the one most frequently used. It works well with the individual who is new to the field and who requires ample guidance and input. The supervisor carries the more dominant role and exercises more control. The supervisee takes a more passive and subordinate role. This model takes less time and is easier for the supervisor. There is no collaboration. It is effective when it is used appropriately to facilitate the growth of the supervisee.

2. In the *collaborative* style, the supervisor and the supervisee work together and make mutually agreeable decisions. The supervisee has more involvement in and ownership of the process.

3. In the *consultative* style, the supervisee sets goals, continues to search for appropriate professional growth activities, and identifies personal strengths and weaknesses. The supervisor is an active listener, helps in problem solving, and gives direct clinical assistance as asked or as deemed necessary.

Throughout the supervision process, the relationship changes between the supervisor and the supervisee. As the individual moves from dependence to independence, the supervisor should move from direct to indirect supervision. Research indicates that this does not always happen. Unfortunately, some supervisors have one style of supervision, and that style does not necessarily facilitate the growth and professional development of the supervisee.

ASHA Statements

In 1978, the ASHA Committee on Supervision in Speech-Language Pathology and Audiology defined *supervisors* as individuals who engage in clinical teaching through observation, conferences, review of records, and other procedures related to the interaction between a clinician and a client and to the evaluation or management of communication skills. The implication of clinical teaching as an integral part of supervision is critical.

In 1985, the ASHA Committee on Supervision outlined 13 tasks that it believed basic to effective clinical teaching in the distinct area of practice that comprises communication disorders (ASHA, 1985). When students, speech-language pathologists, and audiologists investigate the tenets of the supervision process under which they must function, they can measure it against these 13 tasks:

1. establishing and maintaining an effective working relationship with the supervisee

2. assisting the supervisee in developing clinical goals and objectives

3. assisting the supervisee in developing and refining assessment skills

4. assisting the supervisee in developing and refining clinical management skills

5. demonstrating for and participating with the supervisee in the clinical process

6. assisting the supervisee in observing and analyzing assessment and treatment sessions

7. assisting the supervisee in the development and maintenance of clinical and supervisory records

8. interacting with the supervisee in planning, executing, and analyzing supervisory conferences

9. assisting the supervisee in evaluation of clinical performance

10. assisting the supervisee in developing skills of verbal reporting, writing, and editing

11. sharing information regarding ethical, legal, regulatory, and reimbursement aspects of professional practice

12. modeling and facilitating professional conduct

13. demonstrating research skills in the clinical or supervisory processes

The committee enumerated from 4 to 10 competencies under each task. Knowledge and skill in supervision, as well as in the professions and in the area of practice, are essential for an effective supervisor.

Performance appraisal, sometimes a synonym for *the supervisory process,* was defined by the ASHA Committee on Professional Appraisal in 1992 as "the practice of evaluating job-related behaviors." The position developed by this committee and adopted by the 1992 Legislative Council reads:

It is the position of the American Speech-Language-Hearing Association that professional performance appraisals of speech-language pathologists and audiologists who are engaged in the delivery of clinical services should include an assessment of the clinical skills that are unique to the employee's profession. This component of the performance appraisal should be conducted by people who hold ASHA certification (and licensure where appropriate) in the employee's professional area. In cases in which organizational structure precludes adoption of this position, participatory approaches (peer evaluations and/or self-evaluations) should be instituted as components of the performance appraisal process.

The committee's technical report noted that a good performance appraisal (a) improved the quality of client care, (b) maintained or improved performance, (c) facilitated professional growth and development, and (d) provided feedback about the potential for increased job responsibilities.

Supervision and performance appraisal focus on two kinds of employee behaviors, those relating to general responsibilities and those relating to professional skills. The general responsibilities may include attendance, dependability, meeting participation, adherence to employer policies and procedures, punctuality, and appropriate use of resources. These aspects of professional performance can be effectively evaluated by any competent administrator.

Professional skills, however, involve competencies defined by specific education, knowledge, and experience. A supervisor outside the profession can judge interpersonal skills, ability to control a group, planning skills, and timely submission of reports but would experience difficulty evaluating the ability to select, administer, and interpret diagnostic tasks that lead to differential diagnoses of speech, language, or hearing disorders; the ability to implement specialized treatment strategies, and the ability to document the relationship of the student's educational needs to the need for therapy. These job functions are unique to the professions of speech-language pathology and audiology and must, when possible, be evaluated by persons with the same professional background as the employee.

It is a common occurrence, however, that speech-language pathologists and audiologists who work in an educational agency are supervised by an administrator or supervisor outside the professions. They may be evaluated by special education directors, school principals, occupational or physical therapists, or psychologists. It may therefore fall to the employee to develop or assist in the development of a supervision process that in some manner reflects professional as well as generalized and administrative responsibilities. ASHA's Committee on Performance Appraisal (1993) suggested two add-ons that can help speech-language pathologists and audiologists design discipline-specific programs or units to meld into their supervision process: peer appraisal and self-appraisal.

Peer Appraisal

Peer appraisal (peer coaching, peer partnering, etc.), the process whereby colleagues rate or enhance each other's job performance, is a well-accepted supervisory tool. It was developed to enhance instruction, not to supersede the evaluation process. It facilitates the autonomy of participants by enabling them to improve their ability to self-monitor, self-analyze, and self-evaluate. It fosters independence and decision making. To be effective and efficient, peer partners must be trained in the process, which, of course, has been approved by the administration of the employing agency. Peer partners, with input from the supervisor, must first decide whether they will analyze or coach one another.

- *Peer analysis* involves clarification of therapy/evaluation activities and practices. Peer partners share implementation of strategies and interpretation of results and engage in self-analysis and problem-solving techniques.

- *Peer coaching* strives for the improvement of therapy/evaluation activities and practices. This partnering is usually entered with the express goal of improving a specific skill or process by working with a peer who has mastered that skill or process.

Roles must be clarified to avoid possible conflict. Peer partnering can solidify the skills and expand the repertoires of the partners, and it promotes cooperative problem solving. A preobservation form (Appendix 10–A) can set the scene and facilitate achievement of the session's goal.

Self-Appraisal

Self-appraisal is a process of taking responsibility for developing a program of professional growth, for developing and following professional improvement goals, and for using a wide variety of resources to achieve those goals. One form of self-appraisal is self-directed study or self-managed professional development. It is encouraged by advocates of coaching and mentoring, and it is indicated by the changing standards and criteria of educational evaluation, by the increased and more complex roles and responsibilities in which providers in the schools are involved, and by research in the fields of education, psychology, business management, religion, and self-help. It must become an integral part of the professional development of speech-language pathologists and audiologists, whatever their practice site. It allows an employee to enter into a contract with him- or herself to study new facts, acquire a specific skill in a particular domain of practice, keep abreast of current research and literature, and, when applicable, meet state certification and licensure continuing-education requirements. In addition to measuring one's own growth, the process and the results can and should become part of the supervision process. The self-directed process is defined in four steps (Papir-Bernstein, 1995):

1. formulation of an open-ended list of potential professional growth objectives
2. completion of a professional growth plan (Appendix 10–B) that includes both a self-evaluation and targeted areas for growth
3. completion of an action plan that breaks down areas into performance objectives, methods, resources, and time lines needed to achieve the objectives
4. completion of a summative conference or self-evaluation (Appendix 10–C).

There are many sources of information on and resources for self-directed study. They include undertaking independent studies under the sponsorship of ASHA or many state professional associations, participating in workshops and conferences, taking for credit or auditing a course, forming or joining a journal study club, engaging in computer searches on relevant topics, joining a Special Interest Division (SID) through ASHA, and taking self-study "courses" through journals such as *Topics in Language Disorders*. Most of these activities are or can be designed to be eligible for ASHA continuing-education units (CEUs). Acquisition of seven CEUs earns an Award for Continuing Education (ACE) from ASHA. Following issuance of the award, the ASHA national office sends a letter to the recipient's supervisor or employer lauding the accomplishment.

Continuous learning is not optional. The proliferation of journals and research in the professions of speech-language and audiology, the increasing client base, the multiple service delivery models, and the expanding role of the speech-language pathologist and audiologist in the schools require continuous learning to remain current. Self-managed study is an excellent method of accomplishing this goal. And if speech-language pathologists and audiologists in schools are supervised by individuals outside the professions, self-directed study, incorporated into the supervision process with the approval of that supervisor, is an excellent way of educating the supervisor and keeping discipline-specific activities in the supervisory process.

A Model Process

In 1992, in response to concerns regarding the existing supervision process expressed by staff and administrators at the Monroe #1 Board of Cooperative Education Services (BOCES) in upstate New York, a volunteer committee was organized to look at the role of supervision in the teaching/learning process. The committee was made up of an assistant superintendent, a school principal, a program director, a teacher of the deaf, a speech-language pathologist, a vision teacher, and a classroom teacher. Members met monthly through one school year. The process was piloted in several departments, including the Department of Speech-Language Pathology and Audiology, and in one school building. It was included in union bargaining sessions the following year and was approved as part of the teacher contract.

The stated purpose of the adopted supervision/evaluation structure is the promotion of the ongoing development of each staff member. Such development is possible only when mutual trust and respect exist between those being supervised and evaluated and those who supervise and evaluate. It was the goal of the committee to create a structure that makes possible productive, constructive interactions between professionals, both peers and supervisors. The process is based on eight components of professional behavior (Chirico et al., 1992). (Components 7 and 8 are considered *part of a staff member's daily routine, and not the focus of the formalized observation.*)

1. *Communication.* Professionals understand that communication is a two-way process that involves both verbal and nonverbal components. They question and answer openly, and they accurately impart specific knowledge, information, and/or emotion.

2. *Understanding and Knowledge of the Field.* Professionals are proficient in their particular discipline and in learning theory. They avail themselves of resources, internal and external, to increase knowledge and to improve the practice of their professions. They know the purpose of the organization that employs them and the range of services offered within that organization.

3. *Management of the Professional Environment.* Professionals are well organized and consistent, as is their environment. They make good use of time, act independently, and use available resources.

4. *Planning.* Professionals understand that planning is a process that precedes instruction and therapy and involves long-term goals as well as short-range objectives. Planning includes a determination of strategies and resources and requires knowledge of assessment methods and various learning styles.

5. *Instructional Strategies.* Professionals understand the most productive ways to interact with students/clients. They implement appropriate objectives, provide opportunities for active involvement, continually evaluate progress, incorporate practice, use creative and varied methods, and provide ongoing feedback.

6. *Interpersonal Skills.* Professionals within the schools and the community demonstrate respect and empathy for others and behave in ways that foster collaboration.

7. *Professional Responsibilities.* Professionals execute routine matters such as attending meetings, keeping records, contributing to the organization's positive public relations, and maintaining confidentiality whenever appropriate. Within this component, it is understood that a professional is punctual, reliable, and acts in an ethical manner.

8. *Willingness to Grow.* Professionals stay current with their field and take the initiative to become continually more proficient at their work. Such professionals evaluate their needs, establish clear development goals, seek feedback and support, and are receptive to ideas and suggestions.

The second component, "Understanding and Knowledge of the Field," was included after it was introduced and rationalized by the speech-language pathologist member of the committee. For that component, individual departments, including classroom teachers, are required to develop knowledge-of-field documents for new and for experienced staff. The speech-language pathology and audiology documents (Appendixes 10–D and 10–E) were developed by department committees and form the basis for that part of their supervision process (Babiarz et al., 1991; Greer, Newman, & Towsley, 1991).

At Monroe #1 BOCES, the processes of *supervision* and *evaluation* are kept totally separate.

The purpose of *supervision* is to enhance professional growth through an interactive, ongoing process that focuses upon the components of professional behavior listed previously. In the related services departments, such as speech-language pathology and audiology, the supervision is provided by a certified and/or licensed professional in the same field. Multiple observations occur annually, as agreed upon by the supervisor and supervisee. A preconference prior to an observation is optional, but it is useful to clarify what, specifically, will be observed and discussed. A postconference follows each observation, in which observer and person observed discuss the session with the goal of improving professional competence. The written summary of each observation (Appendix 10–F) is not part of the supervisee's permanent record. Peer coaching is an option for nonevaluation years.

The purpose of *evaluation* is to provide a periodic summative statement of the performance of a staff member based on the same components of professional behavior. It reflects input from both evaluator and evaluatee. Evaluation occurs annually for nontenured staff, and every 3 years for tenured staff. An evaluation conference precedes the writing of an evaluation, and the written evaluation reflects this conference (Appendix 10–G). The written evaluation is in a personal letter format and becomes part of the evaluatee's permanent record.

Mentoring

Mentoring is an informal process of support among coworkers, between professionals, and/or between a supervisor and a supervisee. It is not a supervisory process. It is an alliance that facilitates growth. Mentors must be willing to make a commitment of time to work with an individual new to the department, new to an assignment area, or just wanting additional support. Mentors should have basic conferencing skills, be nonjudgmental and supportive, be able to share information, have experience/expertise in a given assignment area, and maintain confidentiality. Again, mentoring is not supervising.

Matching mentors/mentees is critical to the success of the venture. Allowing professional staff to choose a volunteer mentor for a designated period of time is one way to do it. Sharing a mentor's role before the time period begins is advisable (Appendix 10–H). The mentor should not address issues of performance unless responding to a specific question. The mentor can be involved in assisting the mentee in problem solving by sharing strategies, ideas, and new research; discussing diagnostic batteries; helping administer evaluation tools; developing intervention strategies; scheduling, organizing, and planning; helping the mentee understand agency/department policies and procedures; and sharing information about resources and materials (Huffman & Russell, 1992).

Mentoring can be on a volunteer or paid basis. Some states define and encourage mentoring. Their districts employ full- or part-time paid mentors. The time that mentoring requires will vary depending upon the amount of support a mentee requests or the amount of time a district requires.

Students

Students at both the undergraduate and graduate levels should be keenly aware of supervision requirements necessary for state licensure and ASHA Certificates of Clinical Competence (CCC). Specific standards for supervision of students can and do differ depending on work/practicum site. Students should know at the onset of their work/practicum experience that supervised clinical experiences will satisfy ASHA (CCC) requirements *only* if the supervision is provided by ASHA-certified personnel (ASHA, 1994b).

It is incumbent upon each individual to ask for specific information on the supervision process used in the agency/school where practicum experience and/or employment will occur. As it is understood, it can be used for professional growth and self-improvement. In whatever setting the speech-language pathologist/audiologist works, strategies can be employed to enhance professional knowledge, improve skills, and make supervisors, evaluators, and administrators aware of the professional activities that make up the practice of speech-language pathology/audiology in that setting. These strategies require professional energy, time, and occasionally ingenuity, but they result in a work environment that promotes job satisfaction and allows for professional growth and development.

SUPPORT PERSONNEL

The role of support personnel in speech-language pathology and audiology and the guidelines governing their use in schools, agencies, and hospitals have long been controversial issues. In 1967, John P. Moncur, chair of the first Committee on Support Personnel appointed by ASHA, noted that the question of support personnel was not a future issue but one that needed immediate attention. The ASHA Ethical Practices Board published an Issues in Ethics statement, which became effective in June 1979 (ASHA, 1992a). It highlighted the professional and ethical responsibilities of the supervising professional and emphasized the dependent role of the "communication aide." Werven (1993) noted that the support personnel issue has sparked strong discussion between advocates who cite increased caseloads, underserved populations, and a diminishing professional work force, and opponents, who express concerns about job security, quality of care, and ethics. The debate continues, and the problems proliferate.

Use of support personnel in schools has been declared successful in several states. Many titles are used. They include *associate, communication assistant, paraprofessional, speech/audiology assistant, audiometrist, audiometric technician, communication helper, speech aide*, and many more (ASHA, 1992b). Support personnel's responsibilities may range from clerical work, through data collection, to maintenance of corrected articulation and implementation of a feeding plan. Freilinger (1992) supported use of support personnel as it exists in the Iowa schools. He stated that the Iowa schools' motive was to employ someone to do the routine activities that did not require a person with a master's degree. He believed that the support personnel program was efficient, effective, and economical and could complement a school's speech and language program—if it was well thought through and planned, if goals and responsibilities were clearly articulated, and if the support personnel were carefully supervised.

A 1993 study by Nancy Striffler of the National Early Childhood Technical Assistance System (NEC*TAS) in Chapel Hill, North Carolina, looked at the use of support personnel in Early Childhood and preschool services in 31 states. Several of these states had developed new occupational categories to ensure services to children and parents at this level. Many of these categories were for support personnel. In Illinois, teacher aides, child development associates, developmental education associates, and family support associates work in Early Intervention programs.

In Utah, early intervention aides and three levels of early interventionists are active. Striffler noted that some of the factors that influence the establishment of a new occupational category include (a) a commitment to include parents as service providers and a desire to employ individuals who are responsive to the culture they serve; (b) the need to extend the services of professionals, especially allied health professionals; and, (c) a commitment to provide services in varied environments and service settings, including the home and child care centers.

Striffler (1993) reported that the most severe professional shortages are noted in the areas of the allied health services of occupational and physical therapy and speech-language pathology. But using support personnel to provide services in the areas of motor and language development requires very careful consideration. When, for instance, does one cross the line from appropriate developmental activities to therapeutic intervention? What specific activities, and at what level, violate state licensure laws? Why is it appropriate to give developmental recommendations to parents for implementation but not to support personnel? With no professional service providers in many remote areas throughout the country, how do we meet the needs of individuals and groups within those areas who need speech-language and audiology services?

Both opponents and proponents of the use of support personnel have many concerns. They worry about the qualifications and availability of supervisors, the amount of supervision, and the supervisor/support personnel ratio. They express concern about educational and training standards, scope of practice, ethical considerations, reimbursement issues, and the question of who will monitor the credentialing process.

ASHA Statements

ASHA attempted to clarify the use of support personnel in 1969, when the Legislative Council adopted the first guidelines. ASHA's Rule of Ethics II.D states in part that support services may be provided by uncertified persons only when a certificate holder provides appropriate supervision. That paper was not specific in setting ratios or in delineating activities. In 1981, ASHA's second Committee on Supportive Personnel published "Guidelines for the Employment and Utilization of Supportive Personnel." The issues underlying those guidelines were:

1. The legal, ethical, and moral responsibility to the client for all services provided cannot be delegated; that is, they remain the responsibility of the professional personnel.

2. Support personnel may be permitted to implement a variety of clinical tasks, given that sufficient training, direction, and supervision are provided by the audiologist and/or speech-language pathologist responsible for those tasks.

3. Support personnel should receive training that is competency based in character and specific to the job performance expectations held by the employer.

4. The supervising audiologist and/or speech-language pathologist should also be trained in the supervision of support personnel.

5. The supervision of support personnel must be periodic, comprehensive, and documented to ensure that the client receives the high-quality services needed.

These guidelines allow trained speech-language pathology and audiology support personnel to assist in the delivery of services and to augment program and treatment activities under the direct supervision of ASHA certified speech-language pathologists and audiologists.

Since 1981, the use of support personnel in speech-language pathology and audiology has increased throughout the professions. Several factors have influenced that increase:

- The passage of Public Law No. 94-142 in 1975 increased the mandated responsibilities of the speech-language pathologists in the schools. Children with severe disabilities, formerly evaluated and treated elsewhere, are now mandated to be evaluated and serviced by the speech-language pathologists in the schools.

- The passage of Public Law No. 99-457 in 1986 mandated service to the preschool population. Children's disabilities are now identified and treated earlier.

- Technological advances made possible the mainstreaming and inclusion of students who are severely disabled: that is, students who did not participate in public education at an earlier time. The increase of these students has necessitated the increase of service providers to serve them. The technology necessary to allow these students access to public education demands increased and specific expertise of the service provider.

- Personnel shortages and underserved populations across the country have caused administrators and supervisors to look at alternatives to traditional service delivery.

In 1994, the most current ASHA Task Force on Support Personnel prepared a position statement and guidelines for one category of support personnel. These guidelines included a recognized credentialing process and an outcome-based evaluation system.

The 1994 Legislative Council adopted the position statement (ASHA, 1995) but postponed action on the implementation guidelines, leaving the 1981 guidelines most current. The position statement reads:

It is the position of the American Speech-Language-Hearing Association (ASHA) that support personnel may be used to perform activities adjunct to the primary clinical efforts of speech-language pathologists. ASHA supports the establishment and credentialing of categories of support personnel for the profession of speech-language pathology. Appropriate training and supervision must be provided by speech-language pathologists holding ASHA's Certificate of Clinical Competence in Speech-Language Pathology. Activities may be assigned only at the discretion of the supervising speech-language pathologist and should be constrained by the scope of responsibilities for support personnel. The communication needs and protection of the consumer must be held paramount at all times. Violation of these assumptions shall be considered a breach of the professional ethics of ASHA.

Licensure

In 1988, the National Council of State Boards of Examiners for Speech-Language Pathology and Audiology reviewed the support personnel issue by looking at states that had (a) definitions of support personnel; (b) laws, rules, and regulations on the use of support personnel; and (c) no provisions whatever for the use of support personnel. They proposed the following questions to consider:

- Are communication assistants (CAs) appropriately selected, trained, supervised, and evaluated?

- Are CAs functioning as fully licensed professionals?

- What are the ethical considerations for a CA?

- What skills should the supervising speech-language pathologist and audiologist possess in using a CA?

- In what should the CA be trained?

- What are the legal aspects of using CAs?

- How should the CAs be supervised and evaluated?

While the controversy continued on a national level, individual state licensure boards began looking at support personnel. As of October 1994, 29 states regulated their support personnel in some way (ASHA, 1994a). The common threads through these rules and regulations are training/education and supervision. But the differences are vast. Some states use ASHA's 1981 guidelines. Others do not know that these exist. Some states, like Maine and Delaware, require a bachelor's degree in speech-language pathology. Texas requires a bachelor's degree plus 21 credits in speech-language pathology (New Jersey Speech-Language-Hearing Association, 1993). Some states require only a high school diploma, and still others have only definitions of *support personnel* with no requirements for practice.

Regulated/licensed support personnel perform a variety of roles within a broad range of employment settings. The typical scope of responsibilities includes screening, reinforcement and maintenance of improved or corrected articulation, oral exercises, computer simulation programs and programmed instruction, recording and displaying data that reflect a student's performance, filing clinical records and making progress notes, reporting changes in student behavior to the speech-language pathologist, working with parents on carryover activities, demonstrating select assistive listening devices, creating therapy materials, and maintaining equipment and materials inventory. Prohibited activities are typically those that require the formal education and credentialing of a speech-language pathologist/audiologist, including, but not limited to, diagnostic evaluations, caseload selection, interpretation and dissemination of clinical information, writing reports, determining related services, and dismissal from therapy.

Supervision requirements vary across states according to demographics. Rural areas usually require fewer on-site hours and more readily accept audio- and videotapes and record/report reviews. Most states require that support personnel practice only under the supervision of a licensed, certified speech-language pathologist/audiologist who maintains legal accountability and responsibility for all activities and services provided. Also, in most states where there is regulation of support personnel, a formal plan of supervision is required, and the number of support personnel who can be supervised by one speech-language pathologist/audiologist is specified.

Some who object to the development of support personnel in the professions cite proposals that replace professional personnel with trained "aides." The most radical proposals involve something called *institutional licensure*. Under such a system, an institution would be regulated by a state agency, such as the State Education Department, which could essentially decide who is competent to discharge what duties. Proponents of licensing support personnel say this could not happen if licensure defined their scope of practice. In some states, licensure is not required in schools, or schools are exempt from state

licensure. In these states, licensure would provide no protection.

Pros and Cons

Proponents of the use and regulation of support personnel say that the practice is operational and that it is up to "us" to regulate it so as to avoid abuse. They say:

- As speech-language and audiology professionals, we must regulate our own support personnel or risk the possibility that diverse agencies such as State Education Departments will regulate it for us.

- It frees the speech-language pathologist to perform higher level activities that require the education and expertise of the professional.

- It relieves the professional from routine, clerical, and/or time-consuming tasks that do not require discipline-specific expertise.

- It has proved cost-effective in places where large and diverse populations require service.

- It provides a career ladder both for the support personnel who continue into the professions of speech-language pathology and audiology and for the speech-language pathologist/audiologist wishing to move into an administrative and/or supervisory role.

- It has proved effective in areas where readily available support personnel are used to reinforce or maintain recommended activities.

Opponents to the use and regulation of support personnel are very vocal. They ask:

- Will the use of support personnel downgrade the professional status of speech-language pathology/audiology?

- Will jobs be lost? Will support personnel replace, instead of assist?

- Will consumers be confused over differences in provider qualifications?

- Will schools provide adequate release time for training and supervision?

- Will it be possible to implement supervision by a speech-language pathologist/audiologist in a system that clearly allocates supervision to school administrators?

- Will appropriate supervisor/supervisee ratios be enforced?

- Will quality of service be maintained?

- Will there be adequate training of both the support personnel and the supervisor?

- Will abuses occur, especially in schools where cost containment is critical?

- Will third-party payers accept two different levels of reimbursement?

- Does this profession really need another layer of service provider?

The practice of audiology in the schools is an area that lends itself easily to the use of support personnel. In the educational milieu, many students with hearing loss are mainstreamed. The troubleshooting and management of FM systems and other assistive listening devices are responsibilities that could be performed by individuals other than licensed and/or certified audiologists. Under the supervision of an audiologist, support personnel could be trained to troubleshoot and manage that equipment. Viable activities include listening checks on FM systems and hearing aids; communication with vendors; provision of in-service on troubleshooting techniques; arranging annual service maintenance; making minor repairs; managing records and maintaining files; monitoring service contracts and purchase orders; ordering equipment and parts; and keeping updated information on product lines, parts, and prices. Credentials could be minimal. Money could be saved. The audiologist could be relieved from the performance of tasks that can be done easily and well by less credentialed individuals.

Conclusion

The use of support personnel in speech-language pathology and audiology is here. It is not a future possibility about which we have the luxury of pondering. It is something we need to acknowledge, accept, and integrate as necessary into the practice of our professions. As more support personnel become recognized members of service provision teams, more professionals will be called upon to train and supervise. The role of supervision and the supervisory skills needed to carry out this function are critical. The quality of training, support, and supervision provided to support personnel will influence their success in providing quality services to the children in our schools and to their parents.

Individuals who enter the professions of speech-language pathology and/or audiology see themselves as future professionals. They take on the ethics and responsibilities that go with their chosen professions. They do the right thing whether anyone is watching or not. They think first of the client, of the student. They possess a sense of public responsibility, a code of ethics, a sense of duty beyond self. This can be lost if we place our responsibilities in the hands of assorted support personnel with no unifying philosophy. However, we know that our professions are dynamic. We know they change and grow.

We know that over time they acquire new and more complex responsibilities at the upper end of their scopes of practice, while activities at the lower end tend to drop out of the scope. If we are flexible about recognizing selected responsibilities for which support personnel can be responsible, we are more likely to be taken seriously by policy makers when we object to the delegation of professional duties that exposes our consumers to serious risk.

STUDY QUESTIONS

1. Third-party payments for school services: list some of the advantages, and be prepared to discuss some of the serious obstacles to their use.

2. What has ASHA said about third-party payments?

3. If you work for a school system that bills Medicaid or other third-party payers, what are some of the things that you should know?

4. What is performance appraisal, and how is it related to supervision?

5. Differentiate between *supervision, evaluation,* and *mentoring.*

6. What forces have led to the inclusion of support personnel in school services for children with handicapping conditions?

7. What services do you think would be appropriate for support personnel to perform in speech and language?

REFERENCES

American Speech-Language-Hearing Association. (1978). Current status of supervision of speech-language pathology and audiology. [Special Report] *Asha, 20,* 478–486.

American Speech-Language-Hearing Association. (1981). Guidelines for the employment and utilization of supportive personnel. *Asha, 23,* 165–169.

American Speech-Language-Hearing Association. (1985). Clinical supervision in speech-language pathology and audiology. *Asha, 27,* 57–60.

American Speech-Language-Hearing Association. (1990). Utilization of Medicaid and other third party funds for "covered services" in the schools: Report to the 1990 American Speech-Language-Hearing Association Legislative Council as required by LC 42-89. Rockville, MD: ASHA.

American Speech-Language-Hearing Association. (1991). Utilization of Medicaid and other third-party funds for "covered services" in the schools. *Asha, 33,* (Suppl. 5), 51–58.

American Speech-Language-Hearing Association. (1992a). ASHA policy regarding support personnel. *Asha, 34* (Suppl. 9), 18.

American Speech-Language-Hearing Association Task Force on Support Personnel. (1992b). Support personnel: issues and impact on the professions of speech-language pathology and audiology. A technical report. Rockville, MD: ASHA.

American Speech-Language-Hearing Association. (1992c). Third-party reimbursement in the schools: Teleconference report. ASHA Transcript Series: Focus on School Issues.

American Speech-Language-Hearing Association. (1993). Professional performance appraisal by individuals outside of the professions of speech-language pathology and audiology. *Asha, 35* (Suppl. 10), 11–13.

American Speech-Language-Hearing Association. (1994a) 1994 State licensure issues/activities: Year end report. Rockville, MD: ASHA.

American Speech-Language-Hearing Association. (1994b). Supervision of student clinicians. *Asha, 36* (Suppl. 13), 13.

American Speech-Language-Hearing Association. (1995). Position statement on training, credentialing, use, and supervision of support personnel in speech-language pathology. *Asha, 37* (Suppl. 14), 21.

Babiarz, B., Bergin, M., Corea, M. A., Corwley, E., Hooey, K., Oglia, D. & Parry, K. (1991). *Knowledge and skills in speech-language pathology.* New York: Board of Cooperative Educational Services, First Supervisory District, Monroe County.

Chirico, P., Byrne, P., Cullings, J., Diesenberg, V., Keller, S., Lynch-Nadich, K., O'Brien, M.A., Valentine, A., & Yaeger, P. (1992). *Amended supervision and evaluation process.* New York: Board of Cooperative Educational Services, First Supervisory District, Monroe County.

Cornett, B. S. (1988). Speech-language pathologists, audiologists, and HMOs: Status and outlook. *Asha, 30,* 64–67.

Freilinger, J. J. (1992). Support personnel. *Asha, 34,* 51–53.

Greer, C., Newman, S., & Towsley, M. (1991). Knowledge and skills in audiology. New York: Board of Cooperative Educational Services, First Supervisory District, Monroe County.

Huffman, N., & Russell, L. (1992). *Mentoring: Staff directory for speech-language pathology and audiology.* New York: Board of Cooperative Educational Services, First Supervisory District, Monroe County.

National Council of State Boards of Examiners for Speech-Language Pathology and Audiology. (1988). The use of support personnel: Prospectives on licensure. A report.

New Jersey Speech-Language-Hearing Association. (1993). Getting a perspective on supportive personnel: A special report.

O'Brien, M. A. (1991). Third-party billing for school services: The school's perspective. *Asha, 33,* 43–45.

Papir-Bernstein, W. (1995). Supervision for the twenty-first century: Facilitating self-directed professional growth. New York: NYSSLHA Mini-Seminar.

Striffler, N. (1993). Current trends in the use of paraprofessionals in early intervention and preschool services. A report published by the National Early Childhood Technical Assistance System. Chapel Hill, NC.

Werven, G. (1993). Support personnel: An issue for our times. *American Journal of Speech-Language Pathology,* pp. 9–12.

Wolf, K. E. (1991). Third-party billing for school services: The healthcare provider's perspective. *Asha, 33,* 45–48.

RECOMMENDED READINGS

Belasco, J. A. & Stayer, R. C. (1993). *Flight of the buffalo: Soaring to excellence, learning to let employees lead.* New York: Warner.

Casey, P. L., Smith, K. J., & Ulrich, S. R. (1988). *Self-supervision: A career tool for audiologists and speech-language pathologists* (Clinical Series No. 10). Rockville, MD: National Student Speech-Language-Hearing Association.

Coufal, K. L., Steckleberg, A. L., & Vasa, S. F. (1991). Current trends in the training and utilization of paraprofessionals in speech and language programs: A report on an eleven-state survey. *Language, Speech, and Hearing Services in Schools, 22,* 51–59.

Covey, S. (1989). *The 7 habits of highly effective people.* New York: Simon & Schuster.

Dellogrotto, J. (1991). Program management in schools: Supportive personnel and issues in supervision/evaluation of speech-language pathologists. ASHA Teleconference.

Glatthorn, A. A. (1984). *Differentiated supervision: 1984 yearbook of the Association for Supervision and Curriculum Development.* VA: Association for Supervision and Curriculum Development.

Kreb, R. (1991). *Third party payment for funding special education and related services.* Horsham, PA: LRP.

Neidecher, E. A. & Blosser, J. L. (1993). *School programs in speech-language organization and management.* Englewood Cliffs, NJ: Prentice-Hall.

Senge, P. (1990). *The fifth discipline: The art and practice of the learning organization.* New York: Doubleday.

Trace, R. (1994, December 19). ASHA strives to define role of support personnel as debate continues. *Advance.*

Appendix 10–A

Peer Coaching/Partnering Preobservation Form

SLP/A Name _____

Observer Name _____

Observation Date and Time _____

Location _____

Therapy Objective _____

_____

_____

Special Requests _____

_____

_____

Additional information that the observer might find beneficial

_____

_____

Appendix 10–B

Sample Self-Directed Professional Development Plan for Speech-Language Pathologists/Audiologists in Schools

1. Examine your speech-language pathology/audiology program and list some areas that need improvement or about which you need additional information or increased skill level.

2. Check the areas related to your own professional skills that you would like to target for improvement and/or change (Papir-Bernstein, 1995):

___ adapting techniques/materials	___ organization of professional resources
___ assessment	___ parent/home contact
___ changing mandates	___ classroom collaboration
___ planning for therapy	___ problem solving
___ community integration	___ professional credentials
___ conflict management	___ scheduling
___ documenting student progress	___ staff consultation/training
___ implementing new information	___ therapy techniques
___ interpersonal communication	___ use of materials
___ involvement with professional conferences	___ worksite integration
	___ collaboration
___ goal setting	___ other

3. On the basis of (1) and (2) above, for the next school year formulate two professional development goals that will benefit you and/or your program.

   1.

   2.

4. Outline the methods and resources you plan to use to achieve your goals.

5. Outline how you intend to evaluate the achievement of your goals.

Appendix 10–C

Sample Self-Directed Professional Development Evaluation for Speech-Language Pathologists/Audiologists in Schools

1. To what extent were you able to achieve your goals (Papir-Bernstein, 1995)?

2. What, if any, were the impediments to your progress?

3. What methods/resources were most useful (Papir-Bernstein, 1995)?

4. What changes have occurred in your program as a result of your professional development work?

5. What knowledge have you gained as a result of your professional development work?

6. Which of your skills have improved as a result of your professional development work? How?

7. Plans for next year ………

Appendix 10–D

Board of Cooperative Educational Services: Knowledge and Skills in Speech-Language Pathology

I. BASIC COMMUNICATION PROCESSES

A. Basic Competencies

Knowledge of…

… normal processes of speech, language, and hearing in infants, children, and adolescents, including anatomic and physiological bases for the normal development and use of speech, language, and hearing

… normal processes of speech, language, and hearing in infants, children, and adolescents, including physical bases and processes of the production and perception of speech and hearing

… normal processes of speech, language, and hearing in infants, children, and adolescents, including linguistic and psycholinguistic variables related to the normal development and use of speech, language, and hearing

… subject areas related to normal processes of human communication, including anatomy and physiology of the speech-hearing mechanism; respiration; neurology and neurophysiology; linguistics, phonology, and phonetics; speech-language development; psycholinguistics; and speech and hearing science/physics/psychoacoustics

II. SPEECH-LANGUAGE DISORDERS: DEVELOPMENTAL AND ACQUIRED

A. Basic Competencies

Knowledge of…

… etiological bases of communicative disorders

… disorders of articulation, including phonological, motor, and perceptual processes

… voice disorders, including phonatory and resonatory disorders

… swallowing disorders and dysphagia

… fluency disorders and the relationship between an individual's dysfluent speech production behavior and other personal and situational variables

… disordered development of language content, form, and use, including the areas of phonology, morphology, syntax, semantics, and pragmatics

… acquired language disorders related to processes, content, form, and use

… the impact of emotional and psychological factors upon communication

… procedures for obtaining valid and reliable information via standardized tests and instruments as well as observation and nonstandardized instruments measuring articulation, voice and resonance, fluency, and language

... screening materials and techniques for high-risk populations

... test construction, including information relative to standardization, reliability, and validity

... prognostic indicators for initiating and terminating treatment

... record-keeping techniques and report writing for evaluation and treatment

... cultural and socioeconomic factors relevant to assessment and treatment, in order to minimize the effects of cultural bias upon evaluation and treatment

... procedures and techniques for the prevention of speech, language and hearing disorders

Skills to...

... select, score, and interpret diagnostic tools appropriate to specific populations

... develop, write, and evaluate measurable and observable treatment plans, including long-term goals, that reflect an understanding of the student's incoming status, needs, and prognosis for change

... select and utilize appropriate intervention strategies and materials for treatment of disorders in articulation, fluency, voice and resonance, and language

... adapt strategies, materials, and instrumentation to stages of treatment and student needs

... develop and implement effective behavior management programs for special populations as related to communication intervention

... maintain documentation of evaluation, ongoing intervention programs, and student progress

... use home, school, employment, and social contacts to assist in treatment and to monitor generalization and maintenance of newly acquired behaviors

B. Advanced Skills

Knowledge of...

... severe communicative impairments and related areas such as prespeech and nonverbal communication, motor and sensory abilities, and cognitive and social interaction skills

... assessment of adequacy of anatomical and physiological systems utilized in speech and language

... alternative and assistive modes of communication

... manual communication systems and use of interpreters and translators

III. RELATED AREAS

A. Basic Competencies

Knowledge of...

... assistive listening devices and basic interpretation of an audiogram

... interdisciplinary interaction and roles of related professionals in the evaluation and treatment of the communicatively impaired

... services offered and information provided by allied health and education professionals that may be relevant to the evaluation and treatment of students with speech, language, and hearing disorders

... treatment options in the community and referral strategies for service

... one's own professional limitations in evaluation and treatment that might necessitate referral to colleagues

... effects of communicative impairment on educational, vocational, social, and psychological status

... local, state, and federal guidelines, regulations, and legislation that affect the handicapped and the delivery of services to them

... identifying characteristics and referral procedures regarding suspected child abuse and substance abuse

... interpersonal skills necessary for effective conferencing with colleagues and parents

... current information regarding standards of professional and ethical conduct

... the purpose of Monroe #1 BOCES, and the range of services offered within this organization

Skills to...

... seek out continuing education in areas related to current professional needs

... utilize available resources through BOCES' Speech-Language Pathology and Audiology Department

B. Advanced Skills

Knowledge of...

... counseling techniques relevant to student-centered issues

... counseling techniques relevant to parent-centered issues

... counseling techniques related to the grieving process

... instructional techniques appropriate for delivery of service in the classroom

... techniques to facilitate collaborative consultation

Skills to...

... select and utilize systems and technology for collecting, storing, retrieving, and analyzing data

... operate computers and instrumentation required by treatment plans

... supervise student teachers and CFY clinicians, including assessing their needs, planning growth experiences, and facilitating self-evaluation

... foster high levels of job satisfaction, productivity, morale, motivation, and organizational cohesiveness at work settings

... implement in-service training and continuing education programs for staff to improve service delivery

Appendix 10–E

Board of Cooperative Educational Services: Knowledge and Skills in Audiology

The Task Force on Knowledge and Skills in Audiology divided the knowledge base of the profession into seven related areas. They are as follows:

A. Testing
B. Counseling
C. Personal/Professional Skills
D. Knowledge of Education/Special Education
E. Habilitation/Rehabilitation
F. Instruction
G. Knowledge of BOCES Organization

A. *Testing* (Includes Pre-Evaluation, Evaluation, Postevaluation/Interpretation, and Report-Writing Skills)

1. Knowledge of strategies for selecting appropriate tests of hearing, given the client's age; socioeconomic status; cultural background; level of auditory, language, and cognitive function; and presenting complaint(s)

   - *Basic/Entry-level Skills to:*
   - Integrate information from various resources when preparing to take a case history.
   - Interview the client and significant others to facilitate assessment planning, to establish the client's past and present status, and to identify potential etiologic factors.
   - Identify individuals at high risk for speech/language and/or hearing deficits through the use of appropriate screening procedures, to facilitate referrals for assessment and treatment.
   - Gather, review, and evaluate information from referral sources, educational, social, psychological, and/or medical records, and prior testing results, to facilitate assessment planning, to establish the client's past and present status, and to identify potential etiologic factors.

Advanced/Acquired Skills to:

   - Use principles and strategies of behavioral management and modification.

2. Knowledge of techniques and materials for assessing central auditory function, hearing sensitivity, nonorganic hearing loss, and middle ear function

Basic/Entry-Level Skills to:

- Select and use behavioral tests for assessment of hearing sensitivity, middle-ear function, or site of lesion.
- Select appropriate tests and structure testing to elicit behavioral responses to auditory stimulation that are appropriate to the unique characteristics of the client, such as developmental level, language ability, etc.
- Assess residual hearing.
- Select and administer screening instruments/materials.
- Assess reliability and validity of auditory test results.
- Establish pass/fail criteria and interpret screening results.
- Apply principles of operant conditioning and appropriate reinforcement schedules.
- Demonstrate proficiency in the operation and effective utilization of available diagnostic and clinical equipment.
- Administer the selected standardized and/or nonstandardized but clinically appropriate screening and assessment measures, to collect reliable and valid data.
- Develop and implement screening programs for children with hearing disorders.
- Select and use behavioral tests for assessment of central auditory function or nonorganic hearing loss.
- Administer nonstandardized tests of auditory function and interpret their results.

3. Knowledge of acoustics and psychoacoustics and their influence/effect on the listener and his/her communication skills.

Basic/Entry-Levels Skills to:

- Evaluate and describe the influences of the acoustics and visual environment on communicative function.

Acquired/Advanced Skills to:

- Evaluate tests of environment acoustic conditions and determine their influence upon communicative skills.

4. Knowledge of state-of-the-art technology in prosthetic amplification, such as hearing aids, cochlear implants, educational amplification, and other assistive devices.

Basic/Entry-Level Skills to:

- Assess earmold acoustics and techniques for making earmold impressions and subsequent modifications.

- Identify potential candidates for the use of assistive listening devices and understand the application of the device in the setting in which it will be used.

- Assess electroacoustic performance of hearing aids and assistive devices.

- Gather and maintain up-to-date information about instrumentation and materials for treatment.

- Use appropriate procedures, materials, instruments, and equipment to select, evaluate, and monitor hearing aids and other assistive devices.

- Evaluate and interpret listener communication performance with amplification.

Advanced/Acquired Skills to:

- Select prosthetic devices for hearing-impaired clients.

- Fit and adjust amplification and/or assistive devices.

5. Knowledge of appropriate follow-up procedures based on results of testing

Basic/Entry-Level Skills to:

- Refer to medical treatment if need is indicated from client's audiologic assessment data.

- Specify potential candidates for the use of hearing aids.

- Develop prognostic statements based on evaluation results.

- Make appropriate referrals for additional evaluative and treatment services, based on results of treatment monitoring.

- Determine the need for further assessment or information, including otologic consultation.

- Make recommendations and referrals based on evaluation results.

- Prepare and maintain accurate and complete individual client records.

- Document the treatment program.

- Write plans that reflect the client's present status, needs, and prognosis for change. Determine monitoring intervals and procedures for reevaluation.

- Determine reliability and validity of test results.

- Record diagnostic results accurately. Interpret diagnostic results appropriately.

- Write an evaluation report that highlights the client's chief complaints, the past history, and the assessment findings relative to current strengths and limitations, as well as the recommendations for future management, to communicate to the client, family, significant others, and other professionals, and provide an available printed record for future reference.

- Interpret results of the evaluation, to establish type and severity of disorder and to generate recommendations.

B. Counseling

1. Knowledge of the grieving process and pertinent counseling techniques

2. Knowledge of impact of various degrees of hearing loss on social skills, vocational decisions, and hearing and listening in various situations

Basic/Entry-Level Skills to:

- Provide counseling and guidance following assessment.

Advanced/Acquired Skills to:

- Provide supportive guidance and counseling for the client, the family, and significant others, related to such areas as acceptance, adjustment, motivational factors, and coping skills.
- Identify the need for and availability of psychological, social, educational, and vocational counseling.

1. Knowledge of information needed by other professionals, referral sources, client, and family to develop treatment plans

Basic/Entry-Level Skills to:

- Develop and maintain a rapport with patients and professionals.
- Communicate with families on a regular basis regarding diagnostic information, therapy goals, and progress.
- Provide informational guidance and counseling, such as information about the disorder, options for treatment, goals, and progress, to the client, family, significant others, and other service providers.
- Communicate results from the evaluation to the client, family, significant others, and referral agencies.

C. *Personal/Professional Skills* (Includes Organizational Skills, Knowledge of Services Provided by BOCES, Knowledge of Services Provided in the Community, Dependability, etc.)

1. Knowledge of community resources, BOCES-wide resources, and service or product delivery programs (both BOCES-wide and community- or statewide) for the communicatively impaired

Basic/Entry-Level Skills to:

- Seek assistance from other persons or agencies to identify individuals at risk for communication disorders and provide quality services for the communicatively impaired.
- Communicate case information to allied professionals and others working with communicatively impaired individuals.
- Work as a team member to establish the need for treatment, to set treatment goals, and to implement treatment program.

Advanced/Acquired Skills to:

- Identify unmet needs, create new programs, or develop links with existing programs.
- Utilize resources outside the employment setting.

2. Knowledge of administrative, marketing, budgetary, and management techniques and systems relevant to speech, language, and hearing programs

Advanced/Acquired Skills to:

- Obtain ideas for one's program from other programs with which that one is in contact.
- Be familiar with billing procedures and fee schedules with regard to services provided by the department.
- Meet administrative requirements with promptness and accuracy, including utilization reports, service statistics, budget requests, and responses to position and policy statements.
- Seek current information regarding the procurement of private, governmental, and third-party financial support.

3. Knowledge of principles and methods of supervision and self-evaluation

Basic/Entry-Level Skills to:

- Cooperate and respond appropriately to supervising clinician and other professionals.
- Respond to feedback from staff regarding program and one's own strengths and weaknesses.
- Respond to supervision and facilitates communication concerning administrative and clinical issues.
- Assess one's own clinical competencies in evaluation.
- Work in a collaborative fashion with others.
- Advanced/Acquired Skills to:
- Supervise CFY or graduate students.

4. Continuing Education

Advanced/Acquired Skills to:

- Use manual/augmentative communication for client interaction.
- Seek out continuing education in areas related to current professional needs, including but not limited to evaluation and treatment techniques.
- Consult professional journals for updating of knowledge of current research.
- Demonstrate an awareness of trends in the profession, education, and allied health professions.

5. Knowledge of computer applications involving data processing and information management

Advanced/Acquired Skills to:

- Use computer technology to improve data collection, storage, retrieval, and manipulation for program management, client care, and program development.

- Use computer/data processor in report writing, letter writing, and any interoffice communication.

6. Knowledge of current information regarding professional standards (PSB, ESB, licensure, teacher certification, etc.) and ethical conduct relevant to supervision, service delivery, and research

Advanced/Acquired Skills to:

- Demonstrate ethical professional attitudes, commitment, and motivation for continued professional growth.

7. Miscellaneous personal/professional knowledge and skills

Basic/Entry-Level Skills to:

- Adjust oral and written communication to ensure comprehension by the receiver.
- Attend professional meetings and relate useful information obtained to other professionals.
- Work independently.

Advanced/Acquired Skills to:

- Effectively plan daily, weekly, monthly, and yearly schedules.
- Coordinate services to provide maximum efficiency in scheduling and services delivery for patients, families, and support agencies.

D. *Knowledge of Education/Special Education* (Knowledge of State and Federal Regulations; Knowledge of Educational Theories and Practices)

1. Knowledge of normal development and disorders of language, speech, and hearing

2. Knowledge of communication impairment and its impact on cognitive, psychosocial, and motor functions and on learning

3. Knowledge of family structure and dynamics and of socioeconomic, ethnic, and cultural variation and their impact on the client's functioning in society

4. Knowledge of laws and regulations and their respective mandates to provide appropriate services to the communicatively impaired

5. Knowledge of New York State hearing screening laws, regulations, and guidelines

Advanced/Acquired Skills to:

- Communicate treatment plan for approval by regulatory agencies when this is called for in state and federal laws and regulations.
- Monitor and adjust program goals and activities to meet philosophical and financial priorities and patterns mandated by foundations and government agencies.
- Interpret laws and regulations, and their respective mandates, to provide appropriate services to the communicatively impaired.

- Demonstrate knowledge of related current state and federal laws, regulations, and standards.
- Promote legislation beneficial to the profession.
- romote legislation and regulations that will ensure an acceptable quality and availability of services rendered while monitoring and opposing legislation harmful to the communicatively handicapped.

E. Habilitation/Rehabilitation

1. Knowledge of educational, vocational, social, and psychological effects of hearing impairment and their impact on the development of a treatment program

Advanced/Acquired Skills to:

- Develop and implement rehabilitation plan based on consideration of the individual's communicative needs.

2. Knowledge of rehabilitation options appropriate to the client's needs and methods for monitoring and determining the effectiveness of treatment

Basic/Entry-Level Skills to:

- Write, prioritize, and implement long-term goals and short-term objectives and a rationale for discharge or continuance of treatment.
- Plan and adapt treatment procedures based on periodic reassessment of patient's needs.
- Monitor on an ongoing basis the degree of client progress in attaining treatment goals.
- Assess changes in client's communication behavior while using prosthetic devices.
- Utilize monitoring information to make appropriate modifications in treatment plans.
- Plan and implement a program to monitor auditory abilities and communicative function during treatment process.
- Follow up on referrals and recommendations made on the basis of treatment monitoring.
- Generate and communicate recommendations resulting from the evaluation processes to the client, family, significant others, and referring agent relative to the need for additional evaluation, treatment, and reevaluation, to coordinate an appropriate treatment plan.
- Use strategies for establishing and maintaining client motivation.
- Discuss with client the various strategies for improving listening skills.
- Determine and describe communicative needs of the hearing-impaired individual.
- Determine auditory and visual speech recognition abilities.

Advanced/Acquired Skills to:

- Design and implement a program for monitoring and maintaining both personal and group amplification systems.
- Use strategies to encourage family involvement in the rehabilitative management of the client.

3. Knowledge of counseling strategies for orientation to, and use of, hearing aids and prosthetic hearing devices

Basic/Entry-Level Skills to:

- Design and implement a plan to instruct clients on the proper use and maintenance of amplification and/or assistive devices.

4. Knowledge of the effects of hearing impairment on the normal development of phonologic, morphologic, syntactic, semantic, and pragmatic aspects of communication

F. Instruction (School-Based and Professional In-Service)

1. Knowledge of development and implementation of in-service training process.

2. Knowledge of principles of learning to apply when designing instruction.

Basic/Entry-Level Skills to:

- Train support personnel to screen hearing.
- Develop and utilize appropriate levels of effective communication with parents, teachers, and other professionals (e.g., presenting reports, in-services, interviews, conferences).
- Integrate and present information regarding potentially deleterious effects of environmental sound, hearing aid use, and sources of trauma on residual auditory function.
- Describe the availability and use of sensory aids, telecommunication systems, and other assistive devices.

Advanced/Acquired Skills to:

- Speak effectively in public/group settings.
- Plan and implement parent-education programs about the management of hearing impairment and resulting communicative disorders.
- Develop and implement educational programs on the prevention of speech, language, and hearing disorders.
- Implement in-service training and continuing education programs for staff to improve service delivery.
- Plan and implement service programs with allied professionals who serve hearing-impaired persons.

G. Knowledge of BOCES Organization

1. Knowledge of the structure of organization of public education

2. Knowledge of the role and function of BOCES and responsibilities for relationships with school districts

3. Knowledge of the mission of BOCES

4. Knowledge of the organization of speech-language pathology and audiology services within the BOCES organization

5. Knowledge of the mission of the Speech-Language Pathology and Audiology Department.

Appendix 10–F

Observation Conference Form

Participants   _____

                  _____

Date: _____

Discussed:

Next Steps:

THIS DOCUMENT IS NOT PART OF THE OFFICIAL RECORD

Appendix 10–G

Professional Staff Evaluation

The evaluation that follows is based upon the eight components of professional behavior: communication, understanding/knowledge of field, management of the professional environment, planning, instructional strategies, interpersonal skills, administrative responsibilities, and willingness to grow. Your signature below signifies receipt of the evaluation. The original, signed evaluation will be placed in your personnel file.

Please sign and return the original to your department chair.

Evaluatee: _____

Evaluator: _____

Department/School: _____

Date: _____

Evaluator Signature: _____

Evaluatee Signature: _____

Comments:

Appendix 10–H

Sample Mentoring Announcement Letter

Dear _____ :

Welcome to your new assignment in Preschool. The Preschool Services Committee has developed a plan for mentoring individuals who are new to Preschool or for whom Preschool is a change in assignment.

Mentoring in the BOCES #1 Speech-Language Pathology and Audiology Department is an informal, voluntary support process. As an adjunct to our Supervision/Evaluation process, I hope you find it helpful for ongoing, on-the-spot problem solving.

Your mentor is _____. (S)he will be in touch with you soon. Feel free to use offered assistance in ways that are most helpful to you.

Please let me know if you have questions, or if additional information would be helpful.

Sincerely,

Chapter 11

Serving Culturally and Linguistically Diverse Students

Dolores E. Battle and Regina B. Grantham

This chapter will provide information that will assist school speech-language pathologists in providing appropriate service to culturally and linguistically diverse students in the public/private schools. It will present cultural and linguistic variables that must be considered in the evaluation and treatment of students from culturally and linguistically diverse backgrounds.

CULTURALLY AND LINGUISTICALLY DIVERSE CHILDREN IN SPECIAL EDUCATION

There are 48.5 million children enrolled in public and private schools in the United States. It is projected that by 2000, at least 33% of these students will be from culturally and linguistically diverse groups. By 2020, almost half of the nation's students will be from these groups. In California, Hawaii, Mississippi, New Mexico, Texas, and the District of Columbia, Caucasians already make up less than 50% of students enrolled in public and private schools (State Legislatures, 1994).

According to the 1990 census, 32 million people in the United States or 13% of the population speak a language other than English at home, the most common being Spanish. As shown in Table 11–1, in 10 states more than half a million students speak a language other than English at home.

According to 1990 census data, 76.4% of the general population is white and 23.6% is minority. As shown in Table 11–2, the largest group is African American (11.5%), followed by Hispanic (8.53%), Asian/Pacific (2.78%), and Native American (0.75%).

Although minorities make up 23.6% of the U.S. population, 32% of all students in schools are minority. Olsen (1991) stated that about 12% of the minority-language population in the United States requires special education. If estimates of the incidence of communication disorders is consistent across this group as in the general population, 4.8 million culturally and linguistically diverse children, or 10% of the nation's children, will require the services of a speech-language pathologist in the public schools. These estimates are generally thought to be conservative because many cultural and linguistic diverse groups have health and social problems particular to their race, ethnicity, or socioeconomic status that increase the likelihood of communication disorders.

There is, for example, a greater incidence of otitis media, or middle-ear disease, among Native Americans (Downs, in press). Pang-

Table 11–1 The 10 States with the Most Residents (Age 5 and Older) Who Speak a Language Other Than English at Home, and the Percentage Increase between 1980 and 1990

State	Non–English Speakers	% Increase
CA	8,619,334	73.6
TX	3,970,304	39.7
NY	3,908,720	18.5
FL	2,098,315	73.5
IL	1,499,112	22.7
NJ	1,406,148	28.3
MA	852,228	21.0
PA	806,876	5.8
AZ	700,287	38.9
MI	569,807	1.5

Source: Reprinted from U.S. Census Bureau.

Ching, Robb, Heath and Takum (1995) reported that 15% of preschool Native American children failed an auditory test battery including tympanometry, acoustic reflecometry, and pneumatic otoscopy. Approximately 9% to 15% failed audiometric and tympanometric tests at each of serial screenings, indicating significant levels of middle-ear infections. These infections may result in fluctuating hearing loss and, in some circumstances, delayed speech or language development. Native Americans and Asians have a higher incidence of orofacial anomalies such as cleft lip and palate (Vanderas, 1987). Persons of African and Mediterranean descent are more likely than other populations to carry a gene for sickle-cell anemia, which can cause blockage of oxygen-enriched blood to the inner ear and brain, thus causing hearing loss and speech, language, and cognitive disabilities (Scott, 1985).

As many as 13 million children born into poverty are urban and multiracial. According to Hodgkinson (1985), these children are far more likely to be judged by teachers to need remedial or special education than children from middle-class families. The U.S. Department of Health and Human Services (DHHS; 1985) reported that economically disadvantaged populations are more likely to be predisposed to causes of disorders related to environmental, teratogenic (causing developmental malformations), nutritional, and traumatic factors than other groups. For example, children from low socioeconomic urban environments are more likely to be exposed to high levels of lead poisoning, which can cause decreased cognitive abilities and associated speech and language disabilities. Approximately 21% of all American children live below the poverty line. When we examine poverty rates among groups, we find that

Table 11–2 1990 Racial/Ethnic Breakdown of Students Receiving Special Education Under Selected Categories

	Native American	Asian	Hispanic	African American	Total Minority
% of all students in school	1	3	12	16	32
Disability Category					
Mentally retarded	1	1	11	34	47
Speech impaired	1	2	9	16	27
Emotionally disturbed	1	1	6	22	29
Specific learning disabled	1	1	11	17	30

Source: Adapted from the Office of Civil Rights, The National and State Summaries of Data from the 1990 Elementary and Secondary School Civil Rights Survey, 1992.

45.9% of African-American and 40.4% of Hispanic children live in poverty. This contrasts dramatically with the 2% of Swedish children and 9% of Canadian children in poverty homes (Huston, McLoyd, & Coll, 1994). Huston et al. speak of poverty as a pervasive stressor, negatively affecting parenting, home environment, family structure, and immediate resources. Walker, Greenwood, Hart, and Carta (1994) found that children from lower socioeconomic backgrounds received less language stimulation and had lower language abilities, which were predictive of lack of school success.

Although cultural/linguistic diversity is not always accompanied by low socioeconomic status, it frequently is, and low socioeconomic status is itself a negative factor in both language development and school success. Even when socioeconomic levels and environment are held constant, persons from racial/ethnic minority groups appear to have higher incidences of lead poisoning than Caucasians (Mayfield, in press). These and other variables, such as child abuse, single-parent families, hopelessness, teen pregnancies, and low educational achievement, may increase the number of individuals in poverty and cultural and linguistically diverse individuals with communication disorders.

EDUCATIONAL POLICIES AFFECTING CULTURALLY AND LINGUISTICALLY DIVERSE STUDENTS

In spite of the large numbers of children from cultural and linguistic-diverse families, until the 19th century, educational policies in most school laws made no mention of language instruction or permitted instruction in a language other than English (Castellanos, 1983). In the early 1900s, some states required English as the medium of instruction. Prohibition of non-English in the school continued until late 1960s when the Bilingual Education Act of 1968 (Pub. L. No. 90-247) was enacted. This act was to provide transitional programs that used the child's native language in conjunction with English instruction before children entered English-only classes. *Lau v. Nichols* (1974) held that schools must devise programs to ensure equality in educational opportunity for speakers of non-English. The Lau Remedies specified that when school districts had 20 or more limited-English-proficient (LEP) students from one language group, the children's native language was to be used for instruction until each child had sufficient English to enter English-only classes. The Individuals With Disabilities Education Act (IDEA; Pub. L. No. 101-476) requires that children not be placed into special services on the basis of their language, culture, socioeconomic status, or lack of opportunity to learn. These legal requirements make it mandatory for speech-language pathologists to be able to assess and provide intervention appropriately for students in their native language and free from cultural bias.

DISTINGUISHING BETWEEN COMMUNICATION DISORDERS, DIFFERENCES, AND DIALECTS

Communication Disorders Culturally Defined

The first consideration for the speech-language pathologist is to determine whether a communication disorder exists. Communication disorders must be defined within the context of culture and must be distinguished from social dialects and variables expected because of normal development. To provide speech-language services appropriately to culturally and linguistically diverse populations, it is necessary to include reference to expectations within the child's cultural and linguistic community concerning the definition of *communication disorder.* Taylor (1986) provided a culturally sensitive revision of Van Riper's classic definition of communication disorder: communication behavior by an individual can only be considered disordered if it

1. deviates sufficiently from the norms, expectations, and definitions of the child's indigenous culture or language group;

2. is considered to be disordered by the indigenous culture of language group;

3. operates outside of the minimal norms of acceptability of that culture or language group;

4. interferes with communication *within* the indigenous culture or language group, or

5. calls attention to itself within the indigenous culture or language group.

Dialects and Cultural Diversity

A *dialect* is a variation within a specific language. Dialects exist within every language in the world. All dialects are intrinsically valid for the group of persons who speak them (Taylor, 1986). Each dialect has its own unique phonological, semantic, morphological, syntactic, and pragmatic characteristics. Speech-language pathologists must be able to distinguish dialects of a language from its disordered production. For example, it is a feature of Spanish dialects to use /s/ where speakers of Standard American English use /z/, resulting in production of /sebra/ for /zebra/. This is normal and appropriate use of phonology for speakers of Spanish-influenced English and is not considered a disorder.

Linguistic variation is not restricted to phonology and syntax. It also extends to other areas of language, such as pragmatics. Throughout their interactions with children, teachers use certain types of speech acts to control behavior and solicit cooperation. These functions vary across contexts, and expectations may vary across cultures. For example, a teacher may ask, "John will you clean the board?", which is an indirect question-command. Not all children are socialized to respond to indirect question-commands. African-American children get into trouble because they respond literally, as if these utterances were requests that could be denied and not commands. Such a response may not be a lack of ability to understand, but rather a cultural interpretation of a statement.

The ASHA *Position Paper on Social Dialects* (1983) stated that it is the position of the ASHA that no dialectal variety of English is a disorder or a pathological form of speech or language. Therefore a child in the schools who uses a social dialect that is appropriate to his or her indigenous community should not be identified as having a communication disorder.

Normal Language Development

It is also important to distinguish normal developmental patterns from disorders and dialect. General patterns of first-language acquisition follow a set of universal principles. Communicative norms within a particular group are the product of cultural values, perceptions, attitudes, and history (Saville-Troike, 1979). They affect all features of language, including phonology, semantics, syntax, morphology, and pragmatics. For example, the use of /f/ for final /θ/ is a commonly recognized feature of Black English vernacular. However, because the final /ə/ is not developed in General American English until age 7, it is not appropriate to identify the use of final /f/ by any child as a disordered pattern before the child is 7 years of age. It is likewise not appropriate to identify the use of the final /f/ for /ə/ by a user of Black English Vernacular as a disorder at any age because this is a normal feature of the particular dialect.

Normal language development may be affected by social status of the family. Social status is determined by combinations of factors including occupation; education of the parents, especially the mother; income; and lifestyle. A number of studies have identified differences in developmental patterns of preschool children across social class of families. This literature demonstrates that young children, universally, are spoken to and learn to listen and talk to others according to the particular values and beliefs of their language community (Heath, 1982; Lynch & Hanson, 1992; Smitherman, 1988; Ward, 1982).

For example, in a study of families in the Piedmont of North Carolina, Heath (1982) showed that children in working-class Caucasian homes were included in adult conversations, as were children in African-American homes. However, language input was not specifically modified for them, topics were not addressed to them, and adults did not ask the children questions to engage them in conversations.

Speech-Language Disorders Versus Normal Second-Language Acquisition in Bilingual Children

Many children in the schools are bilingual; that is, they speak and understand two languages with equal proficiency. Some children speak two languages, but with unequal profi-

ciency. The unequal proficiency may be because the child is in the process of learning the second language or because he or she has a speech-language disorder that restricts the ability to learn either language.

A speech-language disorder in bilingual children is difficult to distinguish from normal second-language acquisition. This distinction must be made when providing service to culturally and linguistically diverse school-aged children. Speech-language pathologists must not only consider particular dialects but also be able to distinguish the effect of second-language learning from disordered production of either language being used by the child.

Simultaneous Versus Sequential Bilingual Language Development

A child can acquire two languages at the same time or one after the other. Simultaneous bilingualism occurs when the child develops two languages from the onset of language. As preschool children learn language simultaneously, they do not seem to know that they are learning two languages and are able to learn the two languages equally well. This is particularly true if the two languages are learned before the age of 3 years and if each significant caretaker or parent is consistent in the use of the languages. The children are able to switch code or alternate the use of the two languages, with a complete separation between the two languages (Kayser, 1993).

Sequential or consecutive bilingualism occurs when the child acquires a second language (L2) early in childhood but after basic linguistic acquisition of the first language (L1) has been achieved (Langdon, 1992). Children who are learning L2 sequentially may be at various stages of acquisition of L2. It is important that the speech-language pathologist understand principles in bilingual language acquisition to distinguish normal second-language acquisition from speech-language disorders.

Language Mixing

Language mixing occurs when entire linguistic units from one language are attached onto units of another language. This type of mixing is illustrated in the sentence "*Pero verdad que* it was worth it" (But the truth is that it was worth it). Words of the dominant language are more frequently used in the sentences of the nondominant or weaker language. The speaker may also use pronunciation, rhythm, intonation, and other suprasegmental features of the dominant language while speaking the other language (Kayser, 1995). There may be mixing of syntax of both languages as well, resulting in a syntactic pattern that is not common to either language. This normal characteristic of language mixing is often misidentified as language disorder by persons not familiar with the languages being used and the effects of language mixing.

Language Loss

An additional concern in identifying language disorders in bilingual school-aged children is the concept of language loss. Language loss is the loss of a first or second language because of lack of use. As children become more involved in the monolingual environment of school, they will use English more often than their first language. Because English is the language of instruction, it becomes dominant in the academic setting. As children use English more to express the concepts learned in school and to communicate with English-speaking peers in school, they will become less proficient in the language of the home. This is called *language loss*. Language loss is a natural phenomenon as children become more proficient in one language and prefer its use in academic and social settings out of the home (Langdon, 1992). Because children become less proficient in their first language as the result of language loss, they are often identified as having a language disorder while they are developing competence in the second language because neither the first language nor the second language is produced according to the development norms. It is important to take a very careful history of language use in both school and home environments and language development in both languages before language disorder can be distinguished from normal second-language acquisition.

Language Interference

Phonological variation between languages also gives the impression that the speaker is showing a speech disorder. All sounds are not present in all languages. The sounds of one language may be used in place of the sounds of another giving the appearance of a speech-disorder. However, these represent normal influence or interference of one language on the production of another.

It is common for speakers of Spanish to use the following sounds in place of the Standard English sounds (Langdon, 1992, pp 154–155):

/s/ for /z/	*sebra* for *zebra*
/S/ for /tS/	*shair* for *chair*
/tS/ for /S/	*chip* for *ship*
/d/ for /ð/	*den* for *then*
/t/ for /θ/	*tief* for *thief*; *bat* for *bath*
/f/ for /v/	*fan* for *van*
/b/ for /v/	*berry* for *very*; *cabe* for *cave*
/u/ for /U/	*pull* for *pool*
/i/ for /I/	*cheap* for *chip*

/ə/ for /ou/   *call* for *coal*

/esp/ for /sp/   *Espanish* for *Spanish*

Word order variations in one language dialect may be different from that in another. As children acquire the second language, they may use the word order from Language 1 as they use the semantics or words from Language 2. For example, the Spanish "*Se ve linda la luna*" is translated as "Looks pretty the moon" in English. It is acceptable also to produce "*La luna se ve linda*" in Spanish for "The moon looks pretty." Flexibility in Spanish syntax is permissible. Variation in word order within noun phases should not be confused with language disorder.

Language interference may also be present in morphology. Morphological and syntactic differences between Spanish and English include the following:

- Omission of the auxiliary *is*: "he going" versus "he is going"
- Transference of the possessive form: "the coat of the boy" (*el abrigo del nino*) versus "the boy's coat"
- Incorrect negative form: "He not playing any more" (*ya no juega*) versus "He doesn't play any more"
- Incorrect interrogative form: "How the story helps?" (*Como ayuda la historia?*) versus "How does the story help?"
- Incorrect use of pronouns: "She is putting the towel on his head" versus "She is putting the towel on her head" (same pronoun for male and female)
- Substitution of some prepositions: *on* for *in*
- Word order with adjectives: "the house red" (*la casa roja*) versus "the red house"
- Lack of agreement of subject and verb: "The girl are playing" versus "The girls are playing"

- Omission of *to* in the second verb: "I want eat" versus "I want to eat"
- Omission of article: "The ant came back to grass" versus "The ant came back to the grass"
- Omission of pronoun: "Then flew back" versus "Then he flew back"
- Addition of pronouns: "The bird he came too" versus "The bird came too"
- Incorrect use of negative: "No help him" versus "Don't help him"

ASSESSMENT OF CULTURALLY AND LINGUISTICALLY DIVERSE CHILDREN

The Individuals With Disabilities Education Act (IDEA: Pub. L. No. 101-476) requires that all assessment for the purpose of determining the need for special education services be racially or culturally nondiscriminatory. There have been several court cases involving discriminatory evaluation practices in special education. One of the earliest cases was *Diana v. State Board of Education* (1970), in which students whose language was Spanish were evaluated in English, using tests developed for and normed on white, English-speaking students. The students scored low, were classified as mentally retarded, and were placed in special education. *Larry P. v. Riles* (1979), *Mattie T. v. Holliday* (1979), *Lora v. Board of Education* (1984), *PASE v. Hannon* (1980), *Marshall v. McDaniel* (1984) concerned disproportionate classification and placement of students in special education classes for students with intellectual abilities based on the results of IQ tests or inappropriate language. The law (*IDEA*, 1991) specifically requires that tests and other evaluation materials must be provided and administered in the child's native language or other mode of communication, unless [it is] clearly not feasible to do so.

Research consistently indicates that students from low-income and minority families score lower on tests of intelligence and achievement than do Caucasian middle-class children (Cohen, 1969; Williams, 1970) and that typical evaluation procedures tend to be biased against students from minority and low-income families (Fuchs & Fuchs, 1986).

Cultural differences have resulted in overrepresentation of students from culturally and linguistically diverse backgrounds in special education. The U.S. Department of Education reported that African-American students, compared with their percentage in the overall student population, are overrepresented in special education programs in 39 states. The 15th Annual Report to the Congress on the Implementation of the Individuals with Disabilities Act (cited in Ayers, 1994) indicated that minorities are enrolled in special education in greater numbers than general population figures would suggest. The analysis found that they are most likely to be overrepresented in special education classes in predominately white school districts. However, in some school districts, neither the number of African-American students nor household demographics accounted for the high percentage of African-American students in special education. The report concluded that the findings tend to support arguments by critics concerning cultural bias in testing and placement procedures rather than any inherently high level of disability (Peters-Johnson, 1995).

For example, as shown in Table 11–2, although 32% of students enrolled in public schools are minorities, 47% of children classified as mentally retarded in the public schools are minorities, as well as 27% of the speech impaired, 29% of the emotionally disturbed, and 30% of the specific learning disabled. Whereas only 14.0% of the children in secondary schools are African Americans, 24.2% of secondary school children in special education are African Americans (Ayers, 1994).

This overrepresentation of minority children in special education is often cited as being the result of overzealous referrals, inappropriate referrals, inappropriate testing and evaluation, and inappropriate consideration of normal but culturally different behaviors.

To conduct speech-language assessment of culturally and linguistically diverse children in the schools appropriately, it is necessary to understand the relationship between culture and language. Cultural variables affect the way children interact with the clinician and their approach to the testing situation. Language will affect the application of norms and the interpretation of behavior that may be quite appropriate for the culture.

Prereferral Cultural Considerations in Prereferral Observations

IDEA requires that children be observed in the classroom prior to being referred for special education evaluation. There must be an indication that the child's ability to function in the classroom is not related to differences in culture. However, many behaviors of children who are culturally or linguistically diverse can be and often are misidentified as indicators of need for special services (Hoover & Collier, 1985).

Children who are culturally different may be withdrawn and nonverbal in the classroom. They may not interact with their peers, preferring to be alone. They may not respond when spoken to by the teacher because they are unsure of their ability to use appropriate language. This is particularly true of students learning a second language and adapting to a new culture. It may also be culturally appropriate for the child not to respond when unsure of the response.

Culturally different children may also appear to be disorganized because they have difficulty keeping their belongings or bringing required materials from home. This may be because the child is not familiar with the supplies necessary for school and may not have the requested materials in the home. The child may appear to waste time, fail to keep schedules, or not complete assignments within the prescribed time period. This behavior may be because the concept of time varies considerably from culture to culture.

Culturally different children may not comply with classroom rules. They may talk to peers in class and provide assistance to class peers. This may be related to their cultural expectation to cooperate and work for group achievement.

In response to cultural differences, some children appear to not care about school activities, to fight or harass other students, to talk back to the teacher, and not to follow the rules of the school or class. This is often a defensive reaction to changes in cultural expectations brought about by anxiety and resistance to change.

Aspects of the Testing Culture

Testing and evaluation in the public schools are rooted in Western culture. Several nonverbal and verbal factors influence testing and the client's response to the testing situation (Westby, 1994).

Perception and Use of Time

Cultures are either .monochronic or polychronic in their perception of time. In monochronic cultures, time perception is linear, with one task being completed before a second task is begun. Polychronic cultures allow several activities to be carried on at the same time, with varying times of completion. If a child is rooted in a monochronic time culture, he will start and finish a task without interruption and will attempt to be the first to complete a task. If a child is rooted in a polychronic culture, several activities may be conducted at the same time. Certain tasks will be left uncompleted while others are begun. There is no direct pressure to complete one task before another is begun. Students who have a polychronic perception of time will be at a disadvantage in timed tests, may leave items uncompleted, and may not maintain attention on a task or test until all items have been completed.

A second difference in the use of time relates to rigid versus fluid time. In Western European cultures, time is more rigid, with specific time lines for beginning and ending tasks. Certain time parameters are established and followed for all activities. Students from more rigid time cultures will begin tasks on time, finish tasks in the appropriate time, and do well on timed tasks. In more fluid non–Western time cultures, such as Hispanic and Middle Eastern cultures, time markers are not rigid. Activities, personal variation, and social situations govern when activities begin and end, without strict adherence to temporal units. Students who are rooted in fluid time cultures do not do well on timed tests or in activities with strict time limitations.

A child who has a cognitive style that requires a longer contemplative response time may be penalized on test items that require a quick response, or if the tester believes that the longer response time indicates that the child does not know the answer. Navaho and Pueblo Indian children prefer a longer wait time before responding. Wait time is the amount of time given by teachers for a student's responses and the amount of time following a student's response before the teacher again speaks. Navaho teachers permit a longer wait time than Caucasian teachers. What Caucasian teachers perceive as a completed response is often intended by the child to be a pause (Harris, 1993).

Learning and Display Learning

In Western European cultures, children are encouraged to display what they know. They are encouraged to guess rather than let it be thought that they do not know. They are used to a trial-and-error format in which they attempt a response, expect to receive feedback about their success, and then make modifications in their response based on the available feedback. Western-culture children are willing to attempt unfamiliar test items or test formats. They are willing to guess when they are uncertain and are likely to change their response if necessary.

Children with cultural roots in non–Western cultures, such as African American, Asian/Pacific, or Native American, prefer not to display what they know until they are certain that they are correct. They are socialized to observe adult models before attempting a task. They are hesitant to attempt unfamiliar tasks, and they resist trial-and-error learning. Non–Western children will resist guessing and will be reluctant to change their answer once they have made a response. Thus they will not perform well on normative tests that depend on obtaining a raw score of correct responses.

Group Versus Individual

Children who are rooted in Western cultures are competitive and strive for individual recognition and achievement. In test situations, they strive to obtain a high score to earn individual recognition. They are concerned about the number that they get correct and are often overly concerned when they are not correct. This is especially true as the child reaches a ceiling and is aware that his or her responses are not correct.

Non–Western children strive for recognition by the group. They will achieve to please the family and to bring honor to the family. Assurance that the parents will be pleased at the success serves as a motivator during testing. At times, a child will not aggressively pursue a higher score because he or she does not want to exceed the score of the group. Assurance that obtaining a higher score will help the group serves as a motivator to achieve.

Sociolinguistic Dimensions

Children in testing situations are also affected by the social relationship between the child and the clinician. Children from some cultures have a conflict between the race and gender of the clinician and their own. Terrell and Terrell (1993) stated that there is general agreement among African–American persons across educational, socioeconomic, gender, and geographical strata that African-Americans do not trust whites. Terrell, Terrell, and Taylor (1981) and Terrell and Terrell (1983) administered an intelligence test to African–American children who had either a high or a low level of mistrust of whites. It was found that individuals with high levels of mistrust obtained lower test scores than persons with low levels of mistrust. It can be expected, then, that children who have mistrust of the clinician will not do well on speech-language tests.

Verbal Aspects of Testing

Several aspects of testing are directly related to students' language use. These differences affect the ability of the culturally and linguistically diverse student to perform in the test situation.

Language Function

The rules for language function vary across cultures. These may affect the child's manner of responding in the testing situation. Preparation for school is a cultural phenomenon. The child's preparation for school and for testing is largely a factor of the type, quality, and quantity of interactions that vary as a result of parents' educational level, home language, ethnicity, and socioeconomic status (Iglesias, 1985). Child-rearing practices vary across cultures.

In many homes, children are passive listeners. Children from working-class homes may look at pictures in books without verbal input from caretakers. Heath (1982) reported that working-class families had as few as 60 verbal interactions with their children in the same period that middle-class families had 1,522 verbal interactions. Farran (1982) and Heath (1982, 1983) reported that children in working-class homes are rarely read to and do not engage in story retelling. Discourse consists primarily of recounting of family history or events rather than fiction or fantasy.

In other homes, children are active verbal participants in the development of literacy. In middle-class homes, parents engage in more sustained conversations with their preschool children. Children are encouraged to look at pictures that parents name. Children are then expected to label pictures, answer questions, and eventually retell the story themselves.

When children from passive or nonliterate homes are asked to engage in picture-naming or picture identification test items in school, there is a communicative mismatch between the child's communication skills and those expected in the testing situation. Children

may not do well on items that depend on their previous preliteracy skill development.

Question behavior is different in working-class and poverty families. Differences in question function must be considered in testing situations.

Genuine questions are those asked when the questioner does not know the answer. Pseudoquestions are those asked when the questioner knows the answer, such as, for example, "What's this?" "Where's Waldo?" and "Who's this?" (Heath, 1982). In genuine questions, the response is intended to provide information unknown to the questioner, usually concerning the social situation: "Where's your brother?" "Do you want more milk?"

According to Heath (1982), there may be cultural differences in the nature of questions in preschool homes. In many literate homes, pseudoquestions are used to engage children in question–answer routines that are intended to teach picture identification and picture-naming tasks. These pseudoquestions are used for instruction and are common activities in homes where the development of literacy is important. Children from such homes come to the testing situation able to identify pictures and to respond to questions as demanded in most standardized tests. The families challenge their children to expand on their answers and respond at a higher level, and they ask for clarification and explanations. Children are encouraged to do event casts and recounts.

According to the work of Heath (1982), working-class children are asked to recount but are usually asked genuine questions. They are not encouraged to elaborate on their answers. Without pseudoquestion experience, children come to school with less practice and experience with the tasks that are needed to be successful in school and are more likely to be considered to require special services.

In addition, the purpose of questions in the child–caretaker relationship may be viewed as an interrogation. The response to a question such as "Who ate the cake?" may result in punishment or anger from guilty peers. If questions from authority figures are viewed as interrogations, the result may be the child's unwillingness to respond.

Children who do not have formal pseudoquestion experiences as preschoolers may not be successful in response to test questions. Children who are rooted in cultures that do not permit students to challenge or question authority figures will not ask questions for clarification during test situations. To ask a question would imply that the clinician did not give adequate instruction. Such an implication would indicate disrespect for the clinician. This is a particular problem when children are exposed to an unfamiliar test format with unfamiliar directions. Test takers may thus not perform the test item correctly and be penalized by obtaining a score that does not reflect true ability.

Language Content

There is cultural variation in the items that are taught to children prior to coming to test situations. The teaching of preacademic skills, such as color names, shapes, numbers, object names, reading routines, and prewriting skills is an important part of Western middle-class upbringing. It is not an important function in some non–Western or poverty homes. In non–Western and poverty homes, such items are expected to be taught in school. The preschool years are focused on socialization skills, group cooperation, and family roles rather than specific content. Such children will not do well on tests that have heavy content in preacademic skills.

Frequently in vocabulary tests, there is bias in the way words and concepts are represented in test items. Certain vocabulary words may not translate easily from one language or dialect to another. For example, the Navaho translation for *construction* is "There is a man hitting a board with a hammer." If a child gave this response, he would be misidentified as using circumlocution or having a word-finding problem.

Vocabulary items may be easily represented and developed early in one culture but not until a later age or differently in a child in another culture. For example, a child living in the rural Midwest may not develop an understanding of vocabulary items more common in cities, such as *hydrant* or *curb*. If color words are not important in a culture, asking the child to define *brown* as on the Test of Language Development P:2, (Newcomer & Hammill, 1991) will be influenced by the child's lack of exposure to the term.

In addition, some non–Western children attempt to find meaning in items themselves. Because they derive meaning from context, when items are decontextualized they have more difficulty. Test items that require following directions out of context, pointing to discrete pictures, describing, and defining words out of context will be difficult for these children and may not indicate their true potential.

Language Organization

The way language is organized differs across languages.

Western narrative style is linear and direct. Non–Western conversation style is asymmetrical or circular. This difference may give the impression that discourse or narrative style is disordered; however, it may follow the rules of cultural thought patterns. Also, non–Western cultures often will provide no response to questions that they are not sure of or personal questions that they prefer not to answer. This too will affect the tester's perception of the client's ability to manage discourse.

Heath (1982), Smitherman and Van Dyck (1988), and Michaels (1981) reported that the literate style of lower or working-class children is organized differently from that of middle-class children. Middle-class children produced topic-centered, linear narratives tightly structured on a single topic or a series of closely related topics, with no major shifts in perspectives. Their narratives contained a high degree of temporal organization, with a temporal or sequential organization that began with a temporal grounding and statement of focus, followed by the introduction of key agents, developed through elaboration of the theme or topic, and ending with a resolution of the problem. The inclusion of precise detail acknowledged a lack of shared knowledge between speaker and listener. The working-class children produced associative narratives that consisted of a series of associated segments implicitly linked by topic, theme, or event. The topics were marked by shifts across segments often marked by changes in pitch and tempo. Because there was presumed shared knowledge, there was considerable less detail. Narratives were longer because of the increased number of themes.

These differences in organization or structure of language across cultures must be considered when evaluating whether the observed behavior is a speech-language disorder, the reflection of normal development, or a reflection of cultural organization of language.

Limitations of Standardized Tests

According to Wolfram (1983), "The more superficial and limited the scope of language capability tapped in a testing instrument, the greater the likelihood that the instrument will be inappropriate for speakers beyond the immediate population on which it was normed" (p. 21). The problems of speech-language assessment do not end with the administration of tests; they continue into test interpretation and analysis. Test norms generally are not applicable to culturally and linguistically diverse students.

To the extent that test norms and content do not adequately represent the characteristics and culture of specific populations, standardized and norm-referenced tests may produce test results that are biased against students of minority groups, those of low socioeconomic status, or those with existing disabilities. To be used appropriately, standardization criteria of normative tests must be representative of the various cultures, including racial/ethnic groups, social class, and geographical regions as well as such variables as age and gender.

Vaughn-Cooke (1983) has developed a set of guidelines that are useful for the evaluation of assessment instruments:

1. Can the procedure account for language variation?

2. Are the assumptions about language that underlie the procedure valid?

3. Does the procedure include an analysis of a spontaneous speech sample?

4. Does the procedure allow the reliable determination as to whether the system is developing normally?

5. Do the results provide principled guidelines for language intervention?

6. Can the procedure provide an adequate description of the child's knowledge of language?

7. Can the test distinguish between those differences that can be attributed to dialect or cultural differences?

8. Can the results of the test be adjusted to account for dialect differences?

9. Would the test be able to distinguish those speakers from a nonstandard-English-speaking community that indicate a true pathology within the context of the indigenous community from those that simply use indigenous community norms?

10. Will the sociological assumptions underlying the social occasion of the testing and the particular elicitation techniques influence the results of the test?

SUGGESTIONS FOR ADAPTING ASSESSMENT TO CULTURALLY AND LINGUISTICALLY DIFFERENT CHILDREN

In spite of the acknowledged difficulty with the use of standardized tests procedures to document a client's disability, schools often require that disability be verified through standardized test procedures. The tests can be used only to determine the child's performance in relation to the group of mainstream age peers. The reason for the child's performance must be interpreted against the sources of cultural bias, lack of opportunity to learn the required material, unfamiliarity with the test item or test format, or difficulty in the social situation of testing. Several methods have been suggested to modify tests to make them more useful; however, caution must be taken not to assume that the use of any or all of these procedures eliminates the bias present in the testing situation itself (Erickson & Iglesias, 1986; Hamayan & Damico, 1991; Vaughn-Cooke, 1986; Westby, 1994).

Using interpreters and translators or translations of tests into a child's dominant language is a common method of accommodating cultural differences. However, it does not solve the problem of inappropriate test standardization (Kayser, 1989). The linguistic differences in languages and differences in specific dialects within a language make translations inappropriate. For example, in Spanish there are differences in honorifics (formal *Usted* vs. familiar *tu*) gender markers (*el* vs. *la*), semantics (*arroz*, tomato-based and spicy grain, vs. *rice*, white or brown grain), structural rules, and registers (Cuban vs. Mexican), as well as social discourse rules. Also, in Vietnamese there are plurals and no possessives. In Spanish, there are few single-syllable words and no spondee words. Many Native American languages do not have gender pronouns, future-tense verbs, or a word for time (Roseberry-McKibbin, 1995). These differences in languages make it impossible for translations to be equivalent to the original test item.

Interpreters may not accurately reflect the intent of the test item, preferring to explain the item's perceived meaning instead of doing a direct translation of the test item or the response. In addition, translations may not take into account differences in the development of linguistic or semantic concepts, nor may they take into account the linguistic complexity differences between languages.

Standardizing existing tests on minority populations also has limitations. Standardized tests are based on mainstream cultures. Attempts to standardize tests on particular racial/ethnic or cultural groups usually are not feasible because of the cost involved in developing a large enough representative sample even within a particular cultural group. To attempt to standardize a test on "minority populations" in general results in the same problems as with standardization of the test on the mainstream population because of the heterogeneity among and across cultural groups.

Use of tests that include a representative sample of minorities in the standardization sample is another possible adaptation. But although most tests attempt to include representative samples of each group within the standardization sample, the resultant standardization sample is representative only of the group that participated in the standardization. It is not representative of a particular culture or the particular child being tested. The results can be used only to compare the child's performance against the group and cannot be used to indicate whether the child has a speech-language disorder within his or her cultural or linguistic community.

The difficulty with *modification of existing tests* is similar to that involved with translators or interpreters. Lack of equivalency across languages and cultures makes test modification difficult.

Use of a language sample and other observations has also been suggested. But the lack of developmental data and data on appropriate cultural communication behavior and expectations within cultural groups makes the evaluation of language samples and other observational data difficult. Without information on acceptable communication behavior within a cultural group, it is not possible to make reliable judgments about the normality of a client's communication behavior within the cultural community.

The *use of criterion-referenced measures* would appear to be a reasonable solution to the limitations incumbent in the use of standardized tests. Criterion-referenced testing requires the establishment of a standard against which to compare the child's performance to determine whether it is minimally adequate. The difficulty comes in determining what the criteria should be and what the order of the criteria should be.

For example, criteria for acceptable speaking and listening skills in kindergarten through first grade might be to speak clearly, to express oneself in grammatically acceptable simple sentences, to follow a set of basic commands, and to retell a simple short story. To determine whether the culturally and linguistically diverse child has met these criteria within his or her culture, it may be necessary to determine whether he can perform these tasks at acceptable levels in relation to his culture and age peers. It may be necessary to go beyond the basal and ceiling limits established for the test to determine additional pockets of knowledge or skills that the child has that may not be shown within the limits of the test. It may be necessary to observe the child's interaction with same-culture age peers or family members to determine whether his or her speech-language ability is appropriate.

Criterion-referenced measures may be helpful to determine whether the child has appropriate speech-language skills. These measures are designed to ascertain the child's level of performance in relation to a specific standard or criterion. Examples of criterion-referenced assessment questions are as follows:

1. Is the child developing receptive skills in the second language faster than expressive skills? Are the child's receptive and expressive language skills in the native language appropriate?

2. Is the child demonstrating soft signs of learning disability? Does the child have difficulty retaining concepts in his or her first language that are culturally appropriate? Does he or she follow directions in the proper sequence? Does he or she show evidence of difficulty with oral/motor functioning?

3. Is the child progressing at the same rate as others in his or her cultural or language group who have similar histories of exposure to the mainstream culture and language?

4. Is the child struggling to communicate in his or her native language? With same-language peers? With family members? Siblings?

5. How does the child attempt to communicate with English-speaking peers? Does the child attempt to adapt and revise his or her communication attempt to express his or her ideas to English-speaking persons?

6. Does the child use language to get attention? Request? Initiate communication? Are his or her attempts or lack of attempts explainable by his or her cultural communication rules?

7. Does the child ask questions or request clarification when he or she does not comprehend the message in English? In the second language?

8. Is the child learning language/literacy at the same rate as same-culture/same-language age peers?

9. How does the child deal with academic material that he or she has had an opportunity to learn versus academic material that he or she has had no opportunity to learn? Is the material that the child is able to learn context embedded or context reduced? Are there cues in the environment, or must the child rely on verbal cues alone?

10. Is there a difference between the child's ability with basic interpersonal communication skills (BICS; i.e., familiar conversation with his or her peers) and his or her cognitive academic language proficiency (CALP; i.e., the ability to use language to analyze, synthesize, and evaluate information within the academic curriculum expectations, as in science, social studies, and language arts)? (Cummins, 1984).

Mattes and Omark (1991) and Kayser (1990) have identified observable communication behaviors for Spanish- and English-speaking language-impaired students. These include the following:

1. Rarely initiates verbal interactions or activities with peers or family members.

2. Does not respond verbally when verbal interactions are initiated by peers or family members.

3. Does not engage in dialogue or conversation with peers or family members outside the classroom.

4. Uses gestures rather than speech to communicate with peers.

5. Peers indicate that they may be having difficulty understanding the child's oral and/or nonverbal communications.

6. Peers rarely initiate verbal interactions with the child.

7. Nonverbal aspects of communication are perceived by peers as inappropriate.

8. Does not attempt to repair communication failures when peers do not understand.

Because of the many difficulties in obtaining nonbiased, culture-free evaluation of culturally and linguistically diverse children in the schools, Westby (1994) has suggested alternate procedures for assessment with these children.

1. Understand the cultural parameters associated with the particular child being evaluated. This is of critical importance before any observation, assessment, or intervention takes place. All judgments and decisions must be made within the cultural context.

2. *Observe normal age peers in natural settings to determine culturally appropriate behavior and communication behaviors.* The settings must be natural to the child and should not be restricted to the classroom. More natural communication is observed in the cafeteria, the playground, the hallway, and the child's community than in the formal classroom. Observation of preschool children should include age peers' use of greeting, requests, describing, directing, recounting, predicting, initiating conversation, turn taking, amount of verbalization, maintaining topics, elaboration, repair, and other pragmatic and conversational discourse strategies. Observation of school-age children should include understanding elements of stories, causes of events, and characters' feelings problems; telling coherent stories, telling imaginative stories; comprehending complex sentence patterns; comprehending assigned texts; writing coherent and cohesive texts; and other tasks appropriate to the child's age.

3. *Observe the child in natural settings similar to those that served as the normal referent.* This will allow an opportunity to observe the child as he or she attempts to communicate with age peers and family members within the cultural linguistic group. It will allow the observation to be compared to the behaviors observed by normal children in similar situations.

4. *Involve parents and families in the assessment.* IDEA requires that parents participate in decisions regarding special education services for their children. Parental involvement is particularly important in speech-language services for culturally and linguistically diverse children. The parents may have a different view concerning disability and its treatment.

There is considerable variability across cultures in parental views toward disability and special educational services. In some cultures, the family may believe that the child was given a disability because of disapproval of the spirits. To seek treatment for the disability would be to go against the spirits or would indicate that human beings can have power over nature. In Hispanic families, spiritual healers are often sought to help with a physical disability. In some Hispanic families, it is believed that children will approach tasks when they are developmentally ready. In some Native American cultures, there is a wide tolerance of disability, with some groups not even having a word for the concept of disability. In Chinese American and Japanese American families, excellence is expected. School failure or the need for special services is thought to bring shame to the family because the family has not done its job of preparing the child for school.

The clinician must not only understand the parents' worldview regarding disability and rehabilitation but also obtain information about the child's language history, the language being used in the home, the goals that the family has for the child, the family's expectations for the child, and which person will be primarily responsible for the child's education at home. Because the dynamics and social roles within families are so diverse, it is important that the clinician become familiar with the family of the client so that ethnographic procedures can be used in interviewing and obtaining parental participation in the referral-assessment-intervention process, including participation in the development of the Individualized Educational Plan (IEP) or the Individual Family Service Plan (IFSP).

Ethnographic procedures have the goal of assisting the clinician in understanding the social situation in which the child lives; how the family perceive, feel about, and understand the child's problem; and the family's role in the treatment process (Westby, 1990).

INTERVENTION FOR CULTURALLY AND LINGUISTICALLY DIVERSE STUDENTS WITH COMMUNICATION DISORDERS

Western versus Non–Western Cultural Values and U.S. Schools

Culture is those behaviors that define who we are, what we think, and how we act. It is what we need to know to be functional members of a community and to regulate interaction with other members of the community (Taylor, 1986). The dimensions of culture include human nature, gender and family roles, the role of the individual versus groups, concepts of time, activity level, and social relations and traditions.

In cultures that have a non–Western tradition, there is a strong sense of community and allegiance to the family. Within the family, there are very strong gender roles, with elder males and authority figures being highly respected. There is a strong orientation to tradition, to the past, and, with less emphasis on the future, which is often considered to be not under human control.

In cultures that have a Western or European tradition, there is more reliance on individuality and independence. Each member of the community or family strives for individual achievement and individual recognition. There is an emphasis on youth and preparation for the future. Although authority figures are recognized, they are often questioned and challenged. The ability to interact with and challenge or question an authority

figure or elder is valued and encouraged.

Education is deeply rooted in culture. Family values, expectations of education, and relationship between students and peers or students and teachers are all determined by culture. Each culture reflects different styles of learning and rules for interaction that affect the academic setting. Kessen (1979) discussed Vygotsky's perspective on child development, one that emphasizes not individualism but "the embeddedness of the developing mind in society" (p. 820). The child, then, any child, cannot be understood adequately without reference to the society from which he or she comes.

Cultural Variation in Learning Style

For many years, educators have been searching for more effective ways to meet the needs of individual students in their classes. During the 1970s considerable attention was paid to the perceived variation in learning style observed by teachers, particularly in the newly integrated schools resulting from the 1964 Civil Rights Act. It was observed that the children from different families had different approaches to learning (Moore, Goodenough, & Cox, 1977). Witkin (1976) developed a theory of individual variation in approaches to learning, or learning styles, based on individuals' perceptions of the world. The research on learning styles, almost without exception, has been done from a Western, white, middle-class perspective and value system (Dunn & Griggs, 1988; Hilliard, 1989). The literature has focused on young children in elementary and secondary school.

Learning style is a preferred strategy for acquiring new information through organization, perception, processing, manipulation, and recall of information. Although individuals may have access to and use different styles, depending on a particular setting, subject matter, or audience, most persons have at least one preferred learning style. The preferred learning style appears to be a learned phenomenon that develops within a cultural context. Among sociocultural factors that influence learning style are cultural values and beliefs, socialization practices such as child rearing and the system of rewards and punishment in the family, and role development. Because social, cultural, and environmental milieus differ, it is logical to assume that these differences are reflected in the cultural/cognitive styles adopted or preferred by individuals.

Dunn and Dunn (1987) developed a model of learning styles based on student preferences for situations in the learning environment and their approach to the world. According to Messick (1976), each individual has a preferred way of organizing all that he or she sees, hears, remembers, and thinks about. These consistent individual differences in the ways of organizing and processing information and experiences have come to be called *cognitive* or *learning styles*. In each culture, reality is conceptualized in implicit and explicit premises and derivative generalizations that together form a coherent whole. Different cultures produce different learning styles as a factor of the socialization process. These cultural influences affect not only learning style but the subtler aspects of perception and cognition as well. People with different cultural histories, different adaptive approaches, and different socialization practices differ in the respective cognitive/learning styles. These differences in cultural roots are built on worldviews or patterns of beliefs and values that define a way of life and a way in which people act, judge, decide, and solve problems.

With the significant increase in cultural diversity in schools of the 1990s, there has been a rebirth of interest in cultural variation in learning style in schools. Belief that differences in learning style were linked to cultural variation led Sandhu (1994a, b) to propose that all children can learn but that they learn differently and learn better when they are taught in their specific learning style.

Recent examinations of the interaction of language and culture have served to underscore the extreme degree to which they are enmeshed. One example is provided by Maynard (1993) in her detailed treatment of discourse in Japanese. Her work stressed the importance of subjectivity, emotion, and social interaction in the Japanese language and noted that the Japanese linguistic conventions to signal important aspects of messages differ from those in English. This inevitably leads to confusion and difficulty in translation. Maynard further stated that differences in language mirror differences in the view of the self. In a paper more related to children specifically, Minami and McCabe (1995) examined narrative structure in Japanese children. They concluded that parental input shapes children's narratives to conform to cultural expectations and values and that the narratives of Japanese children reflect this influence.

In the United States, education and the manner in which it is presented are based on the cultural values of Northern Europe. The educational system serves primarily to prepare Caucasian middle-class children to participate in their own culture (Saville-Troike, 1979, p. 141). However, many of the children in the schools have their roots in cultures other than Northern European. Persons with cultural roots in Northern Europe, especially males, share the cultural view most consistent with that expected in the schools of the United States. Persons from non–Western cultures, such as Native Americans, African

Americans, Asians/Pacific Islanders, and Hispanics, do not share the Western cultural worldview and are thus at a disadvantage in American schools.

Western Cultural Values and Learning Style

Western culture places high value on objects or the acquisition of objects. Cognitively, Western cultures come to know through counting and measuring. Their logic is primarily dichotomous, with either/or choices being demanded. There is a reliance on technology, with data sets that are repeatable and reproducible (Nichols, 1992). Consequently, Western classrooms tend to be analytic and rule driven, requiring memory and recall of facts, with a direct, linear approach to problem solving. They emphasize competition and individual achievement and are time oriented and scheduled, scientific, hierarchical, and deductive (Hilliard, 1989, 1992; Sandhu, 1994a, 1994b).

Ramirez and Castenada (1974), in an analysis of learning style by cultural variation, concluded that persons from Western cultures prefer a *field-independent* learning style. They perceive elements as discrete from their background (Witkin, 1977). This preference affects their social-personal relationships, preferences for instruction, and communication style.

Field-independent learners maintain formal interpersonal relationships with school personnel. They are individualistic, preferring to work alone rather than in groups. They are highly competitive, valuing individual achievement and nonsocial rewards. Their performance is not affected by the performance of others or by criticism from the teacher. They maintain formal relationships with instructors, limiting their interactions

to the tasks at hand. Field-independent students rarely seek or give physical expression of their feelings to teachers in school.

Field-independent students prefer to attempt new tasks without assistance from the teacher. Trial-and-error learning is expected, with modification after appropriate feedback from the instructor. Their cognitive styles facilitate the analytical, mathematical, and scientific concepts in the curriculum through discovery learning. They learn material that is impersonal and in which details of concepts are emphasized. They prefer to finish tasks first in order to obtain nonsocial rewards or good grades.

The communication style of field-independent learners is linear and direct, with heavy emphasis on verbal language. They are able to understand the meaning of language independent of the context and thus are interested in developing a rich vocabulary.

Field-independent learning/cognitive style is synchronous with the expectation of Western cultures and the schools in this country. In Western cultures, students sit in rows in formal classrooms where teachers provide whole-group instruction on a textbook-lecture format, provide strict time limits and expectations for the completion of tasks, expect individual competition and achievement, and reward compliance with classroom rules and expectations with nonsocial rewards and grades.

Non–Western Cultural Values and Learning Style

Non–Western cultures are those with other than European cultural roots, including African, African-American, Hispanic, Arabic, Asian, Asian/Pacific, and Native American. Non–Western learners are thought to be sensitive to others, socially oriented, and cooperative. Non–Western cultures place the highest values on interpersonal relationships and the cohesiveness of the group. Family and group obligations take precedence over educational obligations. There is a greater emphasis on interdependence of thought and mind, with all sets of knowledge being perceived as harmoniously interrelated. Because they are strongly influenced by their surroundings, including peers and authority figures, non–Western students are thought to prefer a *field-dependent* learning style.

Non–Western cultures view the group and group achievement as more important than individual achievement. Field-dependent students like to work with others to achieve a common goal. There is an expectation of group achievement and cooperation. Families and friends are expected to be consulted and to assist in education. High value is placed on social and interpersonal environments. For example, on the Warm Springs Reservation in Oregon, when teachers solicited individual volunteers or when students were called on to respond individually in front of the group, the children did not respond. Participation in the class and responding increased when there was one-to-one interaction with the teacher or when students were asked to respond as part of a small group (Harris, 1993, Phillips, 1983).

Field-dependent students openly express personal feelings and attitudes about others. Although they may not ask questions about content issues, they openly ask questions about the teacher's tastes, personal life, and personal experiences. They expect the instructor to take a personal interest in their lives and to understand their commitment to family and friends. It is important for field-dependent students to have role models in the classroom and educational environment.

Students are expected to be successful and not to attempt a task until they have observed it and are certain that they can be successful. They are hesitant to guess and would prefer not to answer rather than to risk being wrong. Time is relative, with the past being more important than the present or future. In non–Western classrooms, education is formal, with teachers being highly valued. Teachers and adults are highly respected. They are not to be challenged or interrupted. It is expected that factual information rather than fiction will be taught. Harmony and avoidance of confrontation are expected. Students are expected to be humble (Boggs, 1972).

Field-dependent students do best on verbal tasks, especially those with human, social content and those that are presented in a humanized format. They do best when concepts are related to their personal interests and experiences. Their narrative style is more figurative, with symbolic or metaphoric word meanings rather than literal meanings. They derive words' meanings from context rather than assuming that words have explicit meanings embedded in them. Their performance is influenced by an authority figure's expression of confidence in their ability and social rewards, as opposed to nonsocial rewards or grades. They organize their time in holistic units and are not driven by discrete time units of Western cultures. The learning style of non–Western cultures conflicts with that of the traditional Western school environment.

Although in general, students from non–Western cultures show preference for field-dependent learning, not all non–Western cultures share all the learning style attributes described above. There are many differences as well as similarities between the culturally/linguistically diverse groups of students in our schools, as illustrated in Table 11–3.

Table 11–3 Characteristics of Learning Styles of Some Culturally/Linguistically Diverse Groups

Characteristic	African American	Hispanic	Native American	Asian/Pacific Islander
1. Field Dependent	X	X	X	X
2. Group Cooperation, not Competition	X	X	X	X
3. Interpersonal Relationships Stressed	X	X		
4. Nonconfrontational with Authorities		X	X	
5. Emphasis on Family Obligations			X	X
6. Prefer Auditory/Kinesthetic	X			
7. Prefer Visual Processing			X	
8. Longer Response Time		X	X	
9. Prefer Charismatic Teaching	X			
10. Prefer Formality				X
11. Prefer Informality	X			

It is well to emphasize that generalizations about language and culture are difficult to make with precision. As Gallimore and Goldenburg (1993) pointed out, culture is not equivalent to national origin. There is always a degree of variance within groups; everyone does not receive "an equal dose of something called culture" (Gallimore & Goldenburg, 1993, p. 331). It is just as important to view the child from a culturally diverse background as an individual as it is for any other child. Knowledge of and sensitivity to cultural differences, however, can serve as valuable guides.

Field-Dependent/Independent Teaching Style

Because most teachers and speech-language pathologists in American schools have their cultural roots in Western cultures, most teachers are likely to prefer a Western or field-independent teaching style.

Field-independent teachers maintain formal relationships with their students and give their primary attention to instruction and the academic environment. Social–interpersonal relationships are secondary. They encourage independence and individual achievement and foster competition in instruction. Field-independent instructors prefer a lecture/textbook format. They support the analytic preference of students by using charts, graphs, and mathematical formulas when appropriate. They use discovery learning, which fits with the field-independent preference of their students. As they function in a consultant role, they encourage a trial-and-error format, providing feedback to students and expecting students to monitor and correct their performance (Abraham, 1985).

Field-dependent teachers maintain more personal relationships with students, preferring to give verbal and physical signs of approval rather than nonsocial rewards. They encourage cooperation and group achievement and personalized rewards. Field-dependent teachers show confidence in the student's ability to achieve even if the student is not successful on the task. They prefer to instruct by modeling, providing guidance, and personalizing concepts. The curriculum presented focuses on global aspects and context rather than specific details of concepts. The field-dependent teaching style fits better with the field-dependent learning style of non–Western students.

Implications of Cultural Variation in Learning Style for Speech-Language Services

What should a clinician do when confronted with a variety of learning styles among the students receiving services? How is it possible to adapt the clinician's clinical style to meet the needs of all students? It is suggested that the clinician adapt as follows:

1. Understand that all students have a preferred learning style.
2. Understand that preferred differences in learning style may be culturally based.
3. Understand that there is individual variation in preference for learning style within and across cultural groups.
4. Reach out to those students whose needs and values and learning styles differ from the mainstream or whose styles may be nonassertive.
5. Make adaptations in the types of teaching to accommodate to differences in learning style of all students.
6. Use small-group, large-group, *and* individual sessions.
7. Use both analytic and holistic teaching methods, emphasizing both scientific and interpersonal aspects of the clinical session.

8. Respect all student differences in response time, eye contact, and willingness to self-evaluate.
9. Provide opportunities for modeling, demonstrations, and observations to provide solutions to problems.
10. Respect the cultural values of all students in the clinical situation.

Additional information on cultural variation in learning style can play an important role in improving clinical practices. Regardless of the way in which one views learning style, it is important to understand that learning styles are an important dimension in education; learning style is a preference, with individual variation across situations; culture affects cognitive attitude, behavior, and personality; and perceived differences in learning style are not deficits.

Guidelines for Culturally Sensitive Intervention

As our culture becomes more pluralistic and as students in programs in speech-language pathology represent more culturally and linguistically diverse populations, clinicians will have to understand individual differences and adapt their approach to services to accommodate the needs of all students. The following guidelines will be useful in providing culturally sensitive clinical services:

1. Learn the name of the culture as assigned by its members, and use it. Learn to pronounce the names of students, and do not attempt to shorten the names or use nicknames. Do not comment on unusual names or spelling of names, as names are personal and are often a source of great cultural pride.
2. Be certain that the objectives and expected outcomes of intervention pro-

grams are consistent with the expected outcomes of families, teachers, and clients. Involve parents in intervention planning as appropriate to their culture. Families vary greatly in their willingness and ability to carry out suggestions given by school personnel.

3. Become familiar with the culture of students in the school and in the therapy program by spending time in the community or having discussions with cultural informants.

4. Make certain that methods and procedures do not violate the beliefs and cultural values of the clients.

5. Adapt materials and activities to the culture of the client using books, topics, and materials that are culturally relevant. Be aware of books and materials that portray cultures or different groups in a stereotypical manner. Subscribe to culture-focused newspapers and magazines such as *Ebony* and *Jet* so that cultural role models can be incorporated in lessons.

6. Respect the values and religious beliefs of students. Do not schedule therapy during times when children must participate in a religious practice. Be aware of religious practices regarding dress, foods, family role models, holidays, and other cultural variables in lessons.

7. Understand differences in eye contact and other nonverbal communication rules across cultures.

8. Use examples and vocabulary from real-life situations based in the student's culture, including customs and holidays.

9. Preview and review lessons to be certain that the student understands the relevance of the lesson to the academic curriculum. Review previous lessons to be certain that the concepts are retained.

10. Adapt a clinical style that is appropriate to the client. Because some Asian/Pacific Islander clients prefer a more subdued, humble style, it would not be appropriate to be overly exuberant with them. African American and Hispanic clients, however, may prefer a more animated style of instruction.

11. Be aware of the client's learning and cognitive style, remembering that there is heterogeneity among cultural groups and across groups. Accommodate to the learning style of students in groups by using variation in manner of presenting materials and expected responses.

12. Make input comprehensible by slowing down, pausing, speaking clearly, and rephrasing and restating information. Check frequently for comprehension.

13. Encourage participation by giving extra time for processing and encouraging the student's use of his or her first language if necessary to express ideas. Place more emphasis on meaning and concepts than on grammar and pronunciation. (Adler, 1993, Battle, 1993; Roseberry-McKibbin, 1995)

The Culturally Competent Speech-Language Pathologist

Culturally competent speech-language pathologists recognize that there can be conflict in values, beliefs, and elements of communication between the clinician and the student. The culturally competent clinician is sensitive to circumstances that may influence the client–clinician interaction, to his or her own values and beliefs, and to how his or her values and beliefs may affect others. The culturally competent speech-language pathologist recognizes differences and similarities among people and is comfortable with the differences. Above all, the culturally competent speech-language pathologist adapts to the needs of students and both sends and receives messages that are appropriate to the culture and linguistic competence of the student. This requires explicit knowledge and understanding of the generic characteristics of various cultures, as well as explicit knowledge of verbal and nonverbal communication variables of all clients.

STUDY QUESTIONS

1. Why are there more culturally and linguistically different children in special education programs?

2. Why is it important to distinguish between communication disorder, communication development, and social dialects?

3. What variable must the speech-language pathologist consider when doing an assessment on a limited-English-proficient child?

4. What are the factors that the speech-language pathologist must consider when selecting a standardized test for administration to a child from a culturally and linguistically diverse population?

5. What role should parents play in the education of children with speech-language disorders?

6. How should the speech-language pathologist adapt to the learning style of students in intervention programs?

7. How do differences in learning or cognitive style affect speech-language assessment?

REFERENCES

Abraham, R. (1985). Field independent-dependent and the teaching of grammar. *TESOL Quarterly, 20,* 689–702.

Adler, S. (1993). *Multicultural communication skills in the classroom.* Boston: Allyn & Bacon.

American Speech-Language Hearing Association (1983). Position paper on social dialects. *ASHA, 25,* 23–27.

Ayers, G. E. (1994). Statistical profile of special education in the United States, 1994. *Teaching Exceptional Children, 26*(3, Suppl.), 1–4.

Basso, K. (1970). To give up on words: Silence in western Apache culture. *South West Journal of Anthropology, 26,* 213–230.

Basso, K. (1979). *Portraits of the "Whiteman": Linguistic play and cultural symbols among the Western Apache.* London: Cambridge University Press.

Battle, D. (Ed.) (1993). *Communication disorders in multicultural populations.* Newton, MA.: Butterworth-Heinemann.

Blanchard, E. L. (1983). The growth and development of American Indian children and Alaskan native children. In G. J. Powell (Ed.), *The psychological development of minority group children* (pp. 115–130). New York: Brunner/Mazel.

Boggs, S. T. (1972). The meaning of questions and narratives to Hawaiian children. In C. B. Cazden, V. P. John, & D. Hymes (Eds), *Functions of language in the classroom* (pp. 299–327). New York: Teachers College Press.

Bilingual Education Act of 1968. 20 U.S.C. Section 3221 et seq. (Supp. 1989).

Castellanos, D. (1983). *The best of two worlds: Bilingual- bicultural education in the U.S.* Trenton: New Jersey Department of Education.

Cohen, R. A. (1969). Conceptual styles, culture conflict, and nonverbal tests of intelligence. *American Anthropologist. 71,* 828–856.

Cummins, J. (1984). *Bilingualism and special education.* San Diego: College Hill.

Diana v. State Board of Education, C-70-37 RFP (N.D. Cal. 1970).

Downs, M. (in press). Language disorders from hearing loss in multicultural populations. In L. Cole & V. Deal (Eds.), *Communication disorders in multicultural populations.* Washington, DC: American Speech-Language-Hearing Association.

Dunn, R., & Griggs, S. (1988). *Learning styles: Quiet revolution in American secondary schools.* Reston, VA: Northern Association of Secondary School Principals.

Erickson, J., & Iglesias, A. (1986). Assessment of communication disorders in non-English proficient children. In O. Taylor (Ed.), *Nature of communication disorders in culturally and linguistically diverse populations*. San Diego: College Hill Press.

Gallimore, R., & Goldenburg, C. (1993). Activity settings of early literacy. In E. Forman, N. Minick, & C. Stone (Eds.), *Contexts for learning: Sociocultural dynamics in children's development* (pp. 27–42). New York: Oxford University Press.

Hamayan, E., & Damico, J. (1991). *Limiting bias in assessment of bilingual students*. Austin, TX: Pro-Ed.

Harris, G. (1993). American-Indian cultures: A lesson in diversity. In D. E. Battle (Eds), *Communication disorders in multicultural populations* (pp. 78–113.) Stoneham MA: Andover.

Heath, S. B. (1982). What no bedtime story means: Narrative skills at home and school. *Language in Society, 11,* 49–76.

Heath, S. B. (1993). *Ways with words: Language, life and work in communities and classrooms*. New York: Cambridge University Press.

Hilliard, A. (1989). Teachers and cultural styles in a pluralistic society. *NEA Today, 7*(6) 65–69.

Hilliard, A. (1992). Behavioral style, culture, and teaching and learning. *Journal of Negro Education, 6*(3), 370–377.

Hodgkinson, H. L. (1985). *All one system: Demographics of education—kindergarten through graduate school*. Washington, DC: Institute for Educational Leadership.

Hoover, J. J., & Collier, C. (1985). Referring culturally different children: Sociocultural considerations. *Academic Therapy, 20,* 503–509.

Huston, A., McLoyd, V., & Coll, C. (1994). Children and poverty: Issues in contemporary research. *Child Development, 65,* 275–282.

Iglesias, A. (1985). Communication in the home and classroom: Match or mismatch? *Topics in Language Disorders, 5*(4), 29–41

Individuals with Disabilities Education Act of 1990, P.L. 101-476, 20 U.S.C. Section 1400 et seq.

Jacobs, R. L. (1987). *An investigation of the learning style differences among Afro-American and Euro-American high, average and low achievers*. Unpublished doctoral dissertation, Peabody University, LA.

Kayser, H. (1989). Speech-language assessment of Spanish-English speaking children. *Language, Speech, and Hearing Services in the Schools, 20,* 226–244.

Kayser, H. (1990). Social communicative behaviors of language disordered Mexican-American students. *Child Language Teaching Therapy, 6,* 255–269.

Kayser, H. (1993). Hispanic cultures. In D. E. Battle (Ed.), *Communication Disorders in Multicultural Populations*, (pp. 114–157). Stoneham, MA: Andover.

Kayser, H. (1995). *Bilingual speech-language pathology: An Hispanic focus*. San Diego: Singular.

Kessen, W. (1979). The American child and other cultural inventions. *American Psychologist, 34,* 815–820.

Lamphoon, S. (1986). *A comparative study of the learning style of Southeast Asian and American Caucasian college students on two Seventh Day Adventist campuses*. Unpublished doctoral dissertation, Andrew University, MI.

Langdon, H. (1992). *Hispanic children and adults with communication disorders*. Gaithersburg, MD: Aspen.

Larry, P. Riles, 343 F. Supp. 1306.502 F 2nd 963 (1972).

Lau v. Nichols, 94 S.C. 786 (1990), Calif. 414, U.S. 563.

State Legislatures. (1994, August). 20(8). National Conference of State Legislatures: Author.

Lora v. Board of Education of the City of New York, 587 F. Supp. 1572 (E.D. N.Y. 1984).

Lynch, E. W. & Hanson, M. J. (1992). *Developing cross-cultural competence: A guide for working with young children and their families*. Baltimore: Paul H. Brookes.

Marshall v. McDaniel, Civil No. 482-233 (S.D. Ga. 1984).

Mattes, L. J., & Omark, D. R. (1991). *Speech and language assessment for the bilingual handicapped* (2nd ed.). Oceanside, CA: Academic Communication Associates.

Mattie T. v. Holliday, 3 EHLR 551:109 (N.D. Miss. 1979).

Mayfield, S. A. (in press). Excessive lead absorption and language disorders in Black children. In L. Cole & V. Deal (Eds.), *Communication disorders in multicultural populations*. Washington, DC: American Speech-Language-Hearing Association.

Maynard, S. (1993). *Discourse modality: Subjectivity, emotion, and voice in the Japanese language*. Philadelphia: John Benjamins.

Messick, S. (1976). *Individuality in learning*. San Francisco: Jossey-Bass.

Michaels, S. (1981). "Sharing time": Children's narrative styles and differential access to literacy. *Language in Society, 10,* 423–442.

Minami, M., & McCabe, A. (1995). Rice balls and bear hunts: Japanese and North American family narrative patterns. *Journal of Child Language, 22,* 423–445.

More, A. (1990, August). *Learning styles of Native Americans and Asians*. Paper presented at the 89th annual meeting of the American Psychological Association, Boston. (ERIC Document No. ED 330 535).

Newcomer, P. L. & Hammill, D. (1991). *Test of language development-Primary 2*. Austin, Tex.: Pro-Ed.

Nichols, E. (1992). The philosophical aspect of cultural difference. In *Report from the working group: Research and training needs of minority persons and minority health issues* (Appendix C). Bethesda, MD: National Institutes on Deafness and Other Communication Disorders.

Olsen, P. (1991). *Referring language minority students to special education.* Washington, DC: Center for Applied Linguistics.

Pang-Ching, G., Robb, M., Heath, R., & Takum, M. (1995). Middle ear disease and hearing loss in native Hawaiian preschoolers. *Language, Speech, and Hearing Services in the Schools, 26*(1), 33–38.

PASE v. Hannon, 506 F. Supp. 831 (N.D. Ill. 1980).

Peters-Johnson, C. (1995). Action school services. *Language, Speech, and Hearing Services in the Schools, 26*(2), 97.

Philips, S. (1983). *The invisible culture: Communication in classroom and community on the Warm Springs Indian Reservation.* White Plains, NY: Longman.

Public Law 94-142, Education for all handicapped children act of 1975. 20 U.S.C 1401. *Federal Register, 42* (86), 1977.

Ramirez, M., & Castenada, A. (1974). *Cultural democracy, bicognitive development and education.* New York: Academic Press.

Roseberry-McKibbin, C. (1995). *Multicultural students with special language needs: Practical strategies for assessment and intervention.* Oceanside, CA: Academic Communication Associates.

Sandhu, D. (1994a). *Cultural diversity in the classroom: What teachers need to know.* (ERIC Document No ED 370 910)

Sandhu, D. (1994b). *Culturally specific learning styles: Some suggestions for teachers.* (ERIC Document No. ED 370 910)

Saville-Troike, M. (1979). Culture, language and education. In H. T. Trueba & C. Barnett-Mizzahi (Eds.), *Bilingual multicultural education and the professional: From theory to practice* (pp. 139–148). Rowley, MA: Newberry House.

Scott, D. (1985). Sickle-cell anemia and hearing loss. In F. H. Bess, B. S. Clark, & H. R. Mitchell (Eds.), *ASHA Reports No. 16 Concerns for minority groups in communication disorders* (pp. 69–73). Rockville, MD.: American Speech-Language Hearing Association.

Smitherman, G. (1988). Discriminatory discourse on Afro-American speech. In G. Smitherman & T. Van Dijk (Eds.), *Discourse and discrimination* (pp. 144–175). Detroit: Wayne State University Press.

Swisher, K. (1990). Cooperative learning and the education of American/Indian Alaskan native students: A review of the literature and suggestions for implementation. *Journal of American Indian Education, 29*(2), 36–43.

Taylor, O. (1978). Language issues and testing. *Journal of Non-White Concerns 6*(3), 125–133.

Taylor, O. (1983). Black English: An agenda for the 1980's. In J. Chambers (Ed.), *Black English: Educational equity and the law.* Ann Arbor, MI: Karoma.

Taylor, O. (1986). *Nature of communication disorders in culturally and linguistically diverse populations.* San Diego: College Hill.

Terrell, F., & Terrell, S. (1983). The relationship between race of examiner, cultural mistrust, and intelligence test performance of Black children. *Psychology in Schools, 20,* 367–369.

Terrell, F., Terrell, S., & Taylor, J. (1981). Effects of race of examiner and cultural mistrust on the WAIS performance of black students. *Journal of Consulting and Clinical Psychology, 49,* 570–571.

Terrell, S., & Terrell, F. (1993). African-American cultures. In D. E. Battle (Ed.), *Communication disorders in multicultural populations* (pp. 3-37), Newton, Mass.: Butterworth-Heinemann.

U.S. Census Bureau (1990). *Statistical abstract of the United States,* 110th ed. Washington, D.C.: U.S. Department of Commerce.

U.S. Department of Health and Human Services. (1985). *Report of the Secretary's Task Force on Black and Minority Health: Vol. 1. Executive Summary,* (Pub. No. 491-313/44706). Washington, DC: Government Printing Office.

Vanderas, A. O. (1987). Incidence of cleft lip, cleft palate, and cleft lip and palate among races: A review. *Cleft Palate Journal, 24,* 216–225.

Vaughn-Cooke, F. (1983). Improving language assessment in minority children. *ASHA, 25,* 29–34.

Walker, D., Greenwood, C., Hart, B., & Carta, J. (1994). Prediction of school outcomes based on early language production and socioeconomic factors. *Child Development, 65,* 606–621.

Ward, M. C. (1982). Them children: A study of language learning. New York: Irving.

Westby, C. E. (1990). Ethnographic interviewing: Asking the right questions to the right people in the right ways. *Journal of Childhood Communication Disorders, 13,* 101–110.

Westby, C. E. (1994). Multicultural issues. In J. B. Tomblin, H. L Morris, & D. C Spriestersbach (Eds.), *Diagnosis in speech-language pathology* (pp. 29–51). San Diego: Singular.

Williams, R. L. (1970). Black pride, academic relevance, and individual achievement. *Counseling Psychologist, 2,* 18–22.

Witkin, H. A. (1976). Cognitive style in academic performance and in teacher-student relations. In S. Messick & Associates (Eds.) *Individuality in learning.* San Francisco: Jossey-Bass.

Chapter 12

The Future

Pamelia F. O'Connell

The overall aim of this book has been to help prepare the novice school practitioner or the practitioner-in-training to function in today's schools. Effective performance in this setting depends on many things, and among them surely is knowledge. Wisdom, as Chapter 1 has stated, is only possible through experience. But information about the profession and how it has evolved, the kinds of services provided in schools, the expansion of caseloads, and the emergence of the language specialist into the curriculum and the classroom, should assist the beginner. A state-of-the-art account within a historical context has been this book's intent.

Each contributor has presented a part or parts of the complex and interlocking structure that houses school programs in speech, language, and hearing within the edifice of contemporary education. The resulting portrait of school services in these areas reflects current realities. Yet what is current is also subject to change. That has always been true. It is the rate of change that has marked off late-20th-century society from past eras.

As these words have been written, rewritten, revised, and reviewed, the engines of change have not been idle. The past changes that are here discussed have led in the direction of expansion: expansion of the role of

the speech-language pathologist, inclusion of the educational audiologist in the school services team, expansion of eligibility for services to the learning disabled and the severely and profoundly developmentally impaired, and expansion of communication technology for the handicapped. All these events have moved school practitioners in many directions. They have also created a continuing demand for services that has propelled growth of the profession to numbers undreamed of a generation ago. Although many factors contributed to the pattern of expansion, two seem especially worthy of note. They are (a) the movement toward inclusion and empowerment of all individuals with disabilities, which may be viewed as a logical outgrowth of the civil rights movement of the 1960s and (b) the role of the federal government in mandating a free and appropriate public education for all handicapped children, initiated in 1975 and expanded upon in succeeding years. Although general education has been viewed primarily as a state and locally controlled and financed endeavor, the education of students with handicapping conditions, as well as at-risk infants and toddlers, has become, in large measure, a federal responsibility and to some extent may be conceived as an entitlement. It may well be, however, that at some point in the very recent past, perhaps November 1994, the high-water mark of the era of expansiveness was reached.

Surely, in terms of atmosphere, expansive optimism seems to have been replaced by constriction, or a narrowing of concern. The focus has shifted away from needs to be met toward the means required to meet them. Those means have been subject to increasing unwillingness or perceived unwillingness of the taxpayer to provide for them. Multiple accounts in the popular press have pointed out the ever-increasing expenses for all of the special services in schools, and some accounts have questioned their value. After several decades of constantly increasing services for all aspects of special education, the pendulum of change swings in the opposite direction. A recent issue of *Asha*, the national association's professional issues forum, contained such phrases as "retrenchment within special education funding" (Scherg, 1996), "increasingly constrained resources" (Coufal, 1996), "individual and unlimited treatment for clients may be extinct" (Sonies, 1996), and "another critical area is the so-called 'school reform' movement and the reduction in force . . . emerging as the federal government seeks to pass its responsibilities in education to the states" (Butler, 1996). Other concerns mentioned included large caseloads, competitiveness, and cost consciousness.

The reasons for the trend toward a more constricted view of service to the handicapped appear to be philosophical as well as fiscal. Along with cost consciousness has come a distrust of federal mandates and a generalized erosion of support for federally sponsored educational programs, as evidenced by calls for the abolition of the U.S. Department of Education. Also under attack from many quarters are bilingual educational programs, as activities in several states have supported English as the "official" language.

The *ASHA Leader* the national association's newest publication, has documented the struggle to preserve the Individuals With Disabilities Education Act (IDEA), whose funding and programs have been subjected to attack by the current U.S. Congress ("IDEA Under Fire," 1996). IDEA was to be reauthorized in 1996 and has been continued for one additional year. However, reauthorization will be debated in 1997, at which time cuts in funding, in federal requirements for standards, and in research support are feared. The Chair of the Subcommittee on Early Childhood, Youth, and Families, Representative Randy Cunningham (R-CA), has been quoted as seeing "little use for a strong federal role in education" and as stating that legislation such as IDEA "takes money away from the children" ("Subcommittee Chair," p. 3).

The following issues are of primary concern to ASHA and its members:

> maintaining the personnel standards provision requiring the use of the highest requirements in states; an appropriate definition of paraprofessional; changing the definition of *special education* to include related services; reducing paperwork requirements; and prohibiting retaliation and coercion against service providers for exercising professional judgment or advocating on behalf of students with disabilities. ("Position Statements," p.   )

It is too early to know how much influence antifederal positions will eventually attain and how long such attitudes will persist. It is, however, a fairly safe assumption that the immediate future will be characterized by diminishing growth of special educational services of many kinds. But past experience suggests that the genie is never put back in the bottle. It is unlikely that we, as a society, will return to the isolation and neglect of students with special needs that marked the earlier decades of this century. Rather, new initiatives may be blunted, and service providers in our schools as well as in our health care centers may face increasing pressures to limit their activities and to account for their effectiveness. The era of expansiveness may have been superseded by an era of accountability.

These political challenges play out against a background of division and controversy within the field of special education. Critics of special education have cited bureaucracy, empire building, segregation and labeling of students, and educational fads (Kauffman, 1994). Some controversies could affect the very existence of special education, such as those concerning the concepts of the least restrictive environment (LRE) and the regular education initiative (REI). If, indeed, the ultimate LRE is the regular classroom, what is the role of special education? Fuchs and Fuchs (1994) discussed the movement toward full inclusion and the arguments for and against it, concluding that regular and special education need to forge more meaningful connections with each other. It seems that the best way to educate students with special needs has yet to be resolved. With respect to students with mild handicapping conditions, data reviewed by McLesky and Pacchiano (1994) show that the majority of them, especially the learning disabled, are served within regular classrooms, whereas more severely disabled students tend to be served in self-contained classrooms.

As with the larger societal issues, it is too early to know how the divisions within special education will be resolved or the manner in which speech, language, and hearing services will be delivered to students who need

them. But given the atmosphere of political and professional controversy, the attributes of flexibility adaptability, collaboration, and advocacy should stand the beginning practitioner in good stead in the times ahead.

It is even more difficult to foresee the scientific/intellectual changes that will characterize the future. One assumes that they will be numerous, exciting, and sometimes contradictory. Recently, Wallach (1995), viewing the conceptual changes in learning disability over the past 15 years, made several cogent observations. She noted that the field had moved away from "auditory-visual" dichotomies and toward a more unified and realistic view of language and learning. She spoke of the "splinter-skill training" in the isolation of therapy rooms (p. v). She also warned that new panaceas abound and probably always will (p. vi).

Future research will undoubtedly produce additional shifts in conceptualization of the disabilities engaging the field of speech-language pathology. Although increasingly sophisticated technology holds promises for significant advances in many areas, Wallach's skepticism concerning panaceas is a highly recommended companion.

There will be other research, other theories, and other panaceas. The educational/scientific community has experienced high hopes for many innovations that have met with various degrees of disappointment. Such disparate procedures as whole-language reading instruction, facilitated communication, and privatization have failed to sustain the enthusiasm of their initial supporters. Probably there will be other disappointments as well.

The speech-language pathologists and audiologists who serve the nation's schools in the future will meet challenges and changes that cannot be foreseen. But some that may be expected include rapidly expanding technology to support many types of communication, increasing involvement of families in educational programming of all kinds, and continuing debate on the relative merits of inclusion and separation. All in all, it should be an interesting journey. Certainly, no final destination is in sight.

REFERENCES

Butler, K. (1996). Interview with Katharine G. Butler (interviewed by Barbara Goldberg). *ASHA, 38*(1), 30.

Coufal, K. (1996). Executive board candidates. *Asha, 38*,(1), 13.

Fuchs, D., & Fuchs, L. (1994). Inclusive schools movement and the radicalization of special education reform. *Exceptional Children, 60,* 294–309.

Kauffman, J. (1994). Places of change: Special education's power and identity in an era of educational reform. *Journal of Learning Disabilities, 27,* 610–618.

McLesky, J., & Pacchiano, D. (1994). Mainstreaming students with learning disabilities: Are we making progress? *Exceptional Children, 60,* 508–517.

Moore, M. (1996). IDEA under fire. *ASHA Leader, 1*(3),1, 3

Rabins, A. (1996). Subcommittee chair challenges federal role in IDEA. *ASHA Leader, 1*(3),1, 3

Scherg, K. (1996). Executive board candidates. *Asha, 38*(1), 12.

Sonies, B. (1996). Executive board candidates. *Asha, 38*(1), 14.

Wallach, G. P. (1995). Foreword. *Topics in Language Disorders, 16*(1), v–vii.

Index